evaluation in physical education

evaluation in physical education

assessing motor behavior

Margaret J. Safrit
University of Wisconsin

Prentice-Hall, Inc., *Englewood Cliffs, New Jersey*

Library of Congress Cataloging in Publication Data

SAFRIT, MARGARET J
  Evaluation in physical education.

  Includes bibliographies.
  1. Physical fitness—Testing. I. Title.
GV436.S2 1973   613.7'07   72-5427
ISBN 0-13-292227-4

© 1973 by

PRENTICE-HALL, INC.
Englewood Cliffs, New Jersey

10   9   8   7   6   5   4   3   2   1

Printed in the United States of America

PRENTICE-HALL INTERNATIONAL, INC.,   London
PRENTICE-HALL OF AUSTRALIA, PTY. LTD., Sydney
PRENTICE-HALL OF CANADA, LTD., Toronto
PRENTICE-HALL OF INDIA PRIVATE LIMITED, New Delhi
PRENTICE-HALL OF JAPAN, INC.,   Tokyo

Dedicated to

RUTH B. GLASSOW
and
MARIE R. LIBA

preface

This textbook is designed for upper level undergraduate students in measurement and evaluation in physical education, as well as for graduate students who do not have an extensive background in measurement concepts in physical education. It is hoped that the contents of this book will also be helpful to the physical education teacher by suggesting ways in which educational decisions can be made with a greater degree of objectivity.

The first three chapters are oriented to concepts of evaluation in physical education. Since evaluation is defined as the process of determining the degree to which predetermined goals have been met, the goals should initially be specified in the form of behavioral objectives. The process of writing behavioral objectives is described in Chapter 2. Chapter 3 identifies the distinguishing characteristics of two major types of evaluation, formative evaluation and summative evaluation. Chapter 4 deals with basic statistics that are essential to understanding the measurement theory in subsequent chapters. Chapters 5 and 6 are technical chapters on validity and reliability theory applied to measures of motor behavior, topics that have generally received very little attention in the physical education measurement literature. The remaining chapters deal with the more practical issues of assessment in physical education. However, the reader will not find a great number of physical education tests included in this book. Understanding principles of assessing motor behavior will allow the reader to operate independently with regard to the assessment process rather than encouraging him to rely on the sample of tests presented within a given source. However, to assist the reader in locating available tests, the sources for many skill tests in physical education are listed in Appendix A.

I am indebted to the Literary Executor of the late Sir Ronald A. Fisher, F.R.S., and to Oliver & Boyd, Edinburgh for their permission to reprint Table V. A from their book *Statistical Methods for Research Workers*. Gratitude is also expressed to the following publishers for permission to reprint or to modify materials: Allyn and Bacon, Inc.; American Association for Health, Physical Education, and Recreation; Educational Testing Service; Cambridge University Press; John Wiley & Sons, Inc.; David McKay Company; Macmillan Company; McGraw-Hill Book Company; Prentice-Hall, Inc.; and Psychological Corporation. In addition, three colleagues—Peggy A. Anderson, Ann E. Jewett, and Carol J. Widule—kindly granted permission to reprint materials they had developed.

I would like to express my appreciation to several other colleagues for their contributions to this book. William P. Morgan critically reviewed every chapter, and made many helpful suggestions for the revision of the entire book. The expertise of Anne E. Atwater was indispensable in making major revisions of several of the more technical chapters, especially the reliability and validity chapters. Peggy A. Chapman made significant contributions to the evaluation chapters in the first part of the book. Other colleagues who deserve special thanks are Frances Z. Cumbee, Vern D. Seefeldt, and Ina G. Temple. Gratitude is expressed to Carol L. Stamm for her assistance in proofreading the manuscript. For typing the various drafts of the manuscript as well as assisting in the preparation of the manuscript in many other ways, grateful appreciation is extended to Mrs. Richard (Jan) Whelan.

MARGARET J. SAFRIT

contents

ix

tables

Chapter 5

Chapter 6

Chapter 8

Chapter 9

Chapter 10

Chapter 11

Appendix Tables

figures

Chapter 8

Chapter 9

Chapter 10

**evaluation in
physical
education**

1

introduction

As human beings we cannot live without making countless judgments that affect our lives. Although some of our judgments may be based on an objective view of reality, many decisions are made according to our values and thus are made subjectively. When our judgments affect others, there is an obvious need for objectivity and rationality. In situations where our judgments can have far-reaching implications, such as teachers' decisions about students, rationality is essential. Although it is inevitable that, as teachers, we will operate to some extent according to our value systems, we must continually strive to make objective rather than subjective decisions.

The school system is an atmosphere in which constant judgments must be made. The purpose of this book is to explore concepts of assessment in physical education, especially those involving the assessment of student learning in terms of the course objectives, that will enable teachers to approach decision making with greater objectivity. Measurement and evaluation will be considered a part of the teaching-learning process. We evaluate as we teach.

The process of *assessment* involves both measurement and evaluation. *Measurement* is the process of assigning a number to some property of an entity. In physical education, the "entity" is a person, the student. We speak of "properties" of the student because we are not actually measuring the total student, but rather a capacity of the student, such as running speed or arm strength. *Evaluation* is the process of making judgments about the results of measurement in terms of the course objectives. The measure, then, is useless unless evaluated with regard to progress made toward a goal.

Evaluation can be based on methods of assessment other than measurement. By definition, the process of measurement involves the assignment of a number or score. Some evaluation techniques, such as anecdotal records, cannot be classified as measurement, but are nonetheless useful tools.

Purposes of Assessment in Physical Education

Assessment can serve many useful purposes in the school setting. Because most school systems enforce the practice of giving grades, grading is often the foremost reason for assessment. Although grading, in terms of the teaching-learning process, is a legitimate reason for evaluation, it is one of the least useful.

Even if grades were not used, the process of evaluation should still be thorough and meaningful. Some of the purposes of assessment are:

1. To diagnose weaknesses.
2. To classify according to ability.
3. To exempt from aspects of the program.
4. To predict future ability level.
5. To determine achievement level.
6. To specify amount of improvement.
7. To motivate students.
8. To determine grades.
9. To evaluate teaching.
10. To justify programs to administrators.
11. To evaluate the curriculum.

Diagnosis of Weaknesses

When methods of assessment are used in the diagnostic sense, the student's performance of a given skill is examined in order to detect weaknesses. Unless the physical education programs within a school system are coordinated at all levels, a teacher may not have a very precise expectation of his students' skill levels and might measure them at the beginning of a unit so that he can gear future plans to their needs. When assessment techniques are used effectively, the teacher can provide for the diagnosis of student weaknesses throughout a unit. In many instances, the class can be organized so that the students can assist in diagnosing each other.

For maximum utility, the diagnostic process should be accompanied by a corrective prescription. When an assessment tool both diagnoses and prescribes, the process is called *formative evaluation*. The concept of formative evaluation will be discussed in detail in Chapter 3.

Classification According to Ability

Once the students' initial ability levels have been determined, the teacher may wish to separate the students into ability groups for the duration of a unit. The membership of these groups may change several times. For example, a given individual might be able to execute an effective volleyball pass, but he might have difficulty performing the overarm serve. Therefore, he would be a member of the high-ability group when practicing the pass, but would move to the low-ability group when working on the serve. Because a given student may perform different skills at different levels, the maintenance of intact ability groups throughout a unit, although convenient for the teacher, is clearly undesirable for the students. In addition, the teacher may wish to combine low-ability and high-ability students in the same group upon occasion. The high-ability students can help the low-ability students by correcting errors and by providing an opportunity for them to be exposed to well-executed skills.

Exemption from Aspects of the Physical Education Program

If a student already meets the designated objectives of a unit, he might benefit more from the total program if he were exempt from this unit and allowed to elect another. In order to implement an exemption policy, several teaching stations must be available at any given period, or scheduling problems would become unwieldy. Although the use of proficiency tests may not be feasible in some schools, this practice can enhance a physical education program by providing for a variety of individual needs. Since the time allotted to a physical education unit is usually short, complete proficiency testing for all class members during class time would not be practical. However, evaluation at the beginning of a unit could indicate which students have the potential for exemption, and the appropriate proficiency tests could be administered to them after school.

Prediction of Future Performance

Theoretically tests given at the beginning of a unit could be used to predict the future performance of the students. In practice, tests are rarely given for predictive purposes in physical education classes because in most cases not enough is known about the predictive power of tests. In some school systems tests are used to determine initial team membership of an athletic squad, but such tests are usually supplemented by the coach's subjective judgment.

Determination of Achievement Level

Evaluation is essential for providing feedback on the student's level of achievement. There is considerable evidence indicating that students who are provided with knowledge of results learn faster than those students who receive no feedback. Also, the closer to the actual performance the feedback is received, the more effective it is. Thus, students should constantly receive feedback, not just at the end of a unit. Day-to-day evaluation provides the student with information about his present level of achievement as well as ways in which he can correct any weaknesses. If the student knows the standards of achievement set by the teacher, he will know how well he is progressing toward attaining them.

Determination of Improvement

Evaluation provides information on the degree of improvement made by the student over a period of time. However, there are limitations to the amount of information that can be provided by such a score because of the difficulty in interpreting its meaning. For instance, we know that a small improvement made by a highly skilled person may represent more improvement than a similar amount (in actual score value) made by a poorly skilled person. A student's improvement at any skill level is undoubtedly encouraging to him, even though we may have difficulty in interpreting the improvement score.

Motivation of Students

The student who knows how well he is performing and how he can improve is likely to be better motivated than one who receives no feedback. But if a student continues to practice and feels he is not improving, he may become frustrated and discouraged. Assessment devices can be used as motivational tools. The provision of short-term goals for learning a skill might encourage the student to remain motivated because the goals are not far enough apart to seem unattainable. Each student should be able to reach some of the goals even though not all will reach the final ones.

Determination of Grades

Evaluation is essential for determining grades. A teacher should be able to justify every grade with objective evidence. Only by collecting evidence of the students' skills, abilities, and knowledge can the teacher objectively handle this important decision-making process. Because grades are part of a student's permanent record, a teacher's decision can have far-reaching implications. Therefore, no matter what grading system is used, a high level of objectivity is imperative.

Evaluation of Teaching

We commonly assume that learning will take place in a classroom or gymnasium. If no one in class reaches the performance standard for a skill as set by the teacher, either the standard is unreasonable or the teaching methods have not been effective. Of course, a group of students may be unusually poorly skilled and thus might not be able to meet the same standards as a more typical class. However, if the standards were continually not met, the problem could not be attributed to an "atypical" class. The teacher should then reevaluate his teaching methods and substitute methods that are more effective.

Because our primary concern is teaching, it is reasonable to use evaluations of student performance as a means of gauging teacher effectiveness. In fact, this method is probably more effective than evaluation by supervisors because the teacher must engage in a critical appraisal of his teaching methods and change them if they appear to be ineffective. The supervisor's role, then, rather than to make judgments based on a few observations, would be to assess teacher effectiveness based upon the teacher's statement of intended goals, the methods used to attain them, and evidence of their degree of success, provided that the goals and methods are judged to be educationally sound. In this way evaluation of student performance can aid in objectifying the process of assessing teacher effectiveness.

Justification of Physical Education Program to the Administration

As the process of education becomes increasingly expensive, the public continues to question the cost of various educational programs, and to demand justification of their inclusion in the school curriculum. The usual justification is that the projected outcomes are important to the education of youth. However, when decisions are made about continuing such programs, it is not lofty goals, but results that justify a program. Therefore, physical educators should be prepared to submit *objective* evidence, obtained through assessment, of their degree of success.

Evaluation of the Curriculum

The evaluation of students also aids in curriculum evaluation and change when questions such as these arise: As a physical education program continues, do some standards become so easily met that the curriculum needs to be redesigned? Do students' attitudes change toward certain aspects of the curriculum, suggesting the need for curricular changes? If very few students are able to meet the standards, were standards in previous years too lenient, or are present standards too difficult? With objective information regarding the effectiveness and relevance of the existing curriculum, the curriculum planner is in a better position to plan for needed revision and change.

Assessment Needs in Physical Education

The process of evaluation in physical education is hindered by the lack of standardized measures, available testing materials, and trained personnel who can devote their time to developing appropriate measures. On the national scene, we have no way of knowing what motor skills and/or knowledge about motor behavior our school-age youth possess. Unfortunately the National Assessment Project (Womer, 1970), designed to assess knowledge in ten areas of the curriculum, does not include physical education. Only a few physical education testing projects have been conducted on a nation-wide scale. These projects include the American Association for Health, Physical Education and Recreation Youth Fitness Test (1965), the AAHPER Sports Skills Tests (1967), and the AAHPER Cooperative Physical Education Tests (1970), developed with the cooperation of the Educational Testing Service. There is a great need for an organized approach to the development of physical education evaluation tools.

Summary

Assessment involves both measurement and evaluation. *Measurement* is the process of assigning a number to some property of an entity. *Evaluation* is the process of making judgments about the results of measurement in terms of the course objectives. The process of assessment serves many useful purposes, such as aiding the teacher in diagnosing student faults. By evaluating at the beginning of a unit, the teacher can classify students according to ability, exempt students who demonstrate proficiency, and predict the potential performance level of the student. The student's level of achievement can be determined through evaluation. Assessment helps the student determine the amount of improvement he has made and motivates him to strive further. It also aids in the justification of physical education programs and the evaluation of teaching and the curriculum. Although individual teachers can conduct effective assessment programs as a part of the teaching-learning process, the extensive development of measurement and evaluation techniques by trained personnel in physical education is badly needed.

Bibliography

American Association for Health, Physical Education and Recreation. *AAHPER Sports Skills Tests*. Washington, D. C.: American Association for Health, Physical Education and Recreation, 1967.

American Association for Health, Physical Education and Recreation. *Youth Fitness Test Manual*. Washington, D. C.: American Association for Health, Physical Education and Recreation, 1965.

Cooperative Tests and Services. *AAHPER Cooperative Physical Education Tests*. Princeton, N. J.: Educational Testing Service, 1970.

WOMER, F. B. *What Is National Assessment?* Ann Arbor, Michigan: National Assessment of Educational Progress, 1970.

2

preparing objectives
for physical education classes

Teaching physical education requires systematic planning if the students are to achieve the desired results. Such planning begins with statements of the projected effects in the form of educational objectives. Such statements may suggest appropriate learning experiences, aid in developing a sequential program, define the scope of the program, or help direct evaluation. This process of preparing educational objectives is the first step in implementing the concept of accountability, that is, holding a teacher or a school accountable for the results of their programs.

The process of writing objectives in behavioral terms will be examined, and an analysis of opposing viewpoints will be included for a thorough discussion. Also, the three behavioral domains—cognitive, affective, and psychomotor—will be described.

In the next chapter, formative and summative evaluation will be discussed. To simplify the initiation to the process of writing objectives this chapter will be geared to the needs of the physical education teacher, which generally involve formative evaluation. For the purposes of this chapter, however, the distinction is not important.

Clarification of Terms

An educational objective can be defined as a statement of proposed change in the learner (Mager, 1962; Payne, 1968). This change will presumably take place as the result of planned learning experiences. When an objective is stated in terms of the performance or behavior that the student and Payne, 1971, p. 21). The following examples of evaluation objectives are related to curriculum objective 2:

1. Can run using fast and slow speeds.
2. Can run while body is at high and low levels in space.
3. Can run using heavy and light force.
4. Can run with body at different levels in space, using a slow speed and heavy force.

behavioral objectives become increasingly specific and require different ls of decision making. The long-range goals and the curriculum ob- ves, defining the scope and sequence of the program, would most likely eveloped for the total school district. It is at the third level, evaluation ctives, that the teacher would have the greatest degree of decision ng and therefore it will be described in most detail.

Selection of Objectives

writing objectives, the curriculum planner *must* make choices be- would be impossible to cover all aspects of physical education within ool program. The important questions are: What are the bases for ices? Are the choices sound? er recommends using the following information as a basis for making

Data regarding the students themselves, their present abilities, knowledges, kills, interests, attitudes, and needs. Data regarding the demands society is making upon the graduates, pportunities and defects of contemporary society that have significance r education, and the like. uggestions of specialists in various subject fields regarding the contribu- n they think their subjects can make to the education of students (Tyler, 51, p. 50).

ation will probably provide an excessive number of objectives, ecommends making the final choices according to the planner's of education, the school's philosophy, and principles derived ychology of learning. pe of decision making most frequently occurs at the district ves still a number of choices to be made by the teacher as he daily instructional program, and these choices will be influenced

will exhibit when the objective is successfully attained, it is ref
behavioral objective. By stating objectives in terms of stud
rather than teaching material, both the student and teach
precisely what to expect. Also, stating objectives in behavio
to establish evaluation procedures that relate to student pe
has been described.

Education is concerned with both long-range and imm
Long-range objectives usually specify the behavior of tl
person, and are by nature general. To learn whether stu
toward these long-range goals, immediate objectives ar
provide guidance for activities to be incorporated int
objectives can be attained in a relatively short period of

A variety of terms has been used to describe tl
objectives. In this chapter, the terms long-range goals, c
and evaluation objectives will be used to specify thre
objectives that Krathwohl and Payne (1971) have id
link between long-range goals and immediate obj
long-range goals, represents "the long-term global
describe the end product of a complete education"
1971, p. 21). For example:

1. The student shall develop the fundamental n
2. The student shall develop adequate interes
   pation in some sort of physical activity as
3. The student shall become a citizen who
   health issues and is able to use this inforn

The second level, *curriculum objectives,* is
goals into specific behaviors that form the ter
of students successfully completing an instruc
in itself, and, in some instances, a sequenc
Payne, 1971, p. 21). Students completing
will be expected to have met these objectiv

1. Can execute the hop, skip, jump, ru
   patterns.
2. Can execute the above movement
   time, space, and force.

At the third level, *evaluation obj*
unit or course level of specificity a suc
would be a behavior more sophisticat

Th
leve
ject
be
obje
mak

I
cause
the sc
his ch
Ty
choices

1.

2. I
   o
   fo
3. S
   ti
   19

This inforn
and Tyler
philosophy
from the ps
This ty
level and le
plans for his

by his interests and values. In a soccer unit, for example, one must decide what skills to teach, how much time to devote to learning skills, how much time to devote to playing the game, and so on. There are probably some soccer skills that most teachers and coaches would agree are essential to the game. Beyond these, the teacher makes choices based on his values, interests, knowledge of course content and students, as considered in the perspective of the expectations of the physical education staff within a school, and the school district as a whole.

It may be possible for a teacher to use objectives that have been developed by another teacher or a measurement specialist. However, a teacher must usually write his own objectives, because a meaningful objective in one situation might not be meaningful in another. This is not to say that objectives written by a given teacher need not be clear to other teachers. The objectives should be so clearly stated that anyone could read them and understand exactly what is required. However, a teacher's values and situation might cause him to select different objectives, and to refrain from using behavioral objectives because those of another teacher do not seem important or useful is not logical. Each teacher must clarify his own values, set goals, and define standards.

Writing Behavioral Objectives

Writing sound objectives is not an easy task. Experience has shown that even after thorough exposure to instructional materials on writing objectives, it is necessary for the teacher to have considerable practice in writing objectives for them to be effective. Working with other teachers in small groups and receiving frequent feedback from an authority in the area are useful ways of initiating teachers into the process. Ultimately, each individual must go through the process of writing and rewriting objectives until each one can be read and interpreted correctly by anyone in education. Fortunately, the task becomes easier after practice.

Mager identifies three basic steps in writing objectives:

1. Identify the terminal behavior.
2. Further define the desired behavior by describing the important conditions under which the behavior will be expected to occur.
3. Specify the criteria of acceptable performance by describing how well the learner must perform to be considered acceptable (Mager, 1962, p. 12).

In the first step *student behavior,* rather than teacher behavior, is described because what the student will be able to do is of greater concern than the material the teacher will present, which only evolves from it. The second step deals with the surrounding circumstances, and any given behavior could occur under many possible conditions. The third step refers to evidence that the learner has achieved the objective.

The list of objectives included in Table 2–1 represents *incomplete* statements of objectives because only content, one of several necessary attributes, is included. The basic attributes of a good objective are content, behavior, condition, and standard of performance. *Content* is the material to which the learner will be directed. *Behavior* refers to the type of process the learner is expected to use in dealing with the content. (Levels of behavior are elaborated upon in the next section.) *Condition* refers to the situation in which the behavior is expected to occur. *Standard of performance* is the degree to which the learner is expected to meet the objective. Objectives are always written for a specific age group at a specified level of skill.

TABLE 2–1 • Content of a Football Unit

1. Development of skills: pass, catch, punt, place-kick, block, tackle.
2. Development of ability to play game.
3. Knowledge of rules.
4. Knowledge of safety factors.
5. Knowledge of appropriate principles of movement.

If, for example, in a football unit, a teacher plans to teach the skill of passing, he undoubtedly has specific skill goals in mind, such as: How well should the student be able to pass? Under what conditions? As long as there is no statement of learner behavior, many different interpretations of an objective are possible.

It is helpful to think first of the situation in which we as teachers will expect the student to perform. If we are interested in the football pass, are we concerned with pass performance in a practice situation or in a game? Quite often we are interested in both situations. It is reasonable to expect the student to learn to execute the pass with a certain degree of effectiveness in a game situation. If this is what the teacher expects, two objectives are needed.

OBJECTIVE 1. Given the ball and a partner in a practice situation, the student will be able to pass the ball 20 feet to the partner with both speed and accuracy. (In this case, the partner is stationary. An intermediate objective might be desirable where the partner is moving in a practice situation.)

OBJECTIVE 2. Given the ball in a game situation, and assuming that the pass protection is adequate and that a receiver is open, the student will be able to pass the ball over any reasonable distance with accuracy and an optimum amount of force.

Even though these objectives include both content and student behavior, their interpretation might still differ from one teacher to another. In the first, for example, what degree of speed and accuracy is desired? Is every student expected to master the objective? How often should the student be able to meet a given standard? (It would be unreasonable to expect a student to meet a set standard with every attempt.) These questions will be considered in the following paragraphs.

Both of the above objectives refer to the forward overarm pass in football. Other passes might be considered essential in the unit, and would require different objectives. Also, these two objectives are more relevant to some football positions than to others. Will there nonetheless be common objectives for the pass for the whole class? Again, the answer depends upon the philosophy of the teacher and the requirements of the system. Some teachers may believe that every student should experiment with a variety of positions. In this case, both objectives would be important for all students. Other teachers may emphasize refining skills at one or two positions, but may still want all students to be able to perform the fundamentals of football adequately in a practice situation. In the latter case, objective 1 would be important for all students, whereas objective 2 would only be pertinent for some students.

The two objectives as stated would more properly be classified as curriculum objectives because no standard of performance is given. Returning to the question of how fast and how accurately the ball should be thrown in objective 1, it is seen that even the distance of 20 feet is an arbitrary figure. Clearly, another objective needs to be written to incorporate these points. The new objective can be called an *evaluation objective*. The evaluation objective specifies a minimal level of performance that all students should be able to attain.

It would be unrealistic to write evaluation objectives for our two curriculum objectives unless we know the group of students for whom the objectives are being written. Certainly the speed and accuracy requirements of the pass differ for 7th-grade boys and 12th-grade boys. Even the distance requirements would differ. Another important factor is the boys' levels of skill at the beginning of the unit. Let us develop a tentative evaluation objective for objective 1 that might be appropriate for 9th-grade boys ranked as high beginners in football.

OBJECTIVE 1. (First revision) The student will be able to pass the football with a flat arc and with enough accuracy to place the ball in the partner's waist area 8 out of 10 times. The ball will be passed over a distance of 20 feet.

The above evaluation objective might not satisfy some teachers because the determination of a "flat arc" might be difficult, but it could then be further refined.

OBJECTIVE 1. (Second revision) The student will be able to pass the football to the partner's waist area in x seconds, 8 out of 10 times. The ball will be passed over a distance of 20 feet.

A further criticism might be that the "partner's waist area" is not a very specific standard. The teacher might wish to develop a common accuracy goal for the students to work toward in practice situations. The evaluation objective might then be altered as follows:

OBJECTIVE 1. (Third revision) The student will be able to pass the football to the center of a given target in x seconds, 8 out of 10 times. The ball will be passed over a distance of 20 feet.

The specific standards must be set by the individual teacher based on the level of skill of the boys at the beginning of the unit and on the length of time of the unit. Final standards may be set by the school system, in which case the teacher's intermediate standards will be geared toward meeting these standards.

The determination of standards may be difficult for a teacher with little or no teaching experience. Also, the teacher must revise standards that prove to be unrealistic for a particular class. Seldom should a teacher expect an entire class to achieve the standard set in an objective. A teacher might be satisfied if 90 percent of a class met any given standard, and under some circumstances, the expectation might be as low as 70 percent.

Categories of Behavior

Classification schemes, or taxonomies, have been developed for three domains of behavior. These domains are: cognitive (intellectual skills), affective (interests, attitudes, appreciations, and desires), and psychomotor (motor skills). The schema for the cognitive and affective domains are widely known, and are presented in detail in the two *Taxonomies of Educational Objectives* (Bloom et al., 1956; Krathwohl et al., 1964). Although the Bloom taxonomy was selected for inclusion in this chapter, other classification schemes of cognitive behavior have been developed, such as the one by Gagné (1965).

Cognitive Domain

The classification of educational objectives for the cognitive domain is the result of the work of Bloom and his associates (1956). The assumptions underlying the taxonomy are that the categories are hierarchical, and that this hierarchy is cumulative. The hierarchy of intellectual behaviors ranges from a low order of complexity to a higher one. For example, memorizing facts would represent a lower order of behavior than applying these facts in some way. The cumulative aspect of the hierarchy is described as the dependency at each level on mastery of the levels below. For instance, in order to apply facts in some way, one must be able to recall them. Bloom has classified cognitive behavior into six levels: knowledge, comprehension, application, analysis, synthesis, and evaluation. A synopsis of his taxonomy is presented in Table 2–2.

**TABLE 2–2 • Synopsis of the Taxonomy of Educational Objectives:
Cognitive Domain***

Knowledge

1.00   Knowledge. Recall of information.
1.10   Knowledge of specifics. Emphasis is on symbols with concrete referents.
       1.11   Knowledge of terminology.
       1.12   Knowledge of specific facts.
1.20   Knowledge of ways and means of dealing with specifics. Includes methods of inquiry, chronological sequences, standards of judgment, patterns of organization within a field.
       1.21   Knowledge of conventions: accepted usage, correct style, etc.
       1.22   Knowledge of trends and sequences.
       1.23   Knowledge of classifications and categories.
       1.24   Knowledge of criteria
       1.25   Knowledge of methodology for investigating particular problems
1.30   Knowledge of the universals and abstractions in a field. Patterns and schemes by which phenomena and ideas are organized.
       1.31   Knowledge of principles and generalizations.
       1.32   Knowledge of theories and structures (as a connected body of principles, generalizations, and interrelations).

Intellectual Skills and Abilities

2.00   Comprehension. Understanding of material being communicated, without necessarily relating it to other material.
       2.10   Translation. From one set of symbols to another.
       2.20   Interpretation. Summarization or explanation of a communication.
       2.30   Extrapolation. Extension of trends beyond the given data.
3.00   Application. The use of abstractions in particular, concrete situations.
4.00   Analysis. Breaking a communication into its parts so that organization of ideas is clear.
       4.10   Analysis of elements. E.g., recognizing assumptions.

TABLE 2–2 (Continued)

4.20   Analysis of relationships. Content or mechanical factors.
4.30   Analysis of organizational principles. What holds the communication together?
5.00   Synthesis. Putting elements into a whole.
    5.10   Production of a unique communication.
    5.20   Production of a plan for operations.
    5.30   Derivation of a set of abstract relations.
6.00   Evaluation. Judging the value of material for a given purpose.
    6.10   Judgments in terms of internal evidence. E.g., logical consistency.
    6.20   Judgments in terms of external evidence. E.g., consistency with facts developed elsewhere.

*Reprinted from B. Bloom, et al., *Taxonomy of Educational Objectives, Handbook I: The Cognitive Domain* (New York: David McKay Co., Inc., 1956), pp. 201–7, by permission of the authors and publisher.

Note that the domain is broken down into two major categories: knowledge and intellectual skills and abilities. The first category contains only the first level of behavior—knowledge. The remaining five levels fall into the second category. Furthermore, each level is subdivided so that twenty-nine classifications of intellectual behavior are defined. As the behavior increases in complexity, the degree of abstraction also increases. The higher level behaviors depend upon the sequential development of all the behavior in the lower part of the hierarchy.

A teacher can use the taxonomy by first deciding on the levels of cognitive behavior that are important for his class, and then writing objectives for each of the desired levels. A teacher can then avoid over-emphasizing learning at the lowest level of behavior—the learning of factual material. Clear statements of objectives at all levels reduce the probability of using evaluation procedures that measure only the first level of behavior, such as a teacher encouraging learning at several levels of behavior, but giving tests which require only the recall of facts.

As a first step in learning to write objectives at several levels, Popham and Baker (1970 [a], 1970 [b]) suggest learning to recognize cognitive objectives at both a low level (knowledge) and a higher one. An individual can first practice writing objectives at a low and a high level, then attempt to write objectives within subdivisions of the higher level. Some examples of objectives written for different levels of cognitive behavior are given in Table 2–3.

Very little information is available on the validation of the taxonomy for the cognitive domain, but the validation of one aspect of its internal structure has been reported. Smith used a hierarchical syndrome analysis to test the assumption that cognitive processes form a hierarchy (Smith,

TABLE 2-3 • Examples of Cognitive Objectives at Different Levels of Behavior

1.25   Knowledge of kinesiological techniques for studying patterns of motor skill.

2.10   Skill in translating symbolic statements given as statistics into verbal material, and vice versa.

3.00   Ability to describe the important components of a specific construct, such as physical fitness.

4.20   Ability to explain the relationship between test validity and test reliability.

5.20   Ability to plan appropriate evaluation techniques for a learning situation.

6.00   Ability to judge the validity of a test based on criteria for the selection of a good test.

1968). In general, the analysis supported this assumption. The knowledge and evaluation categories were the only ones to behave in a manner inconsistent with the theoretical formulation.

The taxonomy is difficult to validate for reasons noted by Kropp, Stoker, and Bashaw (1966). For example, a taxonomy is designed to measure responses (behaviors) rather than content. If an item is designed to measure a certain response, the teacher has no assurance that it is actually doing so. Although one could ask the student about his response during or after the process is measured, the student may not be able to accurately describe his response. An alternative might be to give the student a list of possible solutions to the problem, and ask him to choose the one most like his own.

Another difficulty noted by Kropp, et al., is that content must remain constant to get at a measure of process. It is unlikely that the teacher will be able to assume that students have had common previous experiences with the content. Perhaps the solution is to provide for student access to the content at the time the response measures are collected.

A further difficulty is failure of some students to respond correctly to knowledge items even when the content is immediately available. It is not reasonable to test at a higher level when students can not handle even the knowledge level adequately.

Affective Domain

The *Taxonomy* for the affective domain was developed by Krathwohl and his associates (1964). The synopsis of this taxonomy is presented in Table 2-4. Note that five levels of behavior have been identified. Again, a hierarchy exists from the first to the fifth levels.

The major characteristics of the affective continuum are as follows: (1) increasing emotional quality of responses; (2) responses become more automatic as one progresses up the continuum; (3) increasing willingness to attend to a specified stimulus; and (4) developing integration of a value pattern at the upper levels of the continuum. The overall organizing principle which theoretically accounts for the affective phenomena in the process of learning and growth is referred to as internalization (Payne, 1968, pp. 19–20)

TABLE 2–4 • Synopsis of the Taxonomy of Educational Objectives: Affective Domain*

1.0   Receiving (Attending). Sensitivity to the existence of certain phenomena and stimuli.
   1.1   Awareness. Learner is conscious of stimuli.
   1.2   Willingness to receive. Involves suspended judgment.
   1.3   Controlled or selected attention. Differentiation of stimulus.

2.0   Responding. Active attention to stimuli, e.g., compliance and commitment to rules and practices.
   2.1   Acquiescence in responding.
   2.2   Willingness to respond.
   2.3   Satisfaction in response.

3.0   Valuing. Consistent belief and attitude of worth held about a phenomenon.
   3.1   Acceptance of a value.
   3.2   Preference for a value.
   3.3   Commitment.

4.0   Organization. Organizing, interrelating, and analyzing different relevant values.
   4.1   Conceptualizing of a value.
   4.2   Organization of a value system.

5.0   Characterization by a value or value concept. Behavior is guided by values.
   5.1   Generalized set.
   5.2   Characterization.

*Reprinted from D.R. Krathwohl, et al,, *Taxonomy of Educational Objectives, Handbook II: The Affective Domain* (New York: David McKay Co., Inc., 1964), Appendix B, by permission of the authors and publisher.

Krathwohl defines internalization as:

. . . the inner growth that occurs as an individual becomes aware of and then adopts the attitudes, principles, codes, and sanctions that become a part of him in forming value judgments and in guiding his conduct (Krathwohl et al., 1964, p. 29).

Writing objectives for affective behaviors is more difficult than writing cognitive and psychomotor objectives. The major problem is the determination of the standard, the evaluation of the affective behavior. Some examples of objectives for the affective domain are given in Table 2–5.

TABLE 2–5 • Examples of Affective Objectives at Different Levels of Behavior

1.3   Observes a modern dance with some recognition of the use of space, time, and force.

2.1   Accepts umpire's decision in a baseball game.

3.3   Encourages team members to work together by setting an example.

4.0   Weighs team tactics against standards of fair play rather than winning at any cost.

5.0   Consistently honorable in observing training rules.

Popham and Baker (1970[a]) recommend the following steps for writing objectives for measurable affective behaviors: For a given affective behavior, think of an individual who possesses the behavior, and an individual who does not. Describe a situation in which the two individuals will react differently with regard to the behavior in question. Use that situation to write the affective objective. For example, physical education teachers are often concerned with the development of sportsmanship in their students. If a teacher wished to write an affective objective for sportsmanship, he would first identify an individual whom he classifies as a "good sport" and one whom he classifies as a "poor sport." Many situations could be described in which the two individuals would probably behave differently. For instance, an individual possessing the attribute of good sportsmanship would probably play by the rules in a game situation while a non-possessor would attempt to break or "stretch" the rules on every possible occasion. An affective objective could then be written incorporating this situation.

Psychomotor Domain

No handbook for the psychomotor domain has been published by Bloom or Krathwohl and their associates.

> Although we recognize the existence of this domain, we find so little done about it in secondary schools or colleges, that we do not believe the development of a classification of these objectives would be useful at present. We would appreciate comments on this point from teachers and other educational workers who are especially interested in the domain of educational objectives (Bloom, et al., 1956, pp. 7–8).

However, the classification of psychomotor objectives is of obvious importance to physical educators. In recent years, several educators have developed tentative classification schemes of psychomotor behavior. Two of these taxonomies, one developed by Simpson and the other by Jewett, are included in this chapter. The interested reader may also wish to examine the Kibler, Barker, and Miles (1970) classification of motor behavior.

Simpson classification of educational objectives: psychomotor domain.
One of the first classification systems for the psychomotor domain was
developed by Simpson (1966), a home economist. It is important to note
that Simpson considers her system to be a tentative one. The Simpson
classification is presented in Table 2–6.

TABLE 2–6 • Simpson's Classification of Educational Objectives:
Psychomotor Domain—A Tentative System*

1.0   Perception. Process of becoming aware of objects, qualities, or relations by way
       of the sense organs.
    1.1   Sensory stimulation. Impingement of a stimulus upon one or more of the
       sense organs.
        1.11   Auditory
        1.12   Visual.
        1.13   Tactile.
        1.14   Taste.
        1.15   Olfactory.
        1.16   Kinesthetic.
    1.2   Cue selection. Deciding to what cues one must respond in order to satisfy
       the particular requirements of task performance.
    1.3   Translation. Relating of perception to action in performing a motor act.

2.0   Set. Set is a preparatory adjustment or readiness for a particular kind of action or
       experience.
    2.1   Mental set. Readiness, in the mental sense, to perform a certain motor act.
    2.2   Physical set. Readiness in the sense of having made the anatomical adjust-
       ments necessary for a motor act to be performed.
    2.3   Emotional set. Readiness in terms of attitudes favorable to the motor act's
       taking place.

3.0   Guided response. The overt behavioral act of an individual under the guidance of
       the instructor.
    3.1   Imitation. The execution of the act as a direct response to the perception
       of another person performing the act.
    3.2   Trial and error. Trying various responses, usually with some rationale for
       each response, until an appropriate response is achieved.

4.0   Mechanism. Learned response has become habitual.

5.0   Complex overt response. The motor act can be carried out smoothly and efficiently,
       that is, with a minimum expenditure of time and energy.
    5.1   Resolution of uncertainty. The act is performed without hesitation of the
       individual to get a mental picture of task sequence.
    5.2   Automatic performance. The individual can perform a finely coordinated
       motor skill with a great deal of ease and muscle control.

*Reprinted from E.J. Simpson, "The Classification of Educational Objectives: Psycho-
motor Domain," Vocational and Technical Education Grant Contract No. OE 5–85–104 (Washington, D.C.: U.S. Department of Health, Education, and Welfare, 1966).

Jewett taxonomy of educational objectives: motor domain. A more recently developed taxonomy for this domain is due to the efforts of Jewett and her associates (1971), and it appears to be of greater value to physical educators than any of the others proposed. Jewett's taxonomy more closely parallels the cognitive and affective ones, in that her categories are hierarchical and deal with process rather than content. The Jewett classification is presented in Table 2–7.

**TABLE 2–7 • Jewett's Proposed Taxonomy of Educational Objectives:
Motor Domain***

1.0   Generic movement. Movement operations or processes which facilitate the development of human movement patterns.

    1.1   Perceiving. Recognition of movement positions, postures, patterns, and skills by means of the sense organs.

    1.2   Imitating. Duplication of a movement pattern or skill as a result of perceiving.

    1.3   Patterning. Arrangement and use of body parts in successive and harmonious ways to achieve a movement pattern of skill.

2.0   Ordinative movement. Meeting the requirements of specific movement tasks through processes of organizing, performing, and refining movement patterns and skills.

    2.1   Adapting. Modification of a patterned movement or skill to meet specific task demands.

    2.2   Refining. Acquisition of smooth, efficient control in performing a movement pattern or skill as a result of an improvement process, e.g.,

        a.   Elimination of extraneous movements

        b.   Mastery of spatial and temporal relations.

        c.   Habitual performance under more complex conditions.

3.0   Creative movement. Processes of inventing or creating skillful movements which will serve the unique purposes of the learner.

    3.1   Varying. Invention or construction of unique or novel options in performing a movement pattern or skill.

    3.2   Improvising. Extemporaneous origination or initiation of novel movements or combinations of movements.

    3.3   Composing. Creation of unique movement designs or patterns.

*Reprinted from A. Jewett et al,. "Educational Change through a Taxonomy for Writing Physical Education Objectives," *Quest* XVI (1971), p. 35, published by NAPECW and NC-PEAM.

When learning to write psychomotor objectives, the physical education teacher might find it easier to write low and high level objectives, as Popham suggests for the cognitive domain. Then the application of the appropriate techniques to the Jewett taxonomy may not seem so complex. Sample ob-

TABLE 2–8 · Sample Objectives for Jewett's "Motor Domain"*

Learning	Behavior	Educational Objective
1.1	Perceiving	Given a series of body positions, identify each as a stretched or curled position.
1.2	Imitating	Assume the tripod position, replicating the movements demonstrated by another pupil.
1.3	Patterning	Demonstrate the softball overarm throw.
2.1	Adapting	Execute a pass from the rear of the volleyball court to a front-line player.
2.1	Adapting	Complete the 600 yard walk-run in_____minutes.
2.2	Refining	Shoot a one-handed push shot in basketball from different positions on the court during a game.
3.1	Varying	Alter the sculling pattern to propel the body in a prone position feet first and head first.
3.2	Improvising	Originate a movement "trick" on the scooter, combining at least two skills demonstrated.
3.3	Composing	Symbolize youth protest in a "living statuary" tableau of 4–10 participants.

*Modified from A.E. Jewett, "Accountability in the Physical Education Curriculum" (Paper presented at the Wisconsin Association for Health, Physical Education, and Recreation, Whitefish Bay, Wisconsin, 1970), by permission of the author.

jectives using Jewett's proposed taxonomy (1970) are given in Table 2–8.

For further clarification of the use of the Jewett taxonomy, let us examine the objective written for the football pass in the preceding section. The objective reads as follows:

> The student will be able to pass the football to the center of a given target in x seconds 8 out of 10 times. The ball will be passed over a distance of 20 feet.

It is assumed that since the objective was written for ninth grade boys, the overarm throw has already been patterned. Now the student is being asked to *adapt* the overarm throw to meet specific task demands, namely force and accuracy. This should suggest to the teacher that when this objective is met, the next step would be to perform the skill under more complex conditions, such as in a game. The student would then be performing at a higher level of behavior that Jewett calls refining.

If the initial assumption concerning the patterning of the overarm throw is not valid for all students, the teacher would have to write an objective at the *patterning* level for those students. One begins to see that, within a single class, students may be working at several different levels, requiring the planning of appropriate learning experiences and standards for each.

Whatever the criticisms of behavioral objectives, emphasis on their connection with the taxonomies has brought about a re-examination of what is being taught in the classroom. The hope is that as the psychomotor domain is developed in a useful way for physical educators, a similar re-examination of what is being taught in the gymnasium will take place. Such a re-examination may reveal that a teacher proceeded through an entire unit patterning basic skills, thus emphasizing a low level of psychomotor learning. If he wrote his objectives in behavioral terms, it would be clear that either he was not dealing with higher levels of psychomotor learning, or, if his objectives in fact included higher levels of behavior, that he was not teaching according to his objectives. This type of information, when carefully analyzed, can lead to improved instruction.

Opposing Viewpoints on Behavioral Objectives

Examination of opposing views on behavioral objectives can be valuable because there are problems associated with their use, although, in most cases, these have logical solutions. However, judgment of the adequacy of the solutions will be left to the reader. It is the view of this author that the advantages of using behavioral objectives outweigh the disadvantages as long as their use is kept within proper perspective.

A common criticism of the use of behavioral objectives is that any set of specific statements will restrict the teacher by forcing him to stay within a rigid framework. According to this view, any situation that occurs during class that is outside the scope of the stated objectives must not be pursued, a view that considers behavioral objectives in their narrowest sense. If a situation arises that is of obvious educational significance, most conscientious teachers would deal with it whether or not it was originally considered one of the course objectives. The point is that the statement of objectives will determine the direction in which the class will proceed. It is possible that enough new situations will occur to warrant a change in direction and, therefore, a new statement of objectives, but the overall goals might remain unchanged. One should never assume that a teacher must be bound to a framework he himself designed when he can logically see that it merits alteration.

Another objection to behavioral objectives is that there is a basic incompatibility between spontaneous originality and planning (Atkin, 1968). Can one write objectives for creative behavior when outcomes should be innovative and are, therefore, unknown? This problem is of special concern to fine arts teachers. Popham (1970) notes that teachers in the fine arts must, and do, make judgments on the quality of performance, therefore using selected criteria for evaluation. The problem, then, is to state these criteria in the form of objectives.

> Perhaps the best answer on both counts (curriculum and classroom creativity) is to question whether planning really acts as a deterrent to creativity or a director of it. All creativity takes place within certain bounds. While it is true that one can prescribe the operations too tightly for some artists, it is truly amazing what artists have done within tight bounds. Consider the creativity that poets have displayed within the limits of tight structure such as sonnets or in writing haiku, or that Bach displayed in his music. Of the latter, existentialist Jean Paul Sartre is said to have observed, "He taught how to find originality within an established discipline; actually —how to live." The discipline of planning through objectives may be too strict for some individuals, but, considering the values to be gained in using this approach, whether it is in fact too strict should be tested rather than a foregone conclusion (Krathwohl and Payne, 1971, p. 40).

A third objection is that trivial learner behaviors are the easiest to describe behaviorally, the more complex objectives being difficult to indentify and, then, define, Therefore, the teacher might emphasize trivial learning because these behaviors lend themselves to delineation. The complex objectives, however, may be the most worthwhile (Atkin, 1968; Ausubel, 1967; Eisner, 1967). Popham (1970) answers this criticism by noting that behavioral objectives make it far easier to attend to important educational goals. If a teacher actually does emphasize trivial learning, it becomes obvious in examining his objectives. Without a statement of objectives, the teacher, however well-meaning, may not realize the limited framework within which he teaches.

A fourth criticism is based on the lack of evidence of a relationship between educational experiences and changes in behavior (Kliebard, 1968), which is a legitimate point, but should not be limited to the method of teaching that incorporates behavioral objectives. No matter what teaching method is used, it is extremely difficult to determine the degree to which long-range goals are met within a short period of time. One can only attempt to predict the degree of progress by using indicators of behavior.

The fifth objection, sometimes projected as a criticism of the process of measurement, is that some results of education cannot be measured (Eisner, 1967). Even though some aspects of educational measurement are in a primitive stage, there are some highly sophisticated measures of complex behavior available. If a teacher rejects the use of measurement because of this difficulty, he will be doing his students a great disservice by failing to provide feedback on learning and achievement.

A sixth criticism is that innovations in teaching are hampered, not helped, by demands for behavioral statements of objectives (Atkin, 1966; Eisner,

1967). If, for example, a group of physical educators was attempting to design a model unit on movement education, the team would certainly include a movement education specialist and a measurement specialist. The measurement specialist, not being an expert in movement education, would never understand the intricacies of content and behavior in movement education as well as the movement education specialist. The language of the measurement specialist with regard to behavioral objectives might be somewhat foreign to the movement specialist. Thus, a communications gap can exist between them. If the measurement specialist presses for a complete set of objectives before initiating the project, the movement specialist may become frustrated. Because this is a very real problem, Krathwohl and Payne (1971) suggest that it is necessary to operate with greater flexibility. In the case of our physical education team, a satisfactory compromise might be to carry out the project without the complete set of objectives, and finish the set after the curriculum is developed. An example of a flexible approach in English is given in the following quotation:

> Nearly all English teachers insist that their students outline their compositions. Yet, how many students find they can write quite excellent pieces without first going through this step. Because of their particular cognitive style the "organize first then perform" paradigm is foreign to their way of working. We all know individuals like this and this was a characteristic of this particular instructor. He was using a modern learning facility and we needed to judge how to use it properly, and to measure its effect, evaluators needed to know his objectives. He flatly refused to be bothered by specifying them. He was obdurate. He did, however, allow a graduate assistant to visit his classes to try inductively to determine his objectives. Over the semester, the assistant did quite well and at its end showed his work in the form of behavioral objectives to the professor. He included in this report the consequences that flowed from these statements in terms of improved learning methods and measuring devices. The professor was simply delighted. While he has not yet been converted to taking the time to specify these objectives himself, he is now an advocate of their value and has made use of them in developing new instructional devices and the evaluation instruments (Krathwohl and Payne, 1971, p. 41).

For a more thorough treatment of criticisms of behavioral objectives, the reader is referred to several articles (Atkin, 1968; Eisner, 1967; Kliebard, 1968). Popham (1970) has written a rebuttal to many of these objections.

Summary

This chapter was devoted primarily to a practical discussion of behavioral objectives and a theoretical discussion of the behavior domains. Even though there have been criticisms of the use of behavioral objectives, most objections are helpful in bringing about a close reexamination of all aspects of this method. The advantages of using behavioral objectives to guide the teaching-learning process at present appear to outweigh the disadvantages. However, further investigations are needed to provide empirical support for the use of both behavioral objectives and the taxonomies.

Bibliography

ATKIN, J.M. "Behavioral Objectives in Curriculum Design: A Cautionary Note," *The Science Teacher,* XXXV (1968), pp. 27–39.

AUSUBEL, D.P. "Crucial Psychological Issues in the Objectives, Organization, and Evaluation of Curriculum Movements," *Psychology in the Schools,* IV (1967), pp. 111–121.

BLOOM, B. (Ed.). *Taxonomy of Educational Objectives. Handbook* I: *The Cognitive Domain.* New York: David McKay Company, 1956.

CLEIN, M.I. and W.J. STONE. "Physical Education and the Classification of Educational Objectives: Psychomotor Domain," *Physical Educator,* XXVII (1970), pp. 34–35.

DRESSEL, P.L. "Measurement and Evaluation of Instructional Objectives," *Seventeenth Yearbook of the National Council on Measurements Used in Education.* New York: National Council on Measurement in Education, 1960, pp. 1–6.

EISNER, E.W. "Educational Objectives: Help or Hindrance," *The School Review,* LXXV (1967), pp. 250–260.

GAGNÉ, R.M. *The Conditions of Learning.* New York: Holt, Rinehart, and Winston, 1965.

GRONLUND, N.E. *Measurement and Evaluation in Teaching.* New York: The Macmillan Company, 1965.

JEWETT, A.E. "Accountability in the Physical Education Curriculum." Speech presented at the Wisconsin Association for Health, Physical Education and Recreation Convention, Whitefish Bay, Wisconsin, November 1970.

JEWETT, A.E., L.S. JONES, S.M. LUNEKE and S.M. ROBINSON. "Educational Change through a Taxonomy for Writing Physical Education Objectives," *Quest,* XV (1971), pp. 32–38.

KIBLER, R.J., L.L. BARKER and D.T. MILES. *Behavioral Objectives and Instruction.* Boston: Allyn and Bacon, Inc., 1970.

KLIEBARD, H.M. "Curricular Objectives and Evaluation: A Reassessment," *The High School Journal,* LI (1968), pp. 241–247.

KRATHWOHL, D.R. et al. *Taxonomy of Educational Objectives. Handbook II: The Affective Domain.* New York: David McKay and Co., 1964.

KRATHWOHL, D.R. and D.A. PAYNE. "Defining and Assessing Educational Objectives," in *Educational Measurement,* ed. R.L. Thorndike. Washington, D.C.: American Council on Education, 1971.

KROPP, R.P., H.W. STOKER and W.L. BASHAW. "The Validation of the Taxonomy of Educational Objectives," *Journal of Experimental Education,* XXXIV, No. 3 (1966), pp. 69–76.

MAGER, R.F. *Preparing Instructional Objectives.* Palo Alto, California: Fearon Publishers, 1962.

PAYNE, D.A. *The Specification and Measurement of Learning Outcomes.* Waltham, Mass.: Blaisdell Publishing Company, 1968.

POPHAM, W.J. "Probing the Validity of Arguments against Behavioral Goals," in *Behavioral Objectives and Instruction,* ed. R.J. Kibler et al. Boston: Allyn and Bacon, Inc., 1970.

POPHAM, W.J. and E.L. BAKER. *Establishing Instructional Goals.* Englewood Cliffs, N.J.: Prentice-Hall, Inc., 1970[a].

POPHAM, W.J. and E.L. BAKER. *Systematic Instruction.* Englewood Cliffs, N.J.: Prentice-Hall, Inc., 1970[b].

SIMPSON, E.J. *The Classification of Educational Objectives, Psychomotor Domain.* Vocational and Technical Education Grant, Contract No. OE 5–85–104, Office of Education, U.S. Department of Health, Education, and Welfare, May 1966.

SMITH, R.B. "An Empirical Examination of the Assumptions Underlying the Taxonomy of Educational Objectives," *Journal of Educational Measurement,* V, No. 2 (1968), pp. 125–28.

TYLER, R.W. "The Functions of Measurement in Improving Instruction," in *Educational Measurement,* ed. E.L. Lindquist. Washington, D.C.: American Council on Education, 1951.

3

formative and
summative evaluation

New developments in the area of evaluation theory may not reach a level of application in physical education for many years; however, certain innovations such as formative and summative evaluation are new in name only to many physical educators. The concept of formative evaluation, for example, was advocated many years ago by Ruth Glassow at the University of Wisconsin. Knowledge and understanding of formative and summative evaluation is useful because evaluation is placed in a broad perspective that discourages teachers from regarding it in the narrow sense of measurement to determine grades.

Examination of Common Beliefs about Evaluation

Formative and summative classification has not been formally applied in the area of physical education even though both types have been used to varying extents. In this section, three statements that reflect commonly held beliefs about evaluation in physical education will be examined. In each case, acceptance of the belief can have restrictive effects on both the teacher and the student because each statement represents a misconception about evaluation.

MISCONCEPTION 1: The appropriate time for the measurement of skills and knowledge in physical education is at the end of a unit.
While evaluation at the end of a unit is important, it is decidedly specific

in purpose and somewhat limited in nature. Evaluation at the end of a unit is called *summative* evaluation. Obviously, it is also possible to evaluate learning during the instructional unit. This type of evaluation is called *formative* evaluation. Although they will be discussed in detail later in the chapter, a general description of each type is appropriate here.

Summative evaluation generally reflects the level of achievement of students in relation to one another. Quite often, it is used to determine student grades. The feedback to the student on the results of summative evaluation may not be very useful. A summative measure that is used to make decisions about individuals, such as determining grades, must have a high level of reliability and validity. These standards may be reduced somewhat if the test results are used to make group decisions, such as where the class as a whole stands at the end of a unit. Summative evaluation objectives might be set by the school district in order to ensure continuity (Bloom, Hastings, and Madaus, 1971).

Formative evaluation is used throughout a unit as an integral part of the learning process. While it is possible to think of setting aside class time for summative-type testing during a unit, such a practice is not a part of the formative evaluation process where a student is evaluated as he learns. He is provided immediate and continual feedback on his performance. Most teachers, if given the opportunity to teach on a one-to-one basis, could provide a student with continual feedback; however, current class sizes do not permit this type of student-teacher interaction. The teacher must provide opportunities for formative evaluation that can be handled by the student, with the help of his classmates (Bloom, Hastings, and Madaus, 1971).

Formative evaluation objectives are usually set by the teacher, rather than the school district, because they reflect the teacher's philosophy about teaching a sport or activity. For example, formative objectives for a swimming teacher who starts beginning swimmers in deep water would clearly be inappropriate for one who prefers shallow water for beginners. Thus, formative objectives would usually be highly individualized, whereas summative objectives would be the same for all teachers within a school district. The teacher, then, is asked to work toward a common goal, but may select the means of achieving this goal according to his personal philosophy. (This assumption can be made only if the methods in question are equally effective.)

MISCONCEPTION 2: Skill tests are limited in their usefulness because in most cases only three or four students can be active at any one time.

Because some tests are such that very few class members can be active at any given time does not mean that this is correct procedure. In fact, it should rarely occur when formative evaluation techniques, which should be designed to have students practice skills in situations that provide feedback, are used. Thus, the number of students that are active depends on the space available for practice and the ingenuity of the teacher in utilizing that space.

MISCONCEPTION 3: Physical education teachers should select tests for class use from those published in the literature.

This statement reflects a misconception about testing in physical education. Teacher-made tests are commonly used in the classroom because such tests can be designed to measure appropriate stages of learning. If Miss Smith first teaches the full swing in golf, she must design evaluation situations that will provide feedback on the success of that swing. If Miss Jones teaches the short shot first, her evaluation situations must differ from Miss Smith's. Therefore, if a golf manual were published that included formative evaluation procedures for beginning golfers, these procedures could only serve as examples for Miss Smith and Miss Jones unless they were based on a philosophy identical to that of either of the two teachers.

If common goals were set within the school district, the summative evaluation procedures would be the same for both Miss Smith and Miss Jones. Even so, the measures described in the literature might not be appropriate for students in different schools, and it might be necessary to develop different summative measures for each. Of course, reliability and validity would have to be established for these measures.

Total reliance on published tests is hazardous because any given test is designed for a specific age range, level of skill, and stage of learning. A test may have a high level of reliability and validity, and yet not be appropriate for one's students. Until a professional testing organization undertakes skill test development, individual teachers and school districts will have to continue developing their own formative and summative measures. This is not to say that teachers will not find some excellent and appropriate tests in the literature, but a test should be utilized only if it fits the purposes of the teacher and the school district.

Mastery Learning

Because the concept of mastery learning is closely tied to that of formative evaluation, it is helpful to examine the mastery learning model before dealing with formative evaluation in detail. The normal curve has been used for many years to determine the student differences which result in grades. As Bloom (1968) has noted, so many teachers have used this principle for so long that we have begun to believe in its irrefutability. Some administrators prefer to see a range of grades from A to F, and a teacher can get into trouble for being "too easy" or "too hard" in grading. Unfortunately, the constant use of the normal curve convinces some students that they can do only C and D work, and leads some teachers to teach as if only a small number of students can master the work.

For many years, educators assumed that mental abilities, or aptitudes, are closely related to academic achievement. In reality, this situation exists only when achievement tests are designed to assure a normal distribution of scores. Mental abilities, as measured by most intelligence tests, are distributed as a normal curve. In 1963 Carroll suggested that aptitude may be related to the amount of time necessary to achieve mastery. If the students' aptitude scores are distributed over a normal curve, and their periods of instruction are equal, their achievement scores will be distributed normally. Carroll's research yielded a correlation of $+0.70$ between aptitude and achievement in mathematics. If, on the other hand, the instruction and amount of time are adjusted for each student according to his needs, the students are not normally distributed on achievement. This distribution is negatively skewed,* and the correlation between aptitude and achievement approaches zero.

If students are normally distributed with respect to aptitude, and if the kind and quality of instruction and the amount of time available for learning are made appropriate to the needs and characteristics of the learner, Bloom (1968) suggests that a large majority—around 90 percent—can achieve mastery. A model for mastery learning has been described by Mayo (1970). The model includes the following steps:

1. Inform students about course expectations, even lesson expectations and unit expectations, so that they view learning as a cooperative rather than as a competitive enterprise.
2. Set standards of mastery in advance; use prevailing standards or set new ones and assign grades in terms of performance rather than relative ranking.
3. Use short diagnostic progress tests for each unit of instruction.
4. Prescribe additional learning for those who do not demonstrate initial mastery.
5. Attempt to provide additional time for learning for those persons who seem to need it (Mayo, 1970, p. 2).

The literature on mastery learning has dealt primarily with academic achievement. However, any experienced physical educator will recognize that the concept of mastery learning, if not the name, is not uncommon in physical education. Nonetheless, the application of mastery learning theory

*In a negatively skewed distribution of scores, most of the scores fall at the upper end of the continuum and very few scores fall at the lower end. That is, many students receive high scores on the test, and few receive low scores.

in physical education needs to be examined, especially the processes of setting standards and developing diagnostic procedures.

Criterion-Referenced Measures and Norm-Referenced Measures

When mastery learning theory is applied in education, the tests which are developed are referred to as *criterion-referenced* measures, a term first used by Glaser in 1963. A criterion-referenced measure is "one that is deliberately constructed to yield measurements that are directly interpretable in terms of specified performance standards" (Livingston, 1970, p. 653). If students are measured according to normal curve theory, the tests are called *norm-referenced* measures. Since one cannot readily distinguish between the two types of measures by examining the tests, Simon (1969) suggests using the term criterion- or norm-referenced *scores* or *measures,* rather than tests. The discriminating factor between the two types of measures is the score and how it is used.

A different type of test development is required for each of the measures. The following procedures describe the development of norm-referenced measures. In this case, the steps are applicable to the development of a written test.

1. Define the objectives to be measured.
2. Write items to sample content and behavior domains of the objectives.
3. Adjust item characteristics with average item difficulty around 50%–60% and maximum discrimination against internal criterion of total test scores.*
4. Interpret performance against a norm (that is, peer) group (Mayo, 1970, p. 3).

In the development of criterion-referenced measures, the first two procedures are identical to those presented for norm-referenced measures. In step 3, the average difficulty is increased to 85 percent or higher, and item-discrimination is no longer an important consideration. Because the test score is absolute and not relative, there is no need to compare a criterion-referenced score with the scores of peers, as in step 4.

Implications of Criterion-Referenced Measurement

Although a strong case has been made for the use of criterion-referenced measures, this emphasis does not negate the value of norm-referenced meas-

---

*Item difficulty and discrimination are described in Chapter 8.

ures. Norm-referenced measures are essential when a degree of selectivity is required by the situation, such as when only a certain number of people can be accepted for a job or admitted to a school, and a measure that tends to spread people out is needed. If one wishes to know whether an individual possesses a particular skill and there are no constraints regarding how many individuals possess it, the use of criterion-referenced measures is appropriate. The American Red Cross life saving tests are good examples of the latter situation.

Very little information on test theory is available that is appropriate to criterion-referenced measures. Do the assumptions of the classical test theory model that are applicable for norm-referenced measures also apply to criterion-referenced measures? Popham and Husek (1969) have noted that although variability is the key factor in developing norm-referenced measures, it is irrelevant to criterion-referenced ones. Although the meaning of a criterion-referenced score does not depend on comparison with other scores, current theory on reliability, validity, and item analysis is based on the desirability of variability among scores. Since content validity does not require the use of a statistic, it is suited to criterion-referenced measures. Negative item discrimination in a criterion-referenced measure is the aspect of item analysis of most concern to the test constructor.

The estimation of reliability presents the major problem in the construction of this type of measure. Livingston (1970) has studied the reliability of criterion-referenced measures using the assumptions of the classical test theory model to develop a theory that parallels the one used for norm-referenced measures. He notes that the basic distinction between the two types is that norm-referenced measures reflect how much an individual score deviates from the mean score of the norm group, while criterion-referenced scores indicate how much an individual score deviates from a fixed standard, the criterion. Thus, Livingston has substituted the criterion score for the mean score, and has redefined the test statistics accordingly. Subsequently, Harris (1971) pointed out that Livingston's accomplishment has been primarily one of carefully spelling out a special case of the classic approach to reliability theory. Therefore, it appears that the problems associated with estimating the reliability of criterion-referenced tests have not been solved at the present time.

Types of Evaluation

The distinguishing characteristics of formative and summative evaluation lie in their purpose (expected uses), the portion of course covered (time), and the level of generalization sought by the items in the examination used to collect data for the evaluation.

Summative Evaluation

Summative evaluation usually takes place at the end of a unit when it is too late to modify either the teaching or the learning process with respect to that unit of work. In some cases, this type of evaluation is also used at intermediate stages within the unit. When frequent evaluation takes place, it is concerned with more direct, less generalizable outcomes, whereas long-range, end-of-unit summative evaluation is concerned with the extent to which desired course results are achieved. The learning process is thought to be completed when this type of evaluation is made. This latter point differentiates intermediate summative evaluation from formative evaluation in which the learning process is thought to be incomplete. Some of the purposes of summative evaluation are assignment of grades, certification of skills and abilities, prediction of success in subsequent courses, determination of initiation point of instruction in a subsequent course, provision of feedback to students, and comparison of outcomes of different groups (Bloom, 1971).

Assignment of grades. Summative measures are designed to spread individuals out over several grade categories. The grade reflects one student's amount or level of learning in relation to other students. Three kinds of standards may be adopted: empirical norms, estimated norms, and criterion-based performance. Empirical norms are most frequently used with published tests. These norms are based upon responses of a sample of the type for whom the test was designed. Estimated norms are based on the same type of relative standing, but without an actual tryout of the test. Rather, the test is taken by experts in the area who are also familiar with the type of student for whom the test was designed. Estimated norms may be developed in this way by an individual teacher. Criterion-based performances are determined by the performance desired for each given task, as when, for example, the degree of mastery that must be achieved for a grade of A, B, C, and so forth, is determined by the instructor.

Certification of skills and abilities. Summative evaluation used for purposes of certification is typical for technical training in the secondary school or junior college. The assumption is that a known level of performance exists above which most students can do the specified job and below which most cannot. This is a question of prediction and should be substantiated by predictive validity research.

Prediction of success in subsequent courses. Prediction in this respect is a familiar concept to most educators. Satisfactory performance in one course as a prerequisite to entry into another course is a policy incorporated into many school curricula.

Determination of initiation point of instruction in a subsequent course. Often, it is helpful for a teacher to know how well students performed before coming into his class, so that he will know where to begin new instruction. Merely having a student's previous grade will not always provide very useful information. If the grade is accompanied by tables of specifications for previous tests and a breakdown of the student's performance on each area of the table, the teacher will have meaningful information on the strengths and weaknesses of students.

Provision of feedback to students. It is possible to think of the result of summative evaluation as providing feedback to students, although the feedback may have little effect in terms of changing student behavior. At any rate, the feedback must be accompanied by information that will direct and encourage the student to make up his deficiencies.

Comparision of outcomes of different groups. Summative evaluation measures may be used when one wishes to compare groups that have been exposed to different instructional methods or curricular materials. In this situation, one must have pretest information for the students, or the students must be randomly assigned to the classes in order to make comparisons between the groups.

Formative Evaluation

The term formative evaluation was first used by Scriven (1967) in relation to the evaluation of curricular innovations. This type of evaluation can intervene during the formative stages of learning, and point to areas needing remedial help so that immediately subsequent instruction and study can be more beneficial (Bloom, Hastings, and Madaus, 1971). Formative evaluation helps to pace students' learning and motivate them toward putting forth the necessary effort.

If a student has mastered a unit, formative tests may reinforce learning, reassure a student that his approach to study and his mode of learning are adequate, and reduce anxiety about course achievement. If a student lacks mastery, the test should reveal the particular points of difficulty. *Diagnosis* should be accompanied by a specific *prescription,* which might refer to particular instructional materials or processes.

Bloom and his associates (1971) believe that neither grades nor quality points should be assigned to formative measures, but that the test should be marked on a mastery or nonmastery basis. A test marked nonmastery should always be accompanied by detailed diagnosis and a prescription for attaining mastery. It is suggested that using grades in this situation prepares students who receive low grades early in the unit for the acceptance of less than mastery. Formative evaluation tests should be regarded as a part of the learning process, and should not be the basis for judgment of the student's capabilities.

Scoring a test according to *levels* of mastery may provide more meaningful information to the student than mastery or non-mastery scores. A student may achieve something less than full mastery, but more than no mastery. Mastery levels could be identified as steps toward achieving the ultimate goal.

The main purpose of formative evaulation is "to determine the degree of mastery of a given learning task and to pinpoint the part of the task not mastered" (Bloom, Hastings, and Madaus, 1971, p. 61). Some sub-purposes are feedback to teachers, quality control, and forecasting summative evaluation results.

Feedback to teachers. Errors made by the majority of students should be regarded as problems within the instructional material or process, and should be corrected by group instructional procedures. Errors made by less than a majority of the class are errors to be corrected by individual students.

Quality control. The test results can be compared with previous student performance on the same measure. If the present results are lower, the teacher should try to determine the difficulties causing the difference.

Forecasting summative evaluation results. The results of formative measures appear to be related to summative test results (Bloom, Hastings, and Madaus, 1971). Thus, the results of formative measures can be used to predict performance on summative measures. The advantage in being able to make such a prediction is that, in the early stages of formative evaluation, one can always change the forecast.

The content of a formative measure should include all of the important elements in a unit, whereas it is possible only to sample items in summative evaluation. Remedial measures for students receiving non-mastery markings include textbooks, workbooks, programmed instruction, films, tutorial assistance, and small group work. Whenever possible, a student should be allowed to take the test (or an alternate form) again and again until minimal mastery level is achieved.

Example of Summative Evaluation Objectives in Physical Education

As an example of summative evaluation, an objective will be presented for the short serve in badminton. The evaluation objective is designed for high school sophomore girls who are in a beginning badminton unit.

INSTRUCTIONAL GOAL: The student will be able to hit the shuttlecock so that it passes close to the net and lands on, or close to, the short service line.

EVALUATION OBJECTIVE: The student will be able to hit the shuttlecock so that it passes between the net and a string one foot above the net, and lands in an area from one inch in front of the short service line to 10 inches in back of the short service line. Eighty percent of the students will be able to meet the objective 8 out of 10 times.

This objective would be appropriate for all high school sophomore girls in the school district. The person who teaches the high school junior girls knows that at least 80 percent of these girls will have satisfactorily met the above objective.

Example of Formative Evaluation Objectives in Physical Education

There are many ways in which a teacher might direct her students toward the previously stated summative goal. The following set of obejctives represents one approach to developing formative objectives for beginning badminton players. In all cases, 80 percent of the students are expected to meet these objectives. If a student can meet these objectives, she will be equipped to work on the summative evaluation objective.

OBJECTIVE 1: The student will be able to hit the shuttlecock in the air 20 consecutive times.

OBJECTIVE 2: The student will be able to hit the shuttlecock to a height of 15 feet, 20 consecutive times.

OBJECTIVE 3: The student will be able to drop the shuttlecock with the nonracket hand and hit it lightly against the wall, repeating this process successfully 15 times.

OBJECTIVE 4: The student will be able to drop the shuttlecock with the non-racket hand and, using a forceful hit with wrist action, hit it against the wall, repeating this process 15 times. (Distance from wall is greater than distance in Objective 3.)

OBJECTIVE 5: The student will be able to execute a short serve, hitting the shuttlecock diagonally across a net, using the proper stance. The shuttlecock should land in the front one-third of the service court 8 out of 10 times.

OBJECTIVE 6: The student will be able to hit the shuttlecock close to the net (between net and a string 1 foot above net) 8 out of 10 times.

The instructor may wish to have each student meet the first objective before going on to the second, and so forth. When Objective 6 has been met, the student is ready to work on the summative evaluation objective presented in the preceding section. It is also possible to use the results of formative evaluation in determining the final grade for a student. The following section includes an example of utilizing formative evaluation procedures to determine final grades.

Formative Evaluation in Golf

The proposed methods of evaluating beginning golfers include ideas from many sources. Anderson (1971) has utilized many of these ideas, plus some of her own, in preparing an innovative plan for instruction in beginning golf. Anderson has described seven objectives that are important for beginning golfers. Tests for each objective are designed so that another student can score them. When the students meet the minimal standard for one goal, they progress to the next goal or objective. Students having difficulty in achieving goals may be given extra help without holding back others in the class. Some of the tests are in the developmental stage, and require further practical experimentation. Anderson's material is included in this chapter to provide an example of the use of formative measures in physical education. These measures are designed to fit Anderson's philosophy of teaching golf. Extensive usage of the measures is necessary before realistic judgments can be made about their value.

Evaluation Procedure

Part I   Grip. Stance and Swing Fundamentals*   % Final Grade 20%

GRIP. To develop a hand position which will enable the clubface to be "square" at contact and that will keep the club from slipping during the swing.

Checkpoints

Left Hand: Line formed between thumb and index finger should be pointed in the general direction between chin and right shoulder.

Right Hand: Line formed by the right thumb and right index finger is closed solidly and points toward the area between chin and right shoulder.

Hands fit snugly together for best cohesion and grip is firm enough to avoid slipping of club during swing.

TEST. Grip and re-grip the club ten times, taking a full swing between each grip. Check yourself on the above points. 1 point each. Perform on

**Reprinted from P. Anderson, "Evaluation Instruments for Measuring Beginning Golf Skill, (Unpublished paper, 1971). By permission of the author.

two separate days and take average score over two day period.

Optimal level of performance: 30 points
Minimal level of performance: 24 points

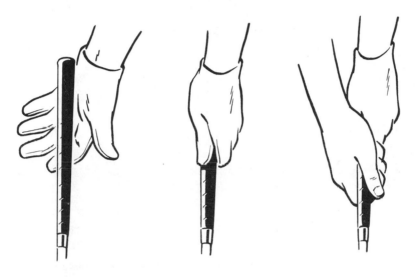

Illustration of Checkpoints (2)

ADDRESS POSITION. To demonstrate ability to take a consistent address position which allows one to swing the club into the backswing, downswing and follow-through keeping swing planes consistent and without losing balance.

Checkpoints

Feet, hips, and shoulders aligned sideways to the target.

Feet should be a comfortable distance apart with left foot toed out slightly.

Knees slightly bent and body bent forward from the waist but with back fairly straight.

Ball should be played from middle of body and clubhead and left arm should form a more or less continuous line from the ball to left shoulder.

TEST. Assume the address position for hitting either practice or regulation balls for a five iron. The address position will be checked during ten trials of the swing. Each checkpoint will receive one point. Perform test on two separate days and take average of score for the two days.

Optimal level of performance: 36 points
Minimal level of performance: 24 points

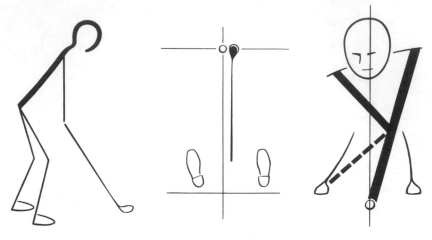

Illustration of Checkpoints

SWING: Developing A Consistent Swing Pattern. To perform a consistent swing pattern so that the clubhead is brought through the ball, a) in a straight line to the target, b) square to the target, and c) as fast as possible.

Checkpoints

Goal 1: To be able to swing the club so that on the backswing the left shoulder swings under the chin and on the forward swing the right shoulder swings under the chin so that during the finish there is a curve in the right side of the body.

Test: Swing a regulation five iron 20 times hitting either practice or regulation balls.

Optimal level of performance: 20 points
Minimal level of performance: 14 points

Goal 2: To be able to swing the clubface straight through the ball towards aiming point and finish with hands high over left shoulder.

Test: Swing a five iron 20 times hitting either practice or regulation balls.

Optimal level of performance: 18–20 points
Minimal level of performance: 12 points

Goal 3: To be able to swing the club so that during the part of the swing when the clubface is in contact with the ball it is aimed square towards the target.

Test: Same as 1 and 2 above.

Optimal level of performance :   16–20 points
Minimal level of performance :   10 points

Goal 4: To be able to swing the clubhead through impact as fast as one can manage while still achieving goals 1, 2, and 3. Action of the downswing should be initiated by the legs, followed by action at the hips, trunk, shoulders arms and clubhead.

Test: Same as those above.

Optimal level of performance :   16–20 points
Minimal level of performance :   10 points

Grip, Address and Swing Fundamentals —   % Final Grade 20%
Levels of Achievement

Excellent   136–150 points
Above Average   115–135 points
Average   94–114 points
Not Acceptable   less than 94 points

Part II   Aspects of a Good Golf Shot For Distance   % Final Grade 20%

To demonstrate the ability to hit a five iron shot for maximal distance so that the ball has an initial trajectory of 23° with the horizontal, travels a minimum of 80 yards on the fly and deviates no more than ten yards to the right or left of the target.

Test**: Swing a five iron club 20 times at a regulation golf ball (2 trials of 10 balls).

Scoring

1. To perform a full swing five iron shot so that the ball passes over a rope set 4 feet high three yards from striking area. (Optimal trajectory for a five iron shot with club loft of 30° is 23° with the horizontal.)

**Field Marking Illustration on page 45.
Suggested Swing Profile chart on page 42.

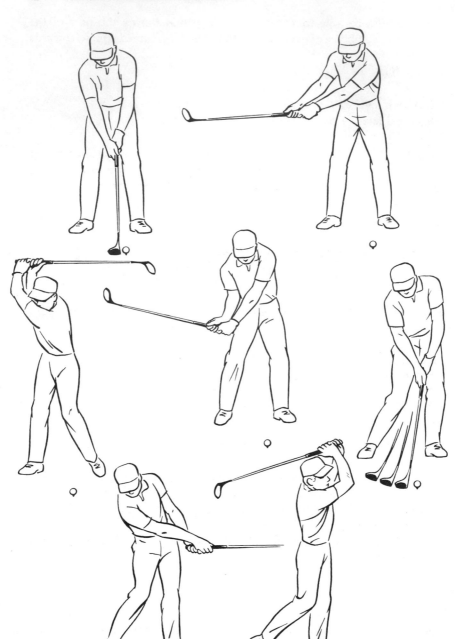

Fundamentals of a Full Swing

3 points: Ball over rope
2 points: Ball on fly under rope
1 point: Topped ball
0 point: Swing and miss

Optimal level of performance: 54–60 points
Minimal level of performance: 36 points

2. To contact the golf ball using a full swing so that it goes a minimum of 80 yards on the fly.

3 points: 100 yards
2 points: 80 yards
1 point: 60 yards

Optimal level of performance: 50-60 points
Minimal level of performance: 35 points

3. To control direction on full swing five iron so that its deviation from landing area does not deviate more than 10 yards in either direction. (left or right)

3 points: Deviations less than 10 yards
2 points: Deviations between 10 and 20 yards
1 point: Deviations greater than 20 yards.

Optimal level of performance: 50-60 points
Minimal level of performance: less than 35 points

Golf shot for Distance: Levels of Achievement   % Final Grade 20%

Excellent   154–180 points
Above Average   136–153
Average   106–135
Not Acceptable   less than   106

Field Markings for 5 iron shot for distance.

Trajectory Rope for 5 Iron Shot   Trajectory Rope for (a) Pitch Shot;
                                          (b) Chip and Run Shot

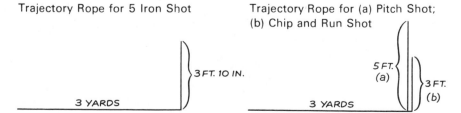

Full Swing Profile Chart**

CLUB_____   TRAJECTORY ANGLE_____   SUGGESTED DISTANCE_____

#	TRAJECTORY					FLIGHT DISTANCE (Yards)					DIRECTION					DEVIATIONS FROM TARGET		
																(Left) 0–10	(Right) 10–20	(yards) 20–30
1	M	Top	LOW	ROPE	HIGH	25	25–50	50–75	75–100	100–125	Str	LF	RT	HK	SL	0–10	10–20	20–30
2	M	Top	LOW	ROPE	HIGH	25	25–50	50–75	75–100	100–125	Str	LF	RT	HK	SL	0–10	10–20	20–30
3	M	Top	LOW	ROPE	HIGH	25	25–50	50–75	75–100	100–125	Str	LF	RT	HK	SL	0–10	10–20	20–30
4	M	Top	LOW	ROPE	HIGH	25	25–50	50–75	75–100	100–125	Str	LF	RT	HK	SL	0–10	10–20	20–30
5	M	Top	LOW	ROPE	HIGH	25	25–50	50–75	75–100	100–125	Str	LF	RT	HK	SL	0–10	10–20	20–30
6																		
7																		
8																		
9																		
10																		
TOTALS																		
1																		
2																		
3																		
4																		
5																		
6																		
7																		
8																		
9																		
10																		
TOTALS																		

Flight Distance = Approximate distance ball is in flight. Contact to initial landing

Direction:
Str = Ball path in line with target
Left = Ball hit to left of target (pull shot) = Deviation in swing plane
Right = Ball hit to right of target (push shot)
Hook = Clubface not square at contact-ball curves left of target
Slice = Clubface not square at contact-ball curves right of target

Key:
Trajectory:
M = Miss
Top = Ball topped
LOW: Ball hit in air under rope
ROPE: Ball clears rope with 10ft
HIGH: Ball popped up into air

**Idea for chart taken from D. Cassidy and M.R. Liba, *Beginning Bowling* (2nd ed.) (Belmont, California: Wadsworth Publishing Company, 1968).

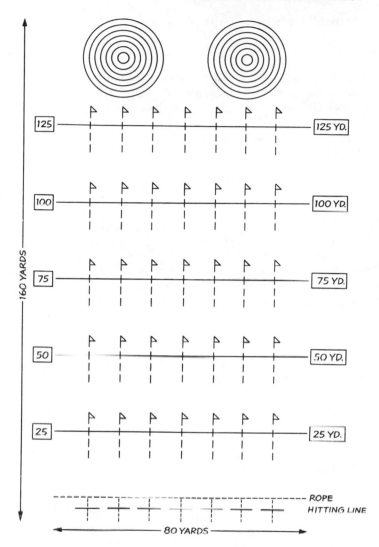

Part III   Aspects of a Good Approach Shot   % Final Grade 15%
40 Yards from Flagstick

To demonstrate the ability to hit a nine iron shot for controlled distance and accuracy so that the ball has an initial trajectory of 29° with the horizontal, travels 30–35 yards in the air and rolls 5–10 yards to target.

Chip and Run Target   Pitch Target
    (Permanent)   (Permanent)

Field Markings (all except dotted lines are permanent—burned in)

TEST. 20 trials of a full swing with the nine iron.

Scoring

To be able to hit a nine iron shot so that the ball passes over a rope set five feet high three yards from striking area. (Optimal trajectory for a nine iron shot with club loft of 45° is 29° with the horizontal.)

3 points: Ball over rope
2 points: Ball on fly under rope
1 point: Topped ball
0 point: Swing and miss

		Weighted Value 2X
Optimal level of performance:	54–60 points	108–120
Minimal level of performance:	36 points	72

To contact the ball using a nine iron so that the ball travels approximately 30–35 yards on the fly and rolls 5–10 yards to target.

Landing points: plotted on score sheet/number of shots landing in same scoring area.

		Weighted Value 7X
Optimal level of performance:	16–20 points	112–140
Minimal level of performance:	8 points	56

Total distance of ball: Score on target where ball finishes: (highest score: 7 points; lowest score; 1 point)

Optimal level of performance:	100–140 points
Minimal level of performance:	60 points

Approach Shot Levels of Achievement   % Final Grade 15%

Excellent	310–400 points
Above Average	255–309 points
Average	188–254 points
Not Acceptable	187 points

Part IV   Aspects of a Good Chip and Run Shot*   % Final Grade 10%

To demonstrate the ability to hit a hooded seven iron shot so that it

---

**Idea for test adapted from Approach Test reported by C. West and J. Thorpe, "Eight-Iron Approach Test," *Research Quarterly*, xxxix (1968), 115-20.

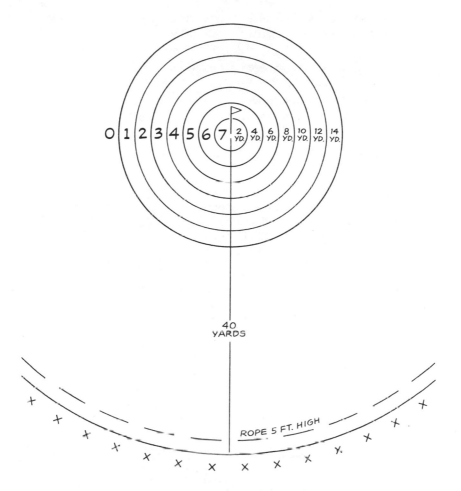

Field Marking for Approach Shot with a Nine Iron

just lands on the edge of the green and rolls up to the cup. The ball should be in the air for approximately one third of the distance (5 yards) and roll two-thirds of the total distance (10 yards or thirty feet). The trajectory of the ball should be less than 23° with the horizontal.

TEST. 20 trials of a chip and run shot with the seven iron.

Scoring

Initial landing points; number of shots landing in same scoring area.

Weighted Value 7X

Optimal level of performance: 17–20 points   119–140
Minimal level of performance: 10 points   70

Final Landing points: Score on target where ball finishes.

Optimal level of performance: 110–140 points
Minimal level of performance: 80 points

Chip and Run Shot Levels of Achievement   % Final Grade 10%

Excellent   229–280 points
Above Average   191–228 points
Average   150–190 points
Not Acceptable   less than 149 points

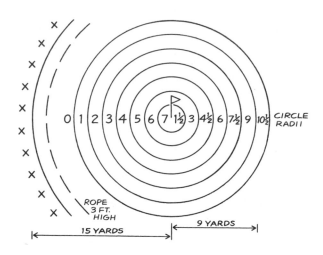

Testing Situation Diagram

Part V   Aspects of Efficient Putting   % Final Grade 20%

1. To develop an efficient putting stroke so that putts of less than 3 feet can be made nine out of ten times; putts of seven feet can be made five out of ten times; and putts of fifteen feet can be made two out of ten times.

Scoring

Total number of putts made in 30 trials

Optimal level of performance: 20–30
Minimal level of performance: 16–30

2. To be able to average a score of 22 (four over par) on four rounds of a putting course where two holes are at least twenty feet long; five holes are between three and twenty feet and two holes are less than five feet long.

Scoring

Average of four nine hole putting scores:

Optimal level of performance: 18 or less
Minimal level of performance: 22

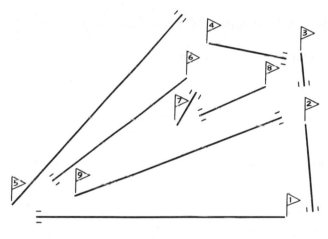

I MM. = 2 YARDS

Suggested Putting Layout

Levels of Achievement   % Final Grade 20%

Distance putting 5%		Putting Course 15%	
Excellent	20+	Excellent	18 or less
Above Average	18–19	Above Average	21–19
Average	15–16	Average	19–18
Not Acceptable	14	Not Acceptable	17

Part VI   Game Score and Written Evaluation   % Final Grade 15%

Ability to demonstrate a student's knowledge or understanding of the game of golf as it is played either on a regulation golf course or on the EOC Short Five Course.

Evaluation will be based upon total score for 18 holes of regulation golf holes or twenty-five holes of the EOC Short Course (Level of Achievement— 10% of grade; Written Evaluation—5% of grade).

Levels of Achievement: Regulation Golf Course (Par 37)

Average score for nine holes

Excellent	45–55 strokes
Above Average	55–65 strokes
Average	65–80 strokes
Not Acceptable	more than 80 strokes

Levels of Achievement: EOC Short Five

Average score for five holes (Par 11)

Excellent	11–13 strokes
Above Average	14–17 strokes
Average	18–20 strokes
Not Acceptable	more than 21 strokes

Written Evaluation. Etiquette; Stroke selection; Fundamentals of Swing; Scoring, etc.

Basic Information

Length of Instruction Unit	11 Weeks
Class periods per week	3
Number of Minutes for Instruction per period	35–40 min
Approximate number of students per class	24–30

Unit Outline: Flexible

Weeks	I-II	Grip, Stance-Swing Fundamentals (includes video taping)
Week	III	5 iron shot for distance
Week	IV	Distance shots with woods and long irons
Week	V	Golf.Game demonstration—Modified game with five iron
Week	VI	Putting
Week	VII	Chip and Run
Week	VIII	Approach Stroking with 9 iron
Weeks	IX, X	Game Play
Week	XI	Written Exam and Playing Evaluation

Summary of Evaluation Procedure

		Percent of total grade
PART I	Grip, Address and Swing Fundamentals	20%
PART II	Golf shot for Distance—5 iron	20%
PART III	Approach Shot From 40 Yards	15%
PART IV	Chip and Run Shot	10%
PART V	Putting	20%
PART VI	Game Score and Written Evaluation	15%
		100%

Summary

Knowledge of the concepts of formative and summative evaluation serves to broaden one's view of the process of evaluation. Formative evaluation takes place during the learning process, while summative evaluation occurs after it has terminated.

The concept of mastery learning is closely tied to that of formative evaluation. If students' aptitude scores are normally distributed in an academic subject and they receive instruction on the subject within the same amount of time, they will be normally distributed on achievement. If the instruction and amount of time are adjusted for each student according to his needs, a majority of students can achieve mastery.

Tests of mastery learning are referred to as criterion-referenced measures. A criterion-referenced measure is constructed so that measurements can be interpreted in terms of specified performance standards. If students are measured according to the normal curve theory, the tests are called norm-referenced measures. A different type of test development is required for each of the two types of measures. A norm-referenced measure is developed so that there is maximum discrimination among students. The criterion-referenced measure is not designed to discriminate since the student's score is compared with an absolute standard, rather than with other students.

Norm-referenced measures are used when a degree of selectivity is required by the situation. If a particular skill is being measured and there are no constraints regarding how many individuals possess the skill, the use of criterion-referenced measures is appropriate.

The distinguishing characteristics of formative and summative evaluation lie in their purpose, the portion of course covered, and the level of generalization that can be made from the scores. Summative evaluation usually takes place at the end of a unit when it is too late to modify either the teaching or the learning process with respect to that unit of work. Some of the purposes of summative evaluation are assignment of grades, certification of skills and abilities, prediction of success in subsequent courses, determination of initiation point of instruction in a subsequent course, provision of feedback to students, and comparison of outcomes of different groups. The main purpose of formative evaluation is to diagnose weaknesses and prescribe ways in which the weaknesses can be corrected. Some sub-purposes are feedback to teachers, quality control, and forecasting summative evaluation results.

Bibliography

ANDERSON, P. "Evaluation Instruments for Measuring Beginning Golf Skill." Unpublished paper, University of Wisconsin, Madison, 1971.

BLOOM, B.S. "Learning for Mastery," *Evaluation Comment,* I, No. 2 (1968), pp. 1–8.

BLOOM, B.S., J.T. HASTINGS and G.F. MADAUS. *Handbook on Formative and Summative Evaluation of Student Learning.* St. Louis: McGraw-Hill Book Company, 1971.

CARROLL, J.B. "A Model of School Learning," *Teachers College Record,* LXIV (1963), pp. 723–33.

CASSIDY, D. and M.R. LIBA. *Beginning Bowling* (2nd ed.). Belmont, California: Wadsworth Publishing Company, 1968.

GLASER, R. "Instructional Technology and the Measurement of Learning Outcomes," *American Psychologist,* XVIII (1963), pp. 519–22.

GLASER, R. and A.J. NITKO. "Measurement in Learning and Instruction," in *Educational Measurement,* ed. R.L. Thorndike. Washington, D.C.: American Council on Education, 1971.

HARRIS, C.W. "An Interpretation of Livingston's Reliability Coefficient for Criterion-Referenced Tests", *Journal of Educational Measurement,* in press.

LIVINGSTON, S.A. "The Reliability of Criterion-Referenced Measures." Report No. 73, Johns Hopkins University, Baltimore, Md.: Center for the Study of Social Organization of Schools, July 1970.

MAYO, S.T. "Mastery Learning and Mastery Testing," *Measurement in Education,* I, No. 3 (1970), pp. 1–4.

POPHAM, W.J. and T.R. HUSEK. "Implications of Criterion-Referenced Measurement," *Journal of Educational Measurement,* VI, No. 1 (1969), pp. 1–9.

SCRIVEN, M. "The Methodology of Evaluation," in *Perspectives of Curriculum Evaluation,* ed. R. Stake. Chicago: Rand McNally and Company, 1967.

SIMON, G.B. "Comments on 'Implications of Criterion-Referenced Measurement'," *Journal of Educational Measurement,* VI, No. 4 (1969), pp. 259–60.

WEST, C. and J. THORPE. "Eight-Iron Approach Test," *Research Quarterly,* XXXIX (1968), pp. 1115–20.

4

basic statistics essential to measurement theory

The primary purposes of this chapter are to cover the statistics that are necessary for an understanding of measurement theory, and to describe procedures that are useful in handling sets of scores. Because the concept of scaling is generally dealt with as an aspect of measurement theory and is an important consideration in selecting statistical techniques, a discussion of scaling will precede the statistics section of this chapter.

The material on statistics in this chapter is not intended to be all-inclusive with regard to elementary statistics. Rather, only the statistics relevant to the measurement theory described in this book are included. In order to organize a set of raw scores, knowledge of the frequency distribution is necessary. To describe accurately a distribution of scores, an understanding of measures of central tendency and measures of variability is essential. The basic transformation of raw scores into z scores is described to aid in clarifying concepts of correlation and standard scores. Knowledge of the use of the correlation coefficient is basic to an understanding of the estimation of validity coefficients. Analysis of variance is included as a prerequisite to the material on the estimation of reliability coefficients. For detailed information on the appropriate statistics for various experimental designs, the reader is referred to statistics texts.

Measurement Scales

Whenever a measurement instrument is used, a score of some sort is obtained. In order to interpret a given set of scores, we must know what the score represents. An accurate interpretation depends in part on the type of scale the score represents. A scale is identified by "a rule for the assignment of numerals to aspects of objects or events" (Stevens, 1951, p. 23). This "rule" is determined primarily by the features of the real number series.

Real Number Series

The real number series consists of three features: order, distance, and origin.

> *Order.* Numbers are ordered.
> *Distance.* Differences between numbers are ordered. That is, the difference between any pair of numbers is greater than, equal to, or less than the difference between any other pairs of numbers.
> *Origin.* The series has a unique origin indicated by the number "zero." An important feature of this origin is that the differences between any pair of numbers containing zero as one member is the number of the other member (Torgerson, 1958, p. 15).

When numbers are assigned to properties (of objects, people, and so forth) so that the relations between the numbers reflect the relations between the properties, the property has been measured. The classification of types of scales is determined by whether the numbers (scores) reflect one, two, or all three of the features of the real number series.

Types of Scales

Although the possibility of an unlimited number of different types of scales exists, four types are commonly described. These are nominal, ordinal, interval, and ratio. A *nominal* scale is a set of mutually exclusive categories. An *ordinal* scale is determined by ranking a set of objects with regard to some specific characteristic. An *interval* scale has equal units of measurement, while a *ratio* scale has the same characteristic plus an absolute zero point. These scales can be characterized not only by the features of the real number series, but also by the range of invariance. Invariance is defined as the kinds of transformations that leave the structure of the scale undistorted (Stevens, 1951).

Nominal. Nominal data contain none of the three features of the real number system. When objects that have attributes in common are grouped into classes, a nominal scale is formed. The classes are mutually exclusive, meaning that no object can fall into more than one class.

Classifying football players by numbers is an example of nominal scaling. A player who is assigned number 42 is not necessarily better than a player who is assigned number 12. *Order* is not a feature of the nominal scale, since membership in any one category does not represent greater or lesser magnitude than membership in any other category. Taking another example, a teacher with five physical education classes might refer to each class according to the period during the school day in which the class is taught. Thus, he may refer to his period two class or his period six class, but these labels are purely for purposes of identification. The period six class is not better (or worse) than the period two class, making order irrelevant even though six is greater than two in the real number system. Since order is not a meaningful factor, neither *distance* nor *origin* can be features of the nominal scale.

The *invariance* range of the nominal scale is one of general substitution. Any one-to-one substitution is legitimate, and does not change the structure of the scale. One might label the defensive and offensive units of a football team in some other way, but the new labels would not change the common properties associated with the persons belonging to each unit.

Because any number used in nominal scaling is not important in terms of magnitude, the nominal scale is not defined as measurement by some writers (Glass and Stanley, 1970; Jones, 1971; Torgerson, 1958). However, since it is impossible to measure human beings in the precise manner of the physical sciences, nominal scales are sometimes useful to educators. Even so, the information that can be obtained from nominal data is limited because only a certain type of statistic is appropriate to them.

Sometimes nominal scales have an underlying order in a gross sense. For example, students might be classified as high, medium, or low on physical fitness. The categories are mutually exclusive, but membership in the high category represents a higher level of fitness than membership in the low category. This type of scale can be referred to as quasi-nominal, something between nominal and ordinal.

Ordinal. Ordinal scales reflect one feature of the real number series, that of *order.* Torgerson (1958) notes that it is possible to have an ordinal scale with a natural origin (meaningful zero point), but unless the existence of a natural origin is noted, the ordinal scale is characterized only by order.

The simplest form of ranking is to order the properties of objects that are of concern, and to assign ranks to these properties. A basketball coach might be asked to rank the basketball teams in a league on the basis of predicted success at the end of the season. If there are ten teams in the league, a rank of one can be assigned to the team that is predicted to win the league title, and a rank of ten to the predicted last team. Since a rank of one is better than a rank of two, *order* is important. However, the first-ranked team may be considerably better than the teams ranked two, three, and four, while the latter three teams might be considered similar in ability. These differences are not reflected in the differences between ranks. Therefore, *distance,* the second feature of the real number series, is not a characteristic of ordinal scales.

Ordinal scales are also used when an attribute is scored rather than ranked, and the differences between the scores have no meaning. When all-star teams are selected by a national press, each sportswriter is asked to vote for the player of his choice. Let us assume that Player F receives 232 votes; Player R, 190 votes; and Player N, 93 votes. It is clear that Player F is considered outstanding by the largest number of sportswriters, but the number of votes does not tell us how much better Player F is than Player R, and so on. Because the *distance* between numbers is not meaningful, these scores are ordinal data. Although the actual number of votes may be published in the newspaper, future reference will usually indicate who was ranked number one, number two, and so on.

Any order-preserving transformation will leave the ordinal scale *invariant.* The number of votes for our football players can be altered in any way we wish as long as the ranking of players remains unchanged. Even though the actual number of votes may be of interest to some people, a player is ranked number one whether he wins by two votes or two hundred. In our example, many players will not receive any votes; however, a zero vote does not reflect an absence of ability in football. Therefore, the third feature of the real number series, *origin,* is also not a characteristic of ordinal scales, except in special cases where the existence of an absolute origin is indicated.

Interval. An interval scale has two features of the real number series: *order* and *distance.* If a zero point exists it is a matter of convention or convenience. A child who scores a zero on a test of ball-throwing accuracy does not totally lack the ability to throw a ball. A flexed-arm hang score of zero does not reflect total lack of arm and shoulder girdle strength. Thus, *origin* is not a characteristic of the interval scale.

In addition to having a meaningful *order,* interval scores have equal *distances* between scores. That is, the difference between 80 degrees and 70 degrees is the same as the difference between 40 degrees and 30 degrees. The difference between 93 and 90 points on a motor performance test is the same as the distance between 53 and 50. (In reality, the latter statement may not always be true. It may be more difficult to gain three points when one's score is 90 than when the score is 50.)

Any linear transformation of the scale is possible without altering the *invariance* of the scale. "Given...that we can...determine differences between different amounts of the property (distances), and the further rule that numbers are to be assigned so that their *differences* reflect the sizes of the corresponding *distances,* the freedom remaining is reduced to the assignment of two members arbitrarily: e.g., the selection of a *unit* and an *origin*"

(Torgerson, 1958, p. 19). Multiplication or division of each value by a specified number merely changes the unit of measurement. Addition or subtraction of a specified number from each value shifts the origin of the number. We cannot take the ratio of any two values on the scale because this would change the property of the scale. Because there is an arbitrary origin rather than an absolute origin, we cannot say that one value is twice as much as another, or one–third as much as another. These kinds of comparisons are possible only when a meaningful zero point exists, that is, when zero represents absence of the attribute being measured.

Ratio. Ratio scales have all three features of the real number series. Ratio data are invariant under somewhat more restricted conditions than interval data. Because an absolute origin is determined, only the unit of measurement is free to vary. Therefore, we cannot add or subtract a given number to each value of the variable without changing the origin and thus losing one of the properties of the ratio scale. Multiplication and division leave the scale invariant.

Ratio data include measures of length, weight, and time, which are frequently used in measuring physical education skills. There are problems associated with some of the underlying assumptions of ratio data when athletic performance is measured. Consider a track and field event, the pole vault. Is the difference between a 17 ft. 1 in. and 17 ft. 2 in. pole vault the same as the difference between a 12 ft. 1 in. and a 12 ft. 2 in. vault? In terms of distance as a pure measure, they are the same. In terms of performance, the difference at 17 feet is much more significant than the difference at 12 feet. Is a vault of 17 feet twice as good as a vault of $8\frac{1}{2}$ feet? In reality, a 17 foot vault is much more than twice as good as an $8\frac{1}{2}$ foot vault. While recognizing the existence of these problems, in practice these types of scores are often treated as interval data even though the assumption of equal distance may be violated (Magnusson, 1966).

Clearly, an attempt to fit all existing data into these four categories is restrictive.

You are likely to get the impression from the works of Stevens, Senders, and Siegel, and others that in some metaphysical way a "scale" underlies certain attributes. A certain set of numbers assigned to a group of objects definitely fits into this one category or that one: the scale is either nominal, ordinal, interval, or ratio; and there is nothing in between. This position can lead to chaos if held to in the face of the less well organized feelings of those who actually perform psychological and educational measurements. Those in the Stevens camp maintain, for example, that IQ scores form an ordinal scale, not an interval scale. Uncritical acceptance of this decree forces one to disregard completely the magnitude of the differences between IQ scores. Suppose Joe has an IQ of 50, Sam an IQ of 110, and Bob an IQ of 112. If IQ is truly an ordinal scale, all that can be said is that Bob is more intelligent than Sam who is more intelligent than Joe. The statement that

Bob and Sam are more alike with respect to IQ than are Sam and Joe would not be defensible. To say that this last statement cannot be made because IQ's are only ordinal would be anarchy. Ask the person who administered the IQ test, and he would have told you before he tested the children that Joe is far less intelligent than Sam and Bob, who are closer together. Try to tell the tester that he must pay no attention to the sizes of the differences between scores, and he will tell you to mind your own business, as he should. Even though an IQ unit is not a completely equivalent unit of measurement at different IQ levels, IQ scores are not on a par with a lowly ordinal scale. The IQ scale defies categorization as strictly ordinal or interval; perhaps it is better to speak of it as "quasi-interval."*

Statisticians such as Hays (1963) and Glass and Stanley (1970) stress the importance of judgment in categorizing the scale of measurement being used. Any statistic can be applied to a set of scores and yield an answer. Whether the answer has any meaning depends upon the type of score used and the meaning attached to the scores.

Normal Curve

Although many theoretical distributions exist, the most commonly known distribution is the normal curve. If the distribution of a set of scores approximates the normal distribution, the known properties of the normal curve provide useful information about the distribution. Actually, few distributions fit all the requirements of normality. However, the normal curve can be closely approximated if the distribution is based on a sufficiently large number of scores.

If a sufficiently large number of random samples of the same size were drawn from an infinitely large population, and the mean (average) was computed for each sample, the distribution formed by these averages would be normal. This is known as the *central limit theorem*. Therefore, a great deal of data used in physical education will approximate the normal distribution. The normal curve is represented by a bell-shaped curve, as shown in Figure 4–1.

The major characteristics of the normal curve are:

1. The curve is symmetrical, that is, the left half of the curve is identical to the right.
2. The space under the curve represents *area*. The area between any given points is determined by the percentage of scores that theoretically would

*Gene V. Glass and Julian C. Stanley, *Statistical Methods in Education and Psychology* (Englewood Cliffs, N.J.: Prentice-Hall, Inc., 1970), p.13.

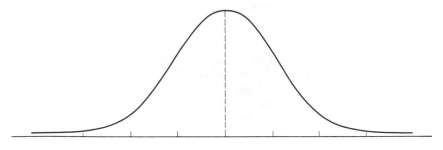

FIG. 4–1   Normal Curve

fall between those points. More scores fall at the middle of the distribution, with fewer and fewer scores falling toward the extremes.

3. The ends of the curve never touch the base line. Theoretically, the distribution includes all possible scores to infinity. Thus, the curve has no upper or lower limits.

4. The shape of the curve changes from convex to concave at specific points above and below the center of the distribution. (These points are one standard deviation above and one standard deviation below the mean.)

If a distribution of scores approximates the normal distribution, parametric statistics may be used. Otherwise, nonparametric statistics are appropriate.

Parametric and Nonparametric Statistics

Certain statistical techniques are used when the assumption can be made that the scores were drawn from a normally distributed population. Since population values are called *parameters,* these statistical techniques are known as *parametric.* If the above assumption cannot be made, "distribution-free" or *nonparametric* statistics may be used. A nonparametric statistical test is a test whose model does not specify conditions about the parameters of the population from which the sample was drawn. Nonparametric statistics are used with nominal and ordinal data, as shown in Table 4–1.

Discrete and Continuous Data

Some scaled scores—such as the number of hits in a baseball game or the number of sit-ups performed by a student—take values only at discrete

**TABLE 4–1 • Four Levels of Measurement and the Statistics
Appropriate to Each Level***

Scale	Defining relations	Examples of appropriate statistics	Appropriate statistical tests
Nominal	(1) Equivalence	Mode Frequency Contingency coefficient	⎫
Ordinal	(1) Equivalence (2) Greater than	Median Percentile Spearman r_s Kendall τ Kendall W	⎬ Nonparametric statistical tests
Interval	(1) Equivalence (2) Greater than (3) Known ratio of any two intervals	Mean Standard deviation Pearson product-moment correlation Multiple product-moment correlation	⎫
Ratio	(1) Equivalence (2) Greater than (3) Known ratio of any two inter-vals (4) Known ratio of any two scale values	Geometric mean Coefficient of variation	⎬ Nonparametric and parametric statistical tests

*Reprinted from Table 3.1 of S. Siegel, *Nonparametric Statistics for the Behavioral Sciences* (New York: McGraw-Hill Book Company, 1965), p. 30, by permission of the author and publisher.

points on a scale. Such scores are known as *discrete* scores. For example, a baseball team might get 16 hits during a game, but never $16\frac{1}{2}$ or $16\frac{1}{4}$ hits. The number of hits is not a variable that can be measured with increasingly greater accuracy. Other examples of discrete data are the number of students in a class, the number of teams in a league, and the number of books in a library.

Other variables, however, can be measured to finer and finer degrees. Measures of these variables are called *continuous* data. The broad jump, for example, can be measured to the nearest foot, the nearest inch, the nearest half-inch, and so on. Continuous variables can have values at every point on a scale. Age, weight, and temperature are examples of continuous variables.

The statistics described in the remainder of this chapter deal with test scores that are considered continuous, since continuous scores can be handled mathematically in ways that discrete values cannot. Discrete scores can be analyzed using nonparametric statistical techniques.

Frequency Distribution

Upon administering a test to a group of students, we are faced with the task of utilizing the scores in the most meaningful way. One of the easiest ways to summarize the data is to build a frequency distribution. A frequency distribution is made up of a set of mutually exclusive classes and the numbers of individuals belonging to each class. Note that the characteristic of "mutual exclusiveness," meaning that a given individual may not belong to more than one class, is also an attribute of nominal data. However, another assumption underlying the use of frequency distribution is that the scores have a meaningful order. Although nominal data meet the criterion of being mutually exclusive, the scores do not have a meaningful order. Therefore, the frequency distribution is not appropriate for nominal scores.

Building A Frequency Distribution

The mutually exclusive classes of a frequency distribution are generally referred to as *intervals*. If an interval contains three scores (5, 6,7), the *score limits* of that interval are 5 to 7. However, a group of scores in the form of a distribution represents area, and if we think of scores as such, in the successive intervals of 5 to 7 and 8 to 10, the area between 7 and 8 is not taken into account. To include all the area represented by the scores, we use the *real limits* of the interval, which are 4.5 to 7.5 and 7.5 to 10.5. (If the score limits are recorded to the nearest whole number, that is 5 to 7, the real limits are set to 0.5, that is, 4.5 to 7.5. If the score limits are recorded to the nearest one-half, that is 1.5 to 2.5, the real limits are set to 0.25, that is 1.25 to 2.75.) The *midpoint* of the interval is halfway between the score limits.

The interval size can be determined by subtracting the lower real limit from the upper real limit, or $10.5 - 7.5 = 3$. The score limits can also be used to determine the interval size. The upper score limit minus the lower score limit plus one equals the interval size. (In our example, $7 - 5 + 1 = 3$.) Note that 5 subtracted from 7 equals 2, but there are clearly three scores in the interval 5 to 7. The reader should guard against the common error of subtracting the lower score limit from the upper score limit without adding one.

In Table 4–2 five intervals of different sizes are identified along with the corresponding score limits, real limits, midpoints, and interval sizes. Intervals containing an odd number of scores are preferred because the midpoint will be a whole number, but intervals of 10 are easy to manipulate, and therefore are an exception. Commonly used interval sizes are 3, 5, 7, and 10. Choice of interval size must be made in conjunction with the choice of the number of intervals to be used. Too few intervals tend to mask the information by compressing the distribution of scores. Too many intervals can spread the distribution so much that it becomes irregular. Generally, between 10 and 20 intervals are recommended.

TABLE 4–2 · Components of the Frequency Distribution

Interval	Score Limits	Real Limits	Midpoint	Interval Size
30–32	30–32	29.5–32.5	31	3
11–15	11–15	10.5–15.5	13	5
10–19	10–19	9.5–19.5	14.5	10
56–62	56–62	55.5–62.5	59	7
80–86	80–86	79.5–86.5	83	7

A sample frequency distribution will be built using a set of scores from a volleyball serve test, along with a step-by-step procedure for building the distribution.

Scores on volleyball serve test. 42, 50, 57, 45, 56, 69, 45, 43, 46, 51, 56, 61, 55, 40, 47, 52, 59, 47, 62, 46, 30, 48, 53, 40, 40, 64, 47, 48, 41, 41, 54, 49, 31, 49, 64, 42, 42, 35, 31, 35, 51, 43, 43, 37, 33, 36, 53, 44, 44, 38, 34, 37, 51, 20, 24, 39, 34, 38, 50, 23, 10, 37, 39, 27, 25, 29, 26.

Step 1.   Determine the range by subtracting the lowest score from the highest score and adding one.

$$\text{Range} = 69 - 10 + 1 = 60$$

Step 2.   Divide the range by the interval size to determine number of intervals. Select an interval size that will yield between 10 and 20 intervals. Try the preferred interval sizes first.

$$60 \div 3 = 20 \text{ intervals}$$
$$60 \div 5 = 12 \text{ intervals}$$

In our example, although 20 intervals would be adequate, 12 intervals are probably more desirable. We will proceed using 12 intervals with interval sizes of 5.

Step 3.   Set up the intervals by score limits, starting the first interval with a multiple of the interval size.

Since our lowest score is 10, that score must be included in the bottom interval. The score of 10 is also a multiple of 5, our interval size, so that the lower score limit of the bottom interval can be set at 10. We can then develop the left-hand column (Intervals) in Table 4–3.

TABLE 4–3 • Sample Frequency Distribution

Intervals	Tally	f	cf	c%
65–69	/	1	68	100%
60–64	////	4	67	99%
55–59	ЖЖ /	6	63	93%
50–54	ЖЖ ////	9	57	83%
45–49	ЖЖ ЖЖ /	11	48	71%
40–44	ЖЖ ЖЖ ///	13	37	54%
35–39	ЖЖ ЖЖ	10	24	35%
30–34	ЖЖ /	6	14	21%
25–29	////	4	8	12%
20–24	///	3	4	6%
15–19		0	1	1%
10–14	/	1	1	1%

$$N = 68$$

Step 4.   Place a tally for each score opposite the interval in which that score falls. Mark off the score once you have tallied it to avoid tallying the same score again.

Step 5.   Add the tally marks for each interval to obtain the frequency of scores within the interval. Label this column f, for *frequency*.

Step 6.   Add up the f column. The total of the frequencies should equal the total number of scores.

Step 7.   Develop the cumulative frequency (cf) column by adding the number of frequencies that fall below the upper limit of any given interval. The top of the cf column will equal the total number of scores. In our example, twenty-four persons had scores falling within or below the interval 35–39, or, twenty-four persons scored below 39.5, the upper real limit of the interval.

Step 8.   Develop the cumulative percent ($c\%$) column. For each interval the cf

is divided by N to obtain the $c\%$.

For interval 35–39, $c\% = \frac{24}{68} = 0.35$ or 35%. In this case, 35% of the sample scored below 39.5.

The cumulative percent can provide useful information in a frequency distribution. It is often valuable to know what percentages of people fall below certain scores in the distribution. A teacher might wish to compare a distribution of scores with some from previous years. By computing cumulative percents, a general comparison can easily be made. Methods for obtaining percentages other than those given in the $c\%$ column will be described in the section on the median.

Graphic Presentations

Graphs of frequency distributions are useful aids for interpreting a distribution of scores. Two types of graphs will be described in this section: the *histogram* and the *frequency polygon*. In each case the vertical axis represents the ordinate of the graph, and the horizontal axis, the abscissa, as depicted in Figure 4–2.

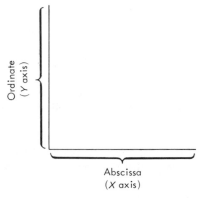

FIG. 4–2   Ordinate and Abscissa

The histogram depicts the number of cases or scores falling in each interval, as shown in Figure 4–3. The scores from Table 4–4 are used to build the histogram. The ordinate of the graph in Figure 4–3 represents the frequencies, or the number of cases, while the abscissa represents the intervals. By marking the midpoint of each interval at the height of the bar and connecting these marks, a frequency polygon is formed. (The bar is the area determined by the number of cases falling in a given interval.) A frequency polygon for the data in Table 4–3 is given in Figure 4–4.

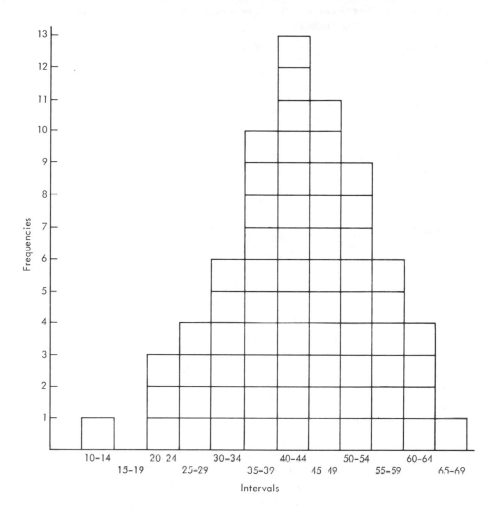

FIG. 4-3   Histogram

Measures of Central Tendency

Given a set of scores either in the form of raw data or organized into a frequency distribution, the distribution of the set can be partially described by determining a score that represents the center of the distribution. We will deal with three measures of central tendency: the *mean,* the *median,* and the *mode.*

TABLE 4–4 • Distribution of Bowling Scores Used for Computation of the Median

Intervals	f	cf
170–174	2	38
165–169	4	36
160–164	3	32
155–159	2	29
150–154	5	27
145–149	7	22
140–144	6	15
135–139	2	9
130–134	4	7
125–129	0	3
120–124	3	3

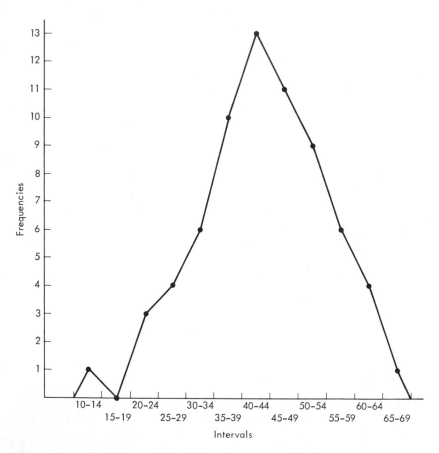

FIG. 4–4   Frequency Polygon

The *mean* is the arithmetic average of the scores. If we are dealing with three scores—20, 30, and 40—the mean, or average, of this set of scores would be 30. The mean is often the preferred measure of central tendency because it is determined by taking all of the scores in a distribution into account. However, an extreme score at either end of the distribution can markedly affect the mean, making it an unrealistic estimate of the center of the distribution, and the median will be the preferred estimate.

The *median* is the middle score in the distribution, and is also known as the 50th percentile, X_{50}, or Q_2. Half of the scores in the distribution fall above the median and half fall below. To obtain the median for a large number of scores, it is convenient to group the scores into a frequency distribution. The mean, however, can be computed from ungrouped as well as grouped data.

Note the following scores made by five individuals shooting four ends in archery:

$$
\begin{array}{ll}
120 & \\
92 & \text{Mean} = 106 \\
98 & \text{Median} = 106 \\
106 & \\
114 &
\end{array}
$$

In this small distribution of scores, the mean and the median are identical. In the next set of scores, only the top score in the distribution is altered.

$$
\begin{array}{ll}
200 & \\
92 & \text{Mean} = 122 \\
98 & \text{Median} = 106 \\
106 & \\
114 &
\end{array}
$$

Although the median has not changed, the mean is 16 points higher. Four of the five scores fall below the mean. In this case, the median should be selected as the measure of central tendency, because the median more accurately represents the middle of the distribution.

The *mode* is the score that occurs most frequently in the distribution. Consider the following set of scores:

9, 11, 11, 12, 12, 13, 13, 13, 14, 15, 15.

The mode of this distribution is 13. The mode, like the median, is determined most easily from a large set of scores by first organizing them into a frequency distribution. The alternative is to arrange the scores in numerical order, which is time consuming when dealing with many scores. Also, the mere ordering of scores serves no other purpose.

Generally, the mode is a less adequate measure of central tendency than the mean or the median. However, if a coach were ordering track, football, or basketball shoes for the coming season, he would want to use the mode from past teams; that is, he would be interested in the most frequently occurring shoe size rather than the mean or median of all shoe sizes. If the largest number of identical scores are clustered at one end of the distribution, clearly the mode does not represent the middle of the distribution. Generally, the mode is a satisfactory measure when most of the scores in a distribution are the same.

Computation of the Median

When scores are grouped into a frequency distribution, the following formula is used for computing the median:

(Formula 4–1)

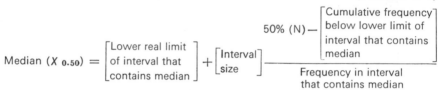

$$\text{Median } (X_{0.50}) = \begin{bmatrix} \text{Lower real limit} \\ \text{of interval that} \\ \text{contains median} \end{bmatrix} + \begin{bmatrix} \text{Interval} \\ \text{size} \end{bmatrix} \frac{50\% \ (N) - \begin{bmatrix} \text{Cumulative frequency} \\ \text{below lower limit of} \\ \text{interval that contains} \\ \text{median} \end{bmatrix}}{\begin{array}{c}\text{Frequency in interval} \\ \text{that contains median}\end{array}}$$

Using the distribution given in Table 4–4, the median for this set of scores is computed.

$$X_{0.50} = [144.5] + [5]\left[\frac{0.50\ (38) - 15}{7}\right]$$
$$= 144.5 + 5[\tfrac{4}{7}]$$
$$= 147.35$$

For a simplified, step-by-step computation of the median using the data in Table 4–4, the following procedures may be followed:

Step 1. Determine 50% of N.
N = 38
0.50(38) = 19   (We now know that the median is the 19th score in in the distribution.)

Step 2. Locate the interval that the median falls in.
The 19th score falls in the 145–149 interval.

Step 3. Identify the *real* limits of the interval found in Step 2.
144.5–149.5

Step 4. Find the number of cases falling below the interval identified above.
15

Step 5. Subtract the number in Step 4 from the number in Step 1.
$19-15 = 4$

Step 6. Identify the number of cases falling *in* the interval containing the median.
7 cases fall in the 145–149 interval.

Step 7. Determine the location of the median in the interval by dividing the number in Step 6 into the number in Step 5.
$\frac{4}{7} = 0.57$

Step 8. Determine the interval size.
$i = 5$

Step 9. Compute the median by multiplying the number in Step 7 by the number in Step 8, and adding the product to the lower *real* limit of the interval.

$$X_{0.50} = 144.5 \qquad\qquad + (0.57) \qquad\qquad (5) = 147.35$$
$$\text{Lower real limit} \qquad\qquad \text{Step 7} \qquad\qquad \text{Step 8}$$

Any percentile may be computed using either the above method or Formula 4 1. Simply substitute the desired percentile for the 50th percentile, and locate the interval in which the percentile falls. If, for example, you wish to determine the 78th percentile ($X_{0.78}$), take 78 percent of N rather than 50 percent of N. For a detailed discussion on percentile ranks, see Chapter 10.

Computation of the Mean

The mean can be computed from ungrouped data using the formula

$$\bar{X} = \frac{\Sigma X}{N}, \quad \text{where } \bar{X} = \text{the mean} \qquad\qquad \textbf{(Formula 4–2)}$$
$$\Sigma X = \text{sum of all scores}$$
$$N = \text{number of scores}$$

The result is the simple average of a set of scores. However, when scores are grouped in a frequency distribution, a different formula is used to determine the mean.

$$\bar{X} = A + \frac{\Sigma x'f}{N} (i), \quad \text{where } A = \text{arbitrary origin} \qquad\qquad \textbf{(Formula 4–3)}$$
$$x' = \text{the rescaled } X \text{ score}$$
$$f = \text{frequency}$$
$$\Sigma x'f = \text{the sum of the product of } x' \text{ times } f \text{ for each interval}$$
$$i = \text{interval size}$$

Since computation of the mean from a frequency distribution must be carried out by hand, the procedure is greatly simplified if we rescale the

X scores. In the first section of Table 4–5, the computation of the mean is demonstrated *without* rescaling the X score. In the second section of Table 4–5, the X scores are rescaled. Note that rescaling reduces considerably the sizes of the numbers with which we must work. Also note that when using data that have been grouped into intervals, the X score used to represent each interval is the midpoint of the interval.

TABLE 4–5 • Computation of the Mean from Grouped Data

Intervals	f	X (midpoint)	fx	f	x'	fx'
63–69	2	66	132	2	4	8
56–62	5	59	295	5	3	15
49–55	6	52	312	6	2	12
42–48	8	45	360	8	1	8
35–41	10	38	380	10	0	0
28–34	9	31	279	9	−1	−9
21–27	7	24	168	7	−2	−14
14–20	4	17	68	4	−3	−12
7–13	3	10	30	3	−4	−12
0–6	2	3	6	2	−5	−10
	$N = 56$		$fx = 2030$			$fx' = -14$

$$\bar{X} = \frac{\Sigma fX}{N} = \frac{2030}{56} = 36.25 \qquad \bar{X} = A + \frac{\Sigma x'f}{N} \ (i)$$

$$= 38 + \frac{-14}{56} \ (7)$$

$$= 38 + (-1.75) = 36.25$$

With large scores and/or large frequencies, the fx column in the first section of Table 4–5 can become unwieldy. The second section demonstrates a systematic rescaling of the X scores to x' scores that are easier to handle. An arbitrary origin, A, of zero is assigned to a designated interval. The zero temporarily replaces the midpoint of that interval, so that in effect the midpoint is rescaled to zero. In our example, the arbitrary origin of zero is substituted for the midpoint 38 in the interval 35 to 41.

The remaining x' scores may then be determined. To keep the numbers as small as possible, use units of $+1$, $+2$, and so on above the arbitrary origin, and -1, -2, and so on below the origin. If the use of negative numbers seems inconvenient, set the arbitrary origin at the midpoint of the bottom interval, and all of the x' values will be positive. Try the latter rescaling procedure on the example in Table 4–5. The mean should be identical to the result given in Table 4–5.

Formula 4–3 takes both the arbitrary origin and the size of the interval into account. The resultant values are thus rescaled back to the original score values in the distribution.

Skewed Distributions

A distribution that is not symmetrical is referred to as a skewed distribution. In a symmetrical distribution, the mean, median, and mode are located at the same point, whereas in a skewed distribution these three measures are located at different points. The mean is affected most by skewness, and moves in the direction of the long tail of the distribution. The median shifts to a position between the mode and the mean. Figure 4–5 shows a positively skewed curve in which the skewness occurs to the right.

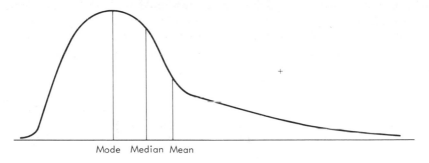

Mode   Median Mean

FIG. 4–5   Positively Skewed Curve

A negatively skewed curve, with the skewness to the left, is depicted in Figure 4–6. The direction of the skewness is determined by the portion of the curve that tapers off into the long tail.

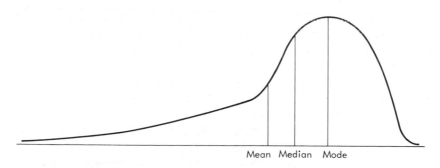

Mean Median   Mode

FIG. 4–6   Negatively Skewed Curve

Since a skewed distribution is nonnormal, a distribution of scores that is markedly skewed should be analyzed using nonparametric statistics. However, as the sample size increases, the distributions of many types of scores tend to approach the normal distribution.

Measures of Variability

After determining a measure of central tendency, further information about the distribution may be obtained by computing a measure of variability. Measures of variability indicate how the scores vary around the measure of central tendency. The measures of variability that will be described are the *range,* the *interpercentile ranges,* and the *standard deviation.*

The *range* is determined by subtracting the lowest score in a distribution from the highest score and adding one. For example, using the data in Table 4–3, 69 (highest) − 10 (lowest) + 1 = range of 60.

If two basketball players recorded the total points each scored during five consecutive games, the following sets of scores might be obtained:

	1	*2*	*3*	*4*	*5*	*Median*	*Range*
			Games				
Player A	18	22	20	28	26	22	11
Player B	22	10	12	29	31	22	22

Notice that the medians for the two sets of scores are identical. By considering only the two medians, it appears that the two players are very similar in shooting ability. However, observing the ranges as well as the medians allows us to make a more accurate appraisal of their abilities. We can see that Player A, with a range of 11, is more consistent in shooting performance than Player B, with a range of 22.

A disadvantage of the range as a measure of variability is that it provides no information about the way in which scores are distributed over a given area. The interpercentile ranges and the standard deviation are better measures of variability than the range.

Interpercentile ranges refer to the ranges between percentiles. Because the median is the 50th percentile, the interpercentile ranges are the measures of variability that are used in conjunction with the median.

The most widely used interpercentile range is the *interquartile range,* or Q_3 to Q_1, or $X_{0.75}$ to $X_{0.25}$, reflecting the difference between the first and third quartiles, or 25th and 75th percentiles. We may choose to use other interpercentile ranges, such as $X_{0.95}$ to $X_{0.05}$, or $X_{0.90}$ to $X_{0.10}$. Notice that the interpercentile ranges cut off equal portions from both ends of the distribution, so that extreme scores cannot distort this measure of variability.

The *standard deviation* is the measure of variability associated with the mean. Whereas measures of central tendency represent points on a distribution, measures of variability represent area within the distribution. In a normal distribution there are six standard deviations, three above the mean and three below. The area between the mean and +1 standard deviation is approximately 34 percent of the distribution; between +1 standard deviation and +2, approximately 14 percent; and between +2 and +3 standard deviations, 2 percent. The same percentages apply to the standard deviations below the mean.

If a normal distribution were developed from a set of 100 scores, thirty-four scores would fall between the mean and +1 (or the mean and –1) standard deviation. Fourteen scores would fall between +1(or –1) and +2 (or –2) standard deviations, and two scores would fall between +2(or –2) and +3 (or –3) standard deviations. Figure 4–7 shows the normal curve divided into standard deviation units.

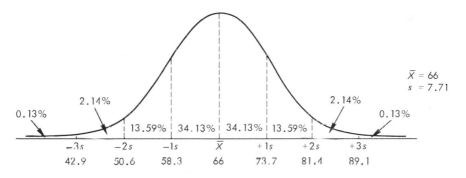

FIG. 4–7   Normal Curve Divided into Standard Deviation Units

Computation of the Standard Deviation
From Ungrouped Data

Variance is the measure of variability based on the deviations from the mean. The standard deviation is the square root of this measure. The symbol for the variance is s^2, and for the standard deviation, s. (The Greek sigma, σ, is used to represent standard deviation and σ^2 is the corresponding symbol for variance when the variability of a population is being computed. The variability of a sample is represented by s and s^2.)

Given a set of five scores, we can compute the variance by (1) subtracting each score from the mean, (2) squaring each deviation, and (3) summing the squared deviations. This sum divided by $N-1$ equals the variance.

Consider the scores in Table 4–6. Note that the sum of the deviations from the mean, $\sum(X-\bar{X})$, is zero. Since this will always be true, the deviations are squared in order to obtain an estimate of the variability. The squared deviations are divided by $N-1$ rather than N to provide an unbiased estimate of the sample variance. Although the computation of the standard deviation using Formula 4–4 clearly demonstrates the processes involved, this method is excessively time-consuming when used with a large number of scores.

TABLE 4–6 · Standard Deviation Computed by Squaring Deviations from the Mean

Scores	$X - \bar{X}$	$(X - \bar{X})^2$
77	77–66 = 11	121
70	70–66 = 4	16
65	65–66 = –1	1
60	60–66 = –6	36
58	58–66 = –8	64

$N = 5$ $\sum(X - \bar{X}) = 0$ $\sum(X - \bar{X})^2 = 238$ **(Formula 4–4)**
$\bar{X} = 66$

$$s^2 = \frac{\sum(X - \bar{X})^2}{N - 1} = \frac{238}{4} = 59.5$$
$$s = \sqrt{59.5} = 7.71$$

With ungrouped data, the standard deviation, like the mean, can be computed using the raw scores. The computational formula is

$$s^2 = \frac{N\sum X^2 - (\sum X)^2}{N(N-1)} \qquad \textbf{(Formula 4–5)}$$

where $\sum X^2 =$ each score squared and summed
$(\sum X)^2 =$ sum of all scores squared

Using the data in Table 4–6, we obtain the same results using the computational formula (For. 4–5) as we did with the formula for deviations from the mean (For. 4–4).

$$s^2 = \frac{5(22018) - 108900}{5(4)} = \frac{1190}{20} = 59.5$$
$$s = \sqrt{59.5} = 7.71$$

Even with a small number of scores, this process is cumbersome to carry out by hand, but simple with the aid of a desk calculator. If it is necessary to compute the standard deviation by hand, grouping the data into a frequency distribution is recommended.

The variance cannot be represented graphically. The standard deviation, however, represents the distance measured along the scale of scores, as shown in Figure 4–7. If the distribution in Table 4–6 were normal (which in reality would not be the case for a set of five scores), the distribution would resemble the one shown in Figure 4–7, where one standard deviation above the mean, $66+7.71$, equals 73.7. Two standard deviations below the mean, $66-(2)$ (7.71), equals 50.6. A student who scores one standard deviation above the mean scores better than 84 percent of the sample. Only 2 percent of the sample falls below a score of two standard deviations below the mean.

Computation of the Standard Deviation from Grouped Data

Formula 4–6 is used to obtain the standard deviation from grouped data. This procedure is described using the data in Table 4–7.

TABLE 4–7 • Computation of the Standard Deviation from Grouped Data

Scores	f	x'	fx'	$f(x')^2$
170–179	1	6	6	36
160–169	2	5	10	50
150–159	4	4	16	64
140–149	5	3	15	45
130–139	8	2	16	32
120–129	9	1	9	9
110–119	10	0	0	0
100–109	7	−1	−7	7
90–99	1	−2	−8	16
80–89	4	−3	−12	36
70–79	0	−4	0	0
60–69	2	−5	−10	50
	$N = 56$		$+35$	345

$$s^2 = (i)^2 \, \frac{N f(x')^2 - (fx')^2}{N(N-1)} \qquad \text{(Formula 4–6)}$$

$$= (10)^2 \, \frac{56(345) - (35)^2}{56(55)}$$

$$= 587.5$$

$$s = \sqrt{587.5} = 24.248$$

In Table 4–7 the X scores are rescaled to X' scores. With the exception of the $f(x')^2$ column, the format of the table is identical to that of Table 4–5 in which the mean is computed from grouped data. The $f(x')^2$ column is obtained by multiplying f times x' times x', or by multiplying the x' score by the corresponding score in the $f(x')$ column. *Do not* square each score in the fx' column to obtain the $f(x')^2$ column.

To check roughly on the accuracy of your computation of the standard deviation, divide the range by the standard deviation. If the resultant value is not between 2.5 and 5.5, it is likely that a computational error has been made. For our example in Table 4–7, the range divided by the standard deviation equals 120/24. 248 = 4.9, indicating that no major computational errors have been made.

Transformation of Raw Scores to z Scores

Although standardized scores will be dealt with in detail in Chapter 10, a brief discussion of z scores is a necessary prerequisite to the section on correlation. In comparing Bill's performances on two track events such as the 50–yd dash and the broad jump, the direct comparison of a time score and a distance score is meaningless. If Bill ran the dash in 5.8 seconds and broad jumped a distance of 7 ft 4 in., is one score better than the other in comparison to performances of other boys his age? If we know the mean and standard deviation for Bill's age group on each skill, we can compare Bill's scores in terms of the distance of his score from the mean. Converting the raw scores to z scores makes direct comparisons possible.

Let us assume that for Bill's age group the mean dash score is 6.9 seconds, and the standard deviation 0.6 seconds. Conversion of the scores on the dash to z scores sets the mean at zero and the standard deviation at one. Whenever scores are converted to z scores, this type of conversion is made. Thus, if the group mean for the broad jump is 7 ft 1 in. and the standard deviation is 8 inches, these figures are converted to z score values of zero for the mean, and one for the standard deviation. Referring to Figure 4–8, we can easily see that Bill's dash score falls slightly below $+2$ z scores, while his jump score falls between the mean and $+1$ z score. Although both scores are above average, the dash score represents the better performance in relation to others in Bill's age group.

The exact z score for each of Bill's raw scores can be computed using the simple formula

$$z = \frac{X - \overline{X}}{s}$$

(Formula 4–7)

Bill's z score for the dash is 5.8–6.9/0.6, which equals $+1.83$, slightly below a z score of $+2$. For the jump, his z score is 7 ft 4 in.–7 ft 1 in./8 in., which equals $+0.38$, slightly less than a $+0.5$ z score. The z score transformation

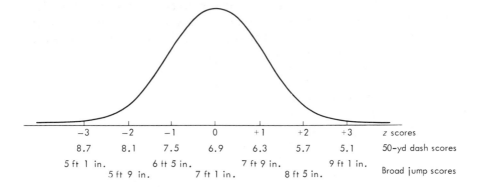

z scores	−3	−2	−1	0	+1	+2	+3
50-yd dash scores	8.7	8.1	7.5	6.9	6.3	5.7	5.1

Broad jump scores: 5 ft 1 in.   5 ft 9 in.   6 ft 5 in.   7 ft 1 in.   7 ft 9 in.   8 ft 5 in.   9 ft 1 in.

FIG. 4-8   Distribution of z Scores

is useful when comparing two sets of scores that have different units of measurement. The z score is also known as a standard score. For more information on standard scores, see Chapter 10.

Correlation

A grasp of the concept of correlation is essential to an understanding of certain aspects of measurement theory. Reliability, validity, and objectivity coefficients are sometimes determined through correlational procedures. This section, then, should be mastered before moving on to the reliability and validity chapters.

The coefficient of correlation reflects the relationship between two variables. It indicates the degree to which individuals retain their standings over two sets of scores. As a simplified example, if five individuals took the same test twice and received the same score each time, the correlation between the two sets of scores would be perfect, or +1.00. If the highest scorer on the first test received the lowest score on the second, the lowest scorer on the first test received the highest on the second and the remaining individuals reversed their scores in the same way, the relationship is still perfect, but *inverse,* and the correlation would be –1.00.

The coefficient of correlation can range from +1.00 to −1.00. Two aspects of the coefficient are of concern: the *size* and the *sign*. The *size* of the coefficient indicates the degree of the relationship between the two variables. A +0.63 coefficient reflects the *same degree* of relationship as a −0.63 coefficient. The *sign* designates the type of relationship, either positive or negative (inverse).

Is a correlation of 0.52 better than a correlation of –0.72? If we are interested in the correlation coefficient that reflects the greater degree of relationship, the –0.72 coefficient is better. The negative sign simply indicates that individuals tend to reverse their standings over two sets of measures. Consider these correlation coefficients:

$r = + 1.00$	perfect positive relationship
$r = + 0.82$	high positive relationship
$r = + 0.23$	low positive relationship
$r = \ \ \ 0$	no relationship
$r = - 0.43$	moderate inverse relationship
$r = - 0.90$	high inverse relationship
$r = - 1.00$	perfect negative relationship

We can expect an inverse relationship when we correlate time scores with other types of scores. For example, as a person runs faster over several trials, his time scores decrease, but as he jumps farther or throws a ball over a greater distance, his scores increase. If persons who perform well on the jump also do well on the dash, and those who are poor on the jump are also poor on the dash, the resultant correlation coefficient will be a negative one. The persons with the higher jump scores will be those with the lower (faster) dash scores.

A few pictorial examples of different sizes of correlation coefficients may be helpful. A graph of the relationship between two variables is determined by plotting the coordinates of the two variables for each individual.. The following scores are used to determine the coordinates in Figure 4–9.

Individuals	One–handed Push Shot	Two–handed Push Shot
A	12	10
B	10	8
C	8	6
D	6	4
E	4	2

The scores of both variables represent the number of baskets made out of 15 tries. The coordinates for each of the five individuals are the scores in parentheses for each individual. In Figure 4–9 there is a perfect linear relationship between the two sets of scores. As the scores on the one-handed push shot *increase,* the scores on the two–handed push shot increase proportionally.

If we reverse the order of the scores on the two–handed push shot, the relationship, although still perfect, is now inverse, as shown in Figure 4–10. Note that as the scores on the one–handed push shot *increase,* the scores on the two-handed push shot *decrease* proportionally.

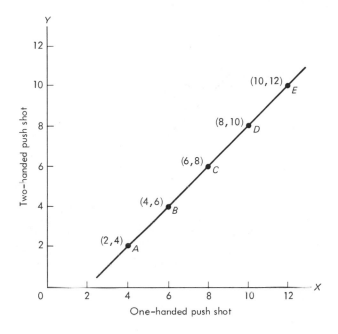

FIG. 4–9 $r = +1.00$

Individuals	One–handed Push Shot	Two–handed Push Shot
A	12	2
B	10	4
C	8	6
D	6	8
E	4	10

If we added 100 points to each of the one–handed push shot scores, the relationship between the two sets of scores would remain the same. In effect, each set of scores is transformed into z scores. If the z scores are identical for each individual, $r = +1.00$. If the z scores are identical except for the sign, $r = -1.00$. As the z scores differ, the correlation decreases. Therefore, the coefficient of correlation can be computed for any two sets of scores for the same individuals because both sets are transformed to a common scale, the z score distribution. In Figure 4–11(a), no relationship exists between the two variables; in Figure 4–11(b), there is a moderate correlation; and, in Figure 4–11(c), a high correlation.

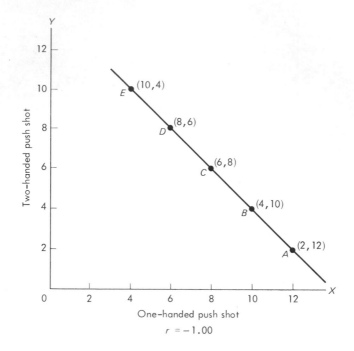

FIG. 4–10 $r = -1.0$

Types of Correlation Coefficients

If the distribution of scores is normal, the coefficient of correlation usually is computed using the Pearson product-moment method. The product-moment correlation coefficient is used with interval scores. For ordinal data, a technique such as Spearman's rho or Kendall's tau may be used. The contingency coefficient and the phi coefficient are appropriate for nominal data. Other coefficients have been developed for combinations of continuous and discrete scores. For descriptions of correlational methods designed for nominal and ordinal data, see the references listed in the bibliography by Siegel (1965) and Conover (1971) on nonparametric statistics.

Interpretation of the Correlation Coefficient

The interpretation of the correlation coefficient is determined in part by the way in which the coefficient is to be used. Up to this point, the only reference to the sizes of coefficients has been in terms of high, moderate, and low. This kind of interpretation is quite general, but more precise

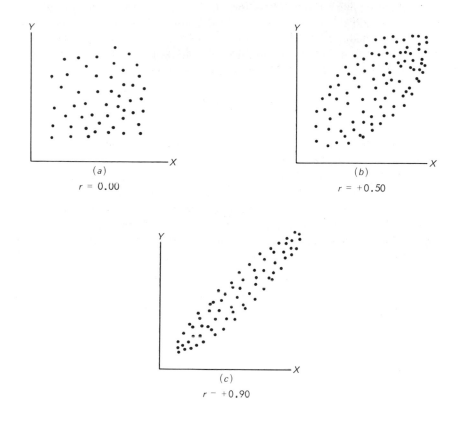

FIG. 4–11   (a) $r = .00$, (b) $r = +.50$, (c) $r = +.90$

methods that yield useful information about the coefficient can be used.

Coefficient of determination. A correlation coefficient is not a proportion. Therefore it is incorrect to say that a correlation coefficient of 0.80 represents twice as much of a relationship between two variables as a coefficient of 0.40. Nor can we say that a coefficient of 0.80 reflects 80 percent of the possible relationship between two variables. However, if we square the correlation coefficient, we can then refer to the proportion of *shared* variance between two variables. Thus, if $r = 0.80$, then $r^2 = 0.64$, and we can say that 64 percent of the variance of the two variables is shared by them. The squared correlation coefficient, r^2, is called the *coefficient of determination.* In some cases, reference is made to the coefficient of non-determination, $1-r^2$, which indicates the variance that is specific to each of the two variables. If $r^2 = 0.64$ or 64 percent, then $1-r^2 = 0.36$ or 36 percent.

Predictive Index. The Predictive Index tells us the degree to which knowledge of one variable (X) improves our ability to predict the value of a second variable (Y) over and above pure chance. In other words, how much does a knowledge of X help us in knowing about Y? Will knowledge of X provide us with more information than we would have purely by chance?

The Predictive Index is computed by the formula

$$P.I. = 1 - \sqrt{1 - r^2} \qquad \text{(Formula 4–8)}$$

The values of the P.I.'s for various correlation coefficients are given in Table 4–8. Coefficient signs are omitted, since squaring the coefficient removes negative signs. Thus a P.I. of 0.046 is the appropriate value for coefficients of both $+0.30$ and -0.30. The information in Table 4–8 indicates the degree to which a given correlation coefficient predicts one variable from another. For example, the P.I. for a correlation coefficient of 0.25 is 3.2 percent better than chance as a predictor, while $r = 0.80$ is 40 percent better than chance.

TABLE 4–8 • Values of the Predictive Index

r	P. I.	r	P. I.
0.05	0.002	0.55	0.165
0.10	0.005	0.60	0.200
0.15	0.012	0.65	0.240
0.20	0.020	0.70	0.286
0.25	0.032	0.75	0.338
0.30	0.046	0.80	0.400
0.35	0.064	0.85	0.474
0.40	0.083	0.90	0.564
0.45	0.107	0.95	0.668
0.50	0.134	1.00	1.000

Statistical significance. Frequent references are made to the significance of a correlation coefficient. If the coefficient is statistically significant, then the coefficient is significantly different from zero, but if the coefficient is not statistically significant, it is for all practical purposes considered the same as zero. Information on statistical significance does *not* help us to assess the degree of relationship that exists between two variables. In fact, when large numbers of scores are obtained, a very small correlation will be significant. Appendix B–2 gives the values of the correlation coefficient necessary for different levels of significance. At the 0.05 level of significance, for example, a correlation of 0.5529 is necessary for statistical significance. (In this example, we are using 11 degrees of freedom. The degrees of freedom,

n, is determined by subtracting one degree for each variable from the total number of individuals being measured. If thirteen people are measured on two variables, $13 - 2 = 11$ degrees of freedom.) For 60 degrees of freedom, a coefficient of 0.2500 is required for significance at the 0.05 level. The information provided in Appendix B–2 is meaningful provided that it is *not* used to determine the degree of relationship between two variables.

Computation of the Correlation Coefficient

The Pearson product-moment coefficient of correlation can be computed in several ways. If a desk calculator is available, the appropriate computational formula is

$$r = \frac{N\sum XY - (\sum X)(\sum Y)}{\sqrt{[N(\sum X^2)-(\sum X)^2]\ [N(\sum Y^2)-(\sum Y)^2]}} \qquad \text{(Formula 4–9)}$$

N = Number of individuals
$\sum XY$ = sum of the products of the X and Y scores for each individual
$\sum X$ = sum of X scores
$\sum Y$ = sum of Y scores
$\sum X^2$ = each X score squared, and summed over all individuals
$(\sum X)^2$ = sum of X scores squared

Note that the square root of the denominator must be taken. Use Appendix B–1 to determine the square root.

Formula 4–9 is used with the data in Table 4–9.

TABLE 4–9 • Computation of Correlation Coefficient by Formula

Individuals	X	X^2	Y	Y^2	XY
1	10	100	6	36	60
2	8	64	9	81	72
3	7	49	5	25	35
4	4	16	7	49	28
5	2	4	3	9	6
	$\sum X = 31$	233	$\sum Y = 30$	200	201
	$(\sum X)^2 = 991$		$(\sum Y)^2 = 900$		

$$r = \frac{5(201) - (31)(30)}{\sqrt{[5(233) - (31)^2]\ [5(200) - (30)^2]}}$$

$$= \frac{75}{\sqrt{[174]\ [100]}} = \frac{75}{\sqrt{17400}} = \frac{75}{131.8} = 0.569$$

When a desk calculator is not available, the correlation coefficient can be computed by hand using a scattergram. For illustrative purposes, scores of two variables will be correlated for ten individuals by the scattergram method. In reality, a correlation coefficient should be computed on a sample of forty or more individuals. We know that as the sample size increases, the distribution tends to approach the normal distribution; therefore, we can place greater faith in a coefficient computed for forty individuals than in one computed for ten individuals. The scattergram is presented in Table 4–10. The step-by-step procedure for developing the scattergram uses the following data:

Individual	X	Y
1	8	14
2	6	13
3	6	12
4	5	10
5	5	9
6	4	9
7	4	8
8	2	6
9	2	2
10	2	3

Step 1. Determine the range and interval size for each variable.
Variable X: Range$=8-2+1=7$
Interval size$=1$
Variable Y: Range$=14-2+1=13$
Interval size$=2$

Step 2. Set up scattergram as in Table 4–10, with the low scores for X in the upper left corner and the low scores for Y in the lower left.

Step 3. Tally each pair of scores in the appropriate column. For example, the scores for the first individual are $8(X)$ and $14(Y)$. Find the X interval that includes a score of 8, and the Y interval that includes a score of 14. Place a tally mark in the square that is associated with both of those intervals. Continue until all pairs of scores are tallied.

Step 4. Sum the tallies for each row and place in the fy column. Sum the tallies by columns, and place in the fx row. Sum both the fy column and the fx row. The answers should be identical, equalling the number of pairs of scores, or N.

Step 5. Estimate the location of the mean for each variable. Usually, the intervals with the greatest frequencies are chosen; however, since the frequencies in our example are small, the middle interval will be chosen for each variable.

Step 6. Determine the x' and y' values. Designate an arbitrary origin of zero for the interval that includes the estimated mean. Label the intervals above

TABLE 4-10 • Scattergram for Computation of Correlation Coefficient

	Low		X Variable		High							High	Low
Y Variable	2	3	4	5	6	7	8	f_y	y'	$f_{y'}$	$f(y')^2$	$\Sigma f_{xy'}$ +	$\Sigma f_{xy'}$ −
13–14	−9	−6	−3		3 1(3	6	9 1(9	2	3	6	18	12	0
11–12	−6	−4	−2		2 1(2	4	6	1	2	2	4	2	0
9–10	−3	−2	−1 1(−1	11	1	2	3	3	1	3	3	0	1
7–8			1					1	0	0	0		
5–6	3 1(3	2	1		−1	−2	−3	1	−1	−1	1	3	0
3–4	6 1(6	4	2		−2	−4	−6	1	−2	−2	4	6	0
1–2	9 1(9	6	3		−3	−6	−6	1	−3	−3	9	9	0
f_x	3	0	2	2	2	0	1	$N = 10$		+5	39	+32	−1
x'	−3	−2	−1	0	1	2	3						
$f_{x'}$	−9	0	−2	0	2	0	3	−6				**+31**	
$f(x')^2$	27	0	2	0	2	0	9	+40					
$\Sigma f_{xy'}$ +	18	0	0	0	5	0	9	+32	**+31**				
$\Sigma f_{xy'}$ −	0	0	1	0	0	0	0	−1					

the mean $+1$, $+2$, and so on, and those below the mean -1, -2, etc.

Step 7. Complete the fx' row by multiplying f by x' for each interval. Sum these values to find $\sum fx'$. Follow the same procedure to find $\sum fy'$.

Step 8. Complete the $(x')^2$ row by multiplying fx' by x' for each interval. Sum these values to find $\sum fx'$. Follow the same procedure for $\sum fy'$.

Step 9. To determine $\sum fx'y'$, the moments are used. These are the values in the upper left-hand corner of the box. The product-moments are determined by multiplying x' by the corresponding y'. For example, the moment for the box in the upper left-hand corner is determined by multiplying y' of 3 by x' of -3. The moment for that box is -9. The column and row over the estimated means have no moment value.

Within each box containing tallies, multiply the moment by the number of tallies. Place this value in the lower right-hand corner of the box. Be sure to include the proper sign ($+$or$-$). These values are the product-moments.

Sum the positive product-moments for each row, and place in the ($+$) column of $\sum fx'y'$. Do the same for the negative product-moments, and place in the ($-$) column of $\sum fx'y'$. Add the ($+$) and ($-$) columns and determine $\sum fx'y'$ by adding the sums of the two columns. As a check, carry out the same procedure for $\sum y'x'$. The results should be identical to those of $\sum x'y'$.

Step 10. Compute the correction factors (Cx'^2 and Cy'^2) for X and Y.

$$Cx' = \frac{fx'}{N} \qquad\qquad Cx' = \frac{-6}{10} = -0.60$$

$$Cy' = \frac{fy'}{N} \qquad\qquad Cy' = \frac{+5}{10} = +0.50$$

Step 11. Compute the standard deviations for X and Y.

$$sx' = \sqrt{\frac{fx'^2}{N} - Cx'^2}$$

$$sy' = \sqrt{\frac{fy'^2}{N} - Cy'^2}$$

$$sx' = \sqrt{\frac{40}{10} - (-0.60)^2} = \sqrt{4.0 - (+0.36)} = \sqrt{3.64} = 1.91$$

$$sy' = \sqrt{\frac{39}{10} - (0.50)^2} = \sqrt{3.9 - (0.25)} = \sqrt{3.65} = 1.91$$

Step 12. Calculate the correlation coefficient.

$$r = \frac{\dfrac{\sum fx'y'}{N} - Cx'Cy'}{sx'sy'} = \frac{\dfrac{31}{10} - (0.50)\,(-0.60)}{(1.91)\,(1.91)}$$

$$= \frac{3.1 - (-0.30)}{3.7481} = \frac{3.4}{3.7481} = 0.907$$

Analysis of Variance

The primary feature of the analysis of variance is that the total sums of squares of a set of measurements composed of several subsets can be broken down into specific parts, each part identifiable with a given source of variation. A simple model of the analysis of variance is described in this section in order to provide a basis for understanding the discussion of the estimation of reliability through analysis of variance procedures in Chapter 6.

In the simple case of the analysis of variance, the total variance is divided into two parts: the variance between subset means and the variance within subsets. Frequently the subsets are samples or groups of individuals that have been assigned to different experimental conditions. The investigator then wishes to ascertain whether or not the mean values of the groups differ after the experimental treatment has been applied. This process is accomplished by analyzing the variance between groups and the variance within groups. Estimates of the population variance are then computed for the sums of squares for the sources of variation. The sum of squares for each source is divided by the degrees of freedom to yield the mean square. A summary table for the sources of variance is given in Table 4–11.

TABLE 4–11 • Summary Table for Analysis of Variance for Independent Scores

Source of Variance	Sum of Squares	Degrees of Freedom	Mean Square	F
Between-groups	SS_{bet}	$k - 1$	MS_{bet}	$\dfrac{MS_{bet}}{MS_{wi}}$
Within-groups (error)	SS_{wi}	$N - k$	MS_{wi}	
Total	SS_{tot}	$N - 1$		

Since the groups are assumed to be random samples from a normal population, the two mean squares are expected to differ only within the limits of random sampling. This hypothesis is tested by dividing the between-groups mean square by the within-groups mean square to get the variance ratio, the F value. If the obtained F value equals or exceeds the tabled values, the difference between the variances is greater than one could expect within the limits of random sampling. Two groups may differ in terms of either means or variances. If the variances of the groups are approximately the same (which is assumed to be the case), a significant difference between groups is attributed to differences in group means.

The degrees of freedom in Table 4–11 are determined by the number of scores free to vary after the mean for the set of scores has been derived. For example, consider a set of three scores. If two of the three numbers are known (2, 4), and the total of the three numbers is 12, the third number must be 6, that is, the third number is not free to vary. In Table 4–11, one score is not free to vary for the total variance, and the appropriate degrees of freedom are $N - 1$. (N equals the total number of scores.) Similarly, the between-groups degrees of freedom are $k - 1$, where k equals the number of groups. The degrees of freedom for the within-groups variance are $k(n - 1)$, where n equals the number of individuals within each group.

When this analysis of variance model is used, it is assumed that the scores are independent of one another. When the analysis of variance is used in estimating the reliability of tests of motor performance, several trials are administered to the same individual, and thus the scores are no longer independent. When a given individual takes repeated measures of the same test, the measures are correlated, or dependent. A modification of the simple model is required so that the correlated scores are taken into account. The total variation can be broken into three component parts: between individuals, between trials, and the interaction of individuals and trials. It is not possible to compute a within-groups source of variance because there is only one score in each cell. Thus, the interaction term is used as the error term. Essentially, the interaction source of variance is a measure of the tendency of subjects to respond differentially over different trials. In this type of analysis of variance model, it is not possible to test the significance of the interaction term because no within-group term can be computed. A summary of the simple analysis of variance model for correlated data is given in Table 4–12, where n equals the number of individuals, t equals the number of trials, and N equals the total number of scores. The F test shown in Table 4–12 is the test for trend described in Chapter 6, where an example of the computation of the analysis of variance for correlated scores is also presented.

TABLE 4–12 · Summary Table for Analysis of Variance for Correlated Scores

Source of Variance	Sum of Squares	Degrees of Freedom	Mean Square	F
Between-individuals (I)	SS_i	$n - 1$	MS_i	$\dfrac{MS_t}{MS_{it}}$
Between-trials (T)	SS_t	$k - 1$	MS_t	
Interaction ($I \times T$)	SS_{it}	$(n - 1)(k - 1)$	MS_{it}	
Total	SS_{tot}	$N - 1$		

Summary

The interpretation of a test score depends in part on the type of scale the scores represent. A scale is described according to the rule by which numbers are assigned to aspects of objects or events. The rule is determined by the number of existing features of the real number series. The three distinguishing features of the real number system are order, distance, and origin. A series of numbers can have a meaningful *order*. The *distance* between any two numbers can be described as greater than, equal to, or less than the distances between any other two numbers. Finally, the series can have a unique *origin* designated by the number "zero".

Four common types of scales are nominal, ordinal, interval and ratio. A *nominal* scale is a set of mutually exclusive categories. Nominal data contain none of the features of the real number system. An *ordinal* scale is determined by ranking a set of objects with regard to some specific characteristic. Ordinal data reflect one feature of the real number series, that of order. An *interval* scale is characterized by equal units of measurement. Interval data have two features of the real number series: order and distance. *Ratio* scales contain an absolute zero point as well as equal units of measurement. Ratio data have all three features of the real number system.

Although there are many theoretical distributions, the most widely known distribution is the normal curve. If the distribution of a set of scores approximates the normal distribution, the known properties of the normal curve provide useful information about that distribution. *Parametric* statistics can then be applied to the data. Even though few distributions fit all the requirements of normality, the normal curve can be closely approximated if the distribution is based on a sufficiently large number of scores. When the assumption cannot be made that the scores were drawn from a normally distributed population, *nonparametric* statistics must be applied to the data. Nonparametric statistics are used with nominal and ordinal data. The statistics described in this chapter primarily apply to interval data describing a normal distribution and are referred to as parametric statistics.

A convenient method of summarizing a set of scores is to build a frequency distribution. A frequency distribution is made up of a set of mutually exclusive classes and the numbers of individuals belonging to each class. The frequency distribution is not appropriate for nominal scores, since an assumption underlying the use of the frequency distribution is that the scores have a meaningful order.

Graphs of frequency distributions are useful aids for interpreting a distribution of scores. Two typical types of graphs are the *histogram* and the *frequency polygon*. The histogram depicts the number of cases falling within each interval. By marking the midpoint of each interval at the height of the bar and connecting these marks, a frequency polygon is formed.

A distribution can be partially described by determining a score that represents the center of the distribution, such as the mean, median, or mode. The *mean* is the arithmetic average of the scores. The mean is often the preferred measure of central tendency because it fits mathematically with other statistics, and is computed by taking all of the scores in a distribution into account. In a distribution that is symmetrical, the mean, median, and mode are all located at the same point. When an extreme score occurs at either end of the distribution (causing the distribution to be skewed), the mean is markedly affected, much more so than the median or mode, and moves in the direction of the skewed end of the distribution. In this case, the median is the preferred measure of central tendency. The *median* is the middle score in the distribution. Half of the scores in the distribution fall above the median and half fall beolw. The *mode* is the score that occurs most frequently in a distribution. Generally, the mode is a less adequate measure of central tendency than the mean or the median.

Measures of variability such as the range, interpercentile range, and standard deviation indicate how the scores vary around the measure of central tendency. The *range* is determined by subtracting the lowest score in a distribution from the highest score and adding one. The range is somewhat limited as a measure of variability because it provides no information about the way in which scores are distributed within a given area. The *interpercentile* range is a better measure of variability because it cannot be distorted by extreme scores. The interquartile range, or Q_3 to Q_1, is the most commonly used interpercentile range. The *standard deviation* is generally the preferred measure of variability since it can be used with many other statistics. When the mean and standard deviation have been determined, a set of raw scores can be converted to z scores. The z score transformation is useful when comparing two sets of scores that have different units of measurement.

The *coefficient of correlation* reflects the relationship between two variables. Correlation coefficients can range from $+1.00$ to -1.00. Two aspects of the coefficient are of concern: the *size* and the *sign*. The size of the coefficient indicates the degree of relationship between the two variables. The sign designates the type of relationship, either positive or negative. A coefficient of correlation can be computed for any two sets of scores for the same individuals, because both sets are transformed to a common scale, the z score distribution.

The correlation coefficient can be interpreted in several ways. The coefficient of determination, that is the square of the correlation coefficient (r^2), indicates the proportion of shared variance between two variables. The Predictive Index is used to determine the degree to which knowledge of one variable (X) improves one's ability to predict a second variable (Y) over and above pure chance. The coefficient of correlation can also be tested for *statistical significance*. Information on statistical significance does not assess the degree of relationship that exists between two variables. Rather, this test determines whether or not the coefficient is significantly different from zero.

The *analysis of variance* is a useful statistical technique in that the total sums of squares of a set of measurements composed of several subsets can be broken down into specific parts. Each part can be identified with a given source of variation. In the simple case of the analysis of variance for independent scores, the total variance is divided into two parts: the variance between groups and the variance within groups. When the scores are correlated, that is, several trials of a given test are performed by the same person, a modification of this simple analysis of variance model is necessary. The total variation is broken into three component parts: between individuals, between trials, and the interaction of individuals and trials. This modified model can be used to determine the reliability estimate for a test.

Problems and Exercises

1. The following scores are velocity scores (rounded off to the nearest whole number) for the underhand softball throw performed by high school girls. Build a frequency distribution for these scores using an *interval size of 3.*
   58, 33, 38, 34, 55, 32, 37, 44, 54, 31, 36, 44, 53, 30, 34, 42, 52, 29, 29, 42, 51, 28, 55, 42, 50, 27, 45, 39, 49, 55, 44, 39, 47, 54, 44, 39, 46, 53, 43, 37, 45, 52, 43, 37, 44, 51, 42, 36, 44, 50, 42, 39, 43, 49, 40, 39, 42, 46, 40, 29, 41, 45, 39, 40, 44, 39, 39, 44, 38, 38, 43, 38, 37, 42, 37, 36, 41, 37, 35, 40, 36, 34, 39, 36.
   a. $N = $ _____
   b. Range $= $ _____
   Show the score limits, real limits, midpoint, and frequency for *each interval.* Show the cumulative frequencies and cumulative percents.

2. Are the following variables discrete or continuous?
   a. The distance one can broad jump. _____
   b. The time necessary to run a mile. _____
   c. The number of pull-ups executed.   _____
   d. The number of books in the library.   _____
   e. The age of a child. _____
   f. The number of boys on baseball team.   _____

3. Obtaining Information from a Frequency Distribution.

Score	Frequency	Cumulative frequency	Cumulative %
70–74	1	53	100
65–69	5	52	98
60–64	9	47	89
55–59	15	38	72
50–54	8	23	43
45–49	6	15	28
40–44	4	9	17
35–39	3	5	9
30–34	2	2	4

   a. Which interval includes the score below which lie 35% of all the scores?
   b. How many scores are smaller than 60?
   c. How many scores are larger than 39?
   d. If one were to regard all scores that rate in the upper 57% as passing scores, how many of the 53 scores would be *failing* scores?
   e. Which interval includes the score below which lie 73% of all the scores?

4. *Computation of the Median and the Interquartile Range.*

Score Intervals	f
100–104	2
95– 99	1
90– 94	3
85– 89	6
80– 84	5
75– 79	10
70– 74	9
65– 69	3
60– 64	2
55– 59	0
50– 54	1
45– 49	2

   a. $N =$ _____
   b. Range = _____
   c. Find the median.
   d. How many cases lie below Q_3?
   e. Determine the interquartile range $(Q_3 - Q_1)$.

5. *Computation of the Mean and the Standard Deviation.*

Score Intervals	f
82–84	2
79–81	8
76–78	6
73–75	8
70–72	8
67–69	12
64–66	5
61–63	6
58–60	2
55–57	5

a. $N =$ _____
b. Range = _____
c. Interval size = _____
d. What is the median of the distribution given above?
e. What is the mean?
f. What is the standard deviation?
g. Suppose four cases are added to the interval 82–84? Which of the two measures of central tendency is least affected by the change?

6. Below are given a score, the mean, and the standard deviation on each of three tests. Compute z scores for each of the three scores. On which test does the score stand highest in relation to the group for which the mean and the standard deviation were computed? On which the lowest?

Test	Mean	Standard Deviation	Score
Wall volley	55	10	60
Repeated set ups	24	8	44
Serve velocity	44	2	42

7. *Computation of the Correlation Coefficient.*

Individuals	X	Y
1	2.7	6.8
2	2.4	6.7
3	2.5	7.1
4	3.2	6.3
5	2.6	7.1
6	3.0	6.2
7	2.9	5.9
8	3.1	5.8
9	2.9	6.9
10	2.9	6.4
11	2.8	6.6
12	3.0	6.9
13	2.8	5.8
14	3.1	5.9
15	3.3	5.9
16	2.5	6.8

X is the time to roll a bowling ball from the foul line to the head pin.
Y is the number of pins knocked down on the first ball in a frame.

a. Compute the correlation coefficient between X and Y.
b. Comment on the sign of the correlation coefficient.

8. Compute the F value from the analysis of variance summary table. Is the F value statistically significant? How should this result be interpreted?

Source of Variance	Sum of Squares	Degrees of Freedom	Mean Square
Between-groups	148.62	2	74.31
Within-groups(error)	1197.00	57	21.00
Total	1345.62	59	

Bibliography

CONOVER, W. J. *Practical Nonparametric Statistics.* New York: John Wiley and Sons, Inc., 1971.

GLASS, G. V. and J.C. STANLEY. *Statistical Methods in Education and Psychology.* Englewood Cliffs, N. J.: Prentice-Hall, Inc., 1970.

HAYS, W. L. *Statistics for Psychologists.* Chicago: Holt, Rinehart, and Winston, 1963.

JONES, L. V. "The Nature of Measurement," in *Educational Measurement,* ed. R. L. Thorndike. Washington, D.C.: American Council on Education, 1971.

MAGNUSSON, D. *Test Theory.* Palo Alto, Calif.: Addison-Wesley Publishing Company, 1966.

SIEGEL, S. *Nonparametric Statistics for the Behavioral Sciences.* New York: Mc-Graw-Hill Book Company, 1965.

STEVENS, S. S. "Mathematics, Measurement, and Psychophysics," in *Handbook of Experimental Psychology,* ed. S. S. Stevens. New York: John Wiley and Sons, Inc., 1958.

TORGERSON, W. S. *Theory and Method of Scaling.* New York: John Wiley and Sons, Inc., 1958.

5

validity

What is meant by the term "validity"? According to Webster, *valid* is defined as "grounded on truth or fact; capable of being justified, supported, or defended; well-grounded; sound" (Webster, 1956, p. 940). A statement can be valid in one set of circumstances but invalid in another. In this chapter, a specific type of validity, the validity of a test, will be discussed. A valid test can be loosely defined as a measure that is sound in terms of the purposes of the test and meets satisfactory criteria for test construction.

If a student is informed of the knowledge and behaviors he is expected to display at the end of a course, he is justified in assuming that his evaluation will be based on the stated goals. If the student evaluation is made on some other basis, the validity of the test is questionable. For example, suppose students in a health class are told that at the end of a course they will be expected to be able to evaluate community health issues, yet the final exam consists of factual material on anatomy, physiology, disease, and so forth. The students may object to the exam because the ability to evaluate community health issues is not measured. In essence, the validity of the test is not considered adequate.

Definition of Test Validity

Validity can be defined as the degree to which a test measures that which it is intended to measure. More broadly, validity is the soundness of the interpretation of the test. This concept is complicated by the diverse definitions and labels used to identify the various aspects of test validity. Even measurement specialists differ in their definitions of the concept. In an attempt at clarification, three types of validity are described in the 1966 *Standards for Educational and Psychological Tests* (American Psychological Association, 1966). These types are *content validity, criterion-related validity,* and *construct validity.* Each type will be discussed in detail in this chapter.

According to Cureton, two aspects of validity must be considered: relevance and reliability (Cureton, 1951). *Relevance* is described as the closeness of agreement between what the test measures and the function that it is intended to measure. *Reliability* refers to the precision and consistency of the measure. Although recognizing the importance of reliability in evaluating validity, the concept of reliability will not be emphasized in this chapter since it is dealt with in Chapter 6.

Validity is restricted by the reliability of a measure in that the validity coefficient cannot exceed the square root of the reliability coefficient, or the index of reliability (Cronbach, 1970; Cureton, 1950 and 1951; Mosier, 1951). However, the idea of expressing validity as a correlation coefficient does not apply outside the realm of criterion-related validity, although correlational techniques may be useful in establishing construct validity. Thus, a coefficient of reliability can always be calculated, but it is not always possible to obtain a coefficient of relevance. When a validity coefficient can not be computed, validity must be interpreted qualitatively rather than quantitatively. The decision regarding interpretation depends upon the nature of the criterion, which is the standard against which the usefulness of the test score is judged. If a criterion score is available, a validity coefficient can be computed; if not, validation is primarily qualitative, or logical. Although qualitative validity is appropriate at some stage in the determination of all three types of validity, it is the primary means of establishing content validity.

Content Validity

According to the 1966 *Standards,* "content validity is demonstrated by showing how well the content of the test samples the class situation or subject matter about which conclusions are to be drawn" (American Psychological Association, 1966, p. 12). This type of validity is appropriate for any written test in education, but a special case known as *logical validity* can be utilized to validate tests of specific sports skills in physical education. Logical validity will be described later in this chapter.

Content validity is used to validate measurements of the type of behavior produced by a specific program of instruction in order to evaluate the effectiveness of that program (Cronbach, 1970). If "type of behavior" can be equated with "process," this description of the purpose of content validity should be acceptable to other measurement specialists (Ebel, 1956; Lennon, 1956). Some writers define this type of validity in specific terms such as curricular validity (Cureton, 1951) and validity by definition (Mosier, 1957). Definitions of other classifications of content validity are presented in a later section.

Determination of Content Validity

One way of determining content validity is to prepare test questions according to the content of the course and the levels of behavior involved. The table of specifications described in Chapter 2 can be used for content validation. For example, two forms of the AAHPER Cooperative Physical Education Tests (Cooperative Tests and Services, 1970) were developed according to the table of specifications presented in Table 5–1. Their content validity should be determined by the degree to which the test items measure the content and behaviors specified in the table. All content areas and levels of behavior are not of equal importance; therefore, some areas and levels are covered to a greater extent than others. The importance of an area or level is determined by its educational value, not by the amount of time spent on learning the content at a certain level of behavior.

The determination of content validity must be distinguished from the process of determining the educational importance of a test. The *content validity* of a test refers to the degree to which the test questions adequately sample the previously described universe. The *educational importance* of a test is being determined when judgments are made about the description of the universe or the suitability of test items. The universe from which the test items are drawn for the AAHPER Cooperative Physical Education Tests is described in Table 5–1. Three content areas (Activity Performance, Effects of Activities, and Factors Modifying Participation in Activities and Their Efforts) and three behavior areas (Knowledge, Understanding, and Thinking) were identified. If the test questions adequately sample this universe, the test has content validity. Note the number of items written for each content area in Form 2A. More than half of the test questions were constructed to measure the content area entitled "Effects of Activities." One might question whether the emphasis on this content area is justified. The test manual gives no information on the relative importance of each of the three content areas. If such information were given and the properties of the test items corresponded with the relative importance of the three content areas of the universe, the test would have content validity. If, however, the content areas are represented equally in the universe, the content validity for both Form 2A and Form 2B would be inadequate.

TABLE 5–1 • Item Classification, Forms 2A and 2B, AAHPER Cooperative Physical Education Tests*

Content	Form 2A				Form 2B			
	Knowledge	Under-standing	Thinking	Numbers of Items	Knowledge	Under-standing	Thinking	Numbers of Items
I. Activity Performance								
Basic sports skills	23, 59	45, 55		2		57		1
Concepts fundamental to movement skills in strategy and activities patterns		10	24	4	9	40, 46	15	4
Body mechanics, rules and procedures, and protective requirements		4, 11, 37	15, 26	5		14, 23, 24, 48	47	5
II. Effects of Activities								
Immediate	1, 2, 12, 16, 25, 47, 52	6, 9, 13, 17, 27, 28, 36, 44, 46	48	17	20, 22, 30, 34, 35, 50, 55	6, 7, 11, 13, 32, 37, 38, 39, 58	8, 12, 59	19
Long term health and appearance	18, 21, 42	5, 29, 30, 50	54	8	2, 25, 31	21, 29, 53, 56	19, 45	9
Capacity for effort	7, 56, 57, 58	3, 31, 32, 40	39	9	4, 10, 18, 60	26, 33, 49, 52		8
III. Factors Modifying Participation in Activities and Their Efforts	8, 20, 41, 51	14, 19, 22, 35, 38, 43, 53	33, 34, 49, 60	15	17, 28, 44	1, 16, 27, 36, 41, 42, 54	3, 5, 43, 51	14
Number of Items	20	30	10	60	18	31	11	60

If we disagree with the test constructor's description of the universe, we are making judgments on the *educational importance* of the test. If the universe contains aspects of content or behavior that are unimportant in regard to educational goals, the educational importance of the test is in question. If the universe omits aspects of content that are important, the question is again one of educational importance. If the relative importance of the content and behavior areas in the universe are clearly described, the suggestion that some areas receive too much emphasis is also a question of educational importance.

The test should measure the goals of instruction, which often are expressed in terms of behavioral objectives. These objectives might include many aspects of learning besides factual material. It cannot be overemphasized that the concept of content validity should not be limited in the test user's mind to the selection of factual course content to be included in a written test.

What is the criterion for content validity? According to Lennon the criterion is the "universe of situations which together constitute the area of concern to the person interpreting the test" (Lennon, 1956, p. 295). Ebel refers to the criterion as a set of goals to be reached (Ebel, 1956). The test user must make careful logical judgments when describing and sampling from the criterion since it is impossible to either measure the entire universe, or, therefore, to compute a validity coefficient.

Controversy about Content Validity

Some measurement specialists feel that judgments about content validity should be restricted to the external, observable side of testing (Melton, 1966). According to this view, making judgments about the subject's internal processes requires stating hypotheses, which leads to empirical construct validation. For example, if one wishes to examine the validity of the Liba and Stauff Volleyball Pass Test (Liba and Stauff, 1963), it is a matter of content (or logical) validity to have a qualified person judge whether the authors did in fact design a measure of the sort they called for in their operational definition. To ask the judge whether high scores on the test reflect a high level of motor behavior is to solicit his speculation about construct validity. Thus, one could make judgments only about the universe description and the test materials, and it would be "content validation," according to those who hold the preceding views.

This concern is a legitimate one because the task of designating desired levels of behavior for any given content has certain inherent problems. Essentially, the problem is that although the test constructor may determine a measure of content for a specific process or level of behavior, in practice the process required may differ for different students (Cronbach, 1971). For example, the skill of dribbling a basketball may be the content area of concern. At a low level of motor behavior, one might wish to measure the ability to dribble without any obstacle; at a low to medium level, the ability to dribble around stationary objects; at a medium level, the ability to dribble around moving objects. Within a given class of high school freshman boys, it is conceivable that a measure of the ability to dribble around moving objects, although designated as a medium-level behavior, may in fact measure a low-level behavior for some boys who are highly skilled and a high-level behavior for some who are poorly skilled. The behavior in question is an inner process, and thus takes on the attributes of a construct. More attention must be devoted to this problem by measurement specialists to provide the expertise needed by teachers in order to make judgments about tests. For a detailed discussion on this problem, see the article by Kropp, Stoker, and Bashaw (1966) listed in the bibliography.

Assessing the Degree of Content Validity

It is inconsistent with sound test construction theory to refer to the validity of a test because although a test may be valid for a specific situation, the validity may not be generalizable to a different type of group or situation. The test, which is used as a measure of the criterion, is considered to be a representative sample of that criterion. The test might be defined as a predictor of a universe of situations; however, the term "prediction" will not be used in the discussion of content validity so that all references to prediction will pertain to a form of criterion-related validity.

Lennon (1956) describes three assumptions underlying the use of content validity. First, the area of concern to the tester can be conceived of as a *meaningful, definable universe of responses,* which is the total of all possible responses that have existed in the past, exist at present, and will exist in the future. Second, *a sample can be drawn from the universe in some meaningful fashion.* Random sampling is usually neither possible nor desirable. Generally, the sample is representative of the essential characteristics of the universe, and includes selected responses that represent those characteristics. Third, *the sample and the sampling process can be defined with sufficient precision to enable the user to judge how adequately the sample performance typifies performance of the universe of responses.*

If we wish to measure knowledge of rules in basketball, the universe would consist of all possible rules. Since measurement of the total universe would be impossible, a representative sample of rules is drawn from that universe. If the sample is randomly drawn, more offensive than defensive rules might be included. This proportion might not be characteristic of the universe. The sample, then, must be developed so that it reflects the appropriate characteristics of the universe. In addition, the levels of behavior in the universe must be identified. When students are first learning the rules, the teacher may wish to construct a test that primarily measures a low level of cognitive behavior. If the rules test is being designed for more experienced players, the teacher may be interested in the degree to which the students can apply the rules, and design test items that measure higher levels of cognitive behavior. A test may consist of items written at several levels of cognitive behavior. Whatever the case, the selection of items should be made according to a systematic plan.

Since the measurement of content validity is not quantitative, some test constructors have relied upon expert judgment to determine the universe or criterion. While the identification of the important elements of a universe by experts may be useful, Gulliksen (1950) warns that judgment by experts is not beyond question, and suggests that the *intrinsic validity* of the universe should be appraised. Intrinsic validity refers to criterion validation that is not dependent on circumstances external to the criterion. One approach to appraising the intrinsic validity of a universe is through the use of factor analytic techniques. In this way, the relationships among various types of tests that sample the universe can be examined, and the effect that training has on the test might be investigated. This information is used to refine the judgment of experts.

Since the degree of content validity cannot be expressed by a validity coefficient, detailed descriptive evidence should be given. First, the criterion and the principles of sampling from it should be stated. Second, the evidence should include an outline of the achievements covered by the test. Third, one should indicate which parts of the test measure what achievement. Lastly, detailed data on the internal analysis of the test should be included.

Cronbach (1971) has described a theoretical method of validating the degree to which the actual test operations correspond to the operational definition of the universe. While this method has not received direct experimentation, it has been approximated by Ebel (1956). Briefly, the method involves duplicate construction of a test. The rules for selecting test content would be described in such detail that there could be no uncertainty as to what domain of tasks is being sampled. Two teams of equally competent writers would work independently on the same test construction problem. These teams would be given the same definition of relevant content, the same sampling rules, the same instructions for reviewers, and the same specifications for tryout and interpretation of data. The resultant two tests should be equivalent. The degree of equivalence would have to be determined through experimentation. The samples, then, would be judged as adequate representations of the universe.

The "duplicate construction" approach suggested by Cronbach can have several limitations. Two teams of equally competent writers would be difficult to obtain, and even if two such teams were available, how would "equal competence" be determined? The Cronbach method, if used successfully, would show that a given universe can be adequately represented, but the results could not be generalized to any other universe. Another limitation is the amount of time that would be required. The value of using this method would have to be weighed against these inherent disadvantages.

Content Validity and Appearance of Validity

The term content validity is sometimes confused with the appearance of validity, that is, when a test looks, but is not necessarily, valid (Ebel, 1961). For example, a test of playing ability in football may include a measure for each important skill (passing, punting, and so forth) and thus may appear to be valid, yet fail to measure the broader aspects of playing ability. Kicking a football through the uprights following a touchdown can only be achieved by a few individuals, but many persons can perform this task well under practice conditions (that is, when it does not count and the opposing linesmen are not charging). The same is true for punting, in that many players can consistently punt a football from 40 to 45 yards in practice. However, there are very few players who have been able to average 40 yards in competition. In short, while the test of place-kicking and punting ability provides indications of performance capacity, the true test of playing ability is whether or not the kicker can perform under game conditions.

The idea of appearance of validity may be important psychologically from the standpoint of a test taker or administrator (Cronbach, 1971). However, a test that is proven valid might not always have the appearance of validity, and this lack is often a source of misunderstanding for laymen who use a test for selection or classification. Nonetheless, the appearance of validity must not be confused with content validity, nor should it be referred to as face validity, a misleading term that should be discarded (Mosier, 1957).

Logical Validity and Tests of Motor Skills

On the surface, it may appear that content validity is appropriate only for the validation of written tests in physical education. This is not true. When a skill test incorporates and directly measures the important components of the skill being evaluated, *logical* validity, which can be considered a special case of content validity, may be claimed. In testing a specific skill it is possible to define the aspects of good performance precisely, and to measure them with great accuracy. This is not the case with measures of playing ability. Even if it were possible to define precisely all of the important components of playing ability, these components would be too numerous to measure. Thus, the validity of measures of playing ability must be determined through a broader type of validation than logical validity.

Although information on the content validity of a playing ability test is important, its validity cannot be determined by defining and measuring all of the significant components of playing ability because too many intangibles exist. Rather, the test constructor should attempt to identify the *most important* components, using such methods as expert opinion, factor analysis, and logical analysis. However, the remainder of this section will be devoted to the testing of individual skills, reserving the measurement of playing ability for later discussion.

When testing specific skills, the test may be validated on logical grounds if good performance is defined and a test is constructed which measures that good performance. In other words, the test is the skill. The concept of logical validity has been applied to physical education measures primarily by Ruth B. Glassow and Marie R. Liba at the University of Wisconsin. There are several good examples of tests which have been validated using logical validity. One of these is a volleyball pass test by Liba and Stauff (1963); another, an eight-iron approach test in golf by West and Thorpe (1968). The general procedure followed in constructing these tests is to define good performance, construct a test according to this definition, and score the test so that the best score represents a performance which closely approximates the definition of good performance.

It might be helpful to examine one of these tests more closely. The West and Thorpe test is designed to measure the eight-iron approach shot 12 yards from the pin. Good performance is defined as follows: "A good approach shot at a distance of twelve yards from the pin has a ball flight which will carry the ball over any intervening water and/or sand hazards, onto the green, and to a position at or near the pin" (West and Thorpe, 1968, p. 1115). The authors refer to two components of successful performance which they feel are important. These components are accuracy (proximity to pin) and vertical angle of projection (angle between ground and path of ball).

Accuracy is measured using a target consisting of six concentric circles surrounding the pin. A restraining line is marked 12 yards from the pin. Accuracy is scored on a scale from one to seven, seven being the score of the inner circle, and one, failure to reach even the outermost circle. The vertical angle of projection, or flight score, is measured on a three-point scale. A topped ball is scored one point. A ball with a low angle of projection, 29 degrees or lower, receives two points. A ball with a high angle of projection, 30 degrees or higher, scores three points.

On the basis of this type of test construction, logical validity is claimed because the test is designed to measure those elements of good performance that are the important components of the skill. This does not mean that the definition of good performance is not open to question, but that such a question is one of *educational importance*. The test user must keep in mind that the test is designed to measure a specific skill in golf, and not to measure overall golf-playing ability, which involves all elements of the game, or a combination of many skills. This test might be used to assess learning in the formative sense or achievement in the summative sense.

In the West and Thorpe study, evidence of construct validity was also given to add support to the claim of logical validity. The test was given to a group of experienced golfers and a group of beginning golfers. The scores for the two groups on the test were significantly different, with the performance of the experienced golfers being significantly better than that of the beginners. In this case, the sample sizes of the two groups were markedly different, which may have accounted for the significant difference. In any case, once a test constructor hypothesizes that two groups of individuals will perform differently on his test and designs an experiment to test this hypothesis, he is exploring the *construct validation* of the test.

Criterion-Related Validity

Criterion-related validity is demonstrated by comparing the test scores with one or more external variables that are considered direct measures of the characteristic or behavior in question. Two general types of validity may be classified as criterion-related: *predictive validity,* dealing with the prediction of future behavior, and *concurrent validity,* which involves the comparison of a given test with another test that has an established validity, but is excessively time-consuming or costly to administer. Criterion-related validity is ultimately determined by statistical methods although content validation techniques may also be useful in constructing the test.

Criterion-Related Validity (Predictive)

Predictive validity is the degree to which a criterion is foretold from predictor scores. A person's expected future performance is predicted from a test or a group of tests. Of primary interest is the *criterion,* the standard against which the usefulness of the test score is judged. *Predictors* are tests or variables that predict criterion behavior. If more than one test is used as a predictor, the statistical technique of multiple correlation is used to select the most effective combination of tests, to determine how they should be weighted in arriving at a final prediction, and to assess the effectiveness of the composite predictor. For example, the ability to broad jump might be predicted by some combination of the following variables: length of thighs, strength of leg muscles, height, and running speed on short dashes. In this case, broad jumping ability is the criterion and the latter four variables are the predictors.

Design for predictive validity study. Theoretically, a predictive study should follow a standard format in which predictive measures are given to an entire group before any selection is made. In other words, if a test is designed to predict membership on a baseball team, the test is given to all individuals trying out for the team. All people, whether qualified for the team or not, are eligible to become team members. A judgment must be made about the overall baseball ability of each member at some point in the future. The criterion measure, overall baseball ability, is obtained for all who took the predictive tests. Only then can statements legitimately be made about how well the predictors predict the criterion. Although it may seem impractical to retain, for a period of time, all persons who try out for the team, this step must be taken to determine true predictive validity.

The criterion score. The score that an individual receives on the criterion measure is the criterion score. In predictive validity, the criterion can only be judged in a logical sense. Either ratings of behavior or a group of tests may be used to measure the criterion. If the criterion is used as a standard for judging the accuracy of the scores from the predictor test, it should always exemplify a measurement procedure clearly superior to the predictor test. Since the criterion cannot be validated statistically, care must be taken to insure that all identifiable sources of criterion bias are removed.

Four classifications of criterion bias have been described by Brogden and Taylor (1950):

> *Criterion deficiency*–the omission of pertinent elements from the criterion.
> *Criterion contamination*–introducing extraneous elements into the criterion.
> *Criterion scale unit bias*–inequality of scale units in the criterion.
> *Criterion distortion*–improper weighting in combining criterion elements.

Criterion deficiency can be determined through an analysis of the situation in which the job behavior occurs. This type of deficiency can result from using only one type of criterion measure, such as ratings or a complex test or production records. Other causes might be the use of a composite criterion (discussed later in this chapter) and failure of raters to consider all the important elements of the criterion.

Criterion contamination occurs during the construction of the measuring instrument. This type of bias includes any source of variance in the criterion, except errors of measurement, that is not a reflection of the criterion. The halo effect is an example of this type of bias. A coach may give an athlete a high performance rating due to a likeable personality rather than superior performance; or, conversely, an athlete may be cut from the squad because of a low rating due to psycho-social factors rather than performance capability. In either case, the halo effect reduces the objectivity of the coach.

Criterion scale unit bias can occur in the selection of a cut-off point for a a set of scores. This bias is commonly found in the use of rating scales, where the high end of the scale is more frequently used than the low. If gymnastic events are rated on a scale of one to ten, and the lowest rating any judge gives is five, criterion scale unit bias is operating.

Criterion distortion has a different meaning for each of the above three biases. In criterion deficiency, distortion occurs when weights of zero are assigned to elements that should have non-zero weights. When only one component of a projectile skill such as the overarm throw is measured, other important components receive zero weights. For example, if both force and accuracy are important components of the overarm throw and only accuracy is measured, a zero weight is assigned to the force aspect of the skill (as well as to any other component that is omitted). In criterion contamination, weights of non-zero are assigned to elements that should have zero weights. If a teacher is influenced by the student's personality when rating him on skill development, elements of personality are indirectly weighted along with elements of skill achievement. In criterion scale unit bias, different weights are assigned to different parts of the continuum of a given element. If judges fail to use ratings 1 and 2 when an event is to be rated on a scale of one to five, ratings 1 and 2 are essentially weighted zero. Or, when a group of students makes the same score on a criterion measure, criterion distortion occurs because a test that does not discriminate necessarily is weighted zero.

Technical aspects of the criterion score. There are inherent disadvantages in combining scores from several tests to form a criterion score for the validation of a test. When this is done, the combination is referred to as a *composite criterion,* and is most simply obtained by converting the criterion scores to standard scores and then averaging them. In essence, it assigns equal weights to each of the tests, implying that each one is of the same importance, and this usually is not the case. Averaging the equally weighted criterion test scores when they should instead be weighted differentially will yield a composite criterion that is identical to the first principal component (factor accounting for the greatest variance) in a principal component analysis. This was demonstrated by Cumbee and Harris (1953). If all the measures making up a criterion score were essentially measures of one general factor, a composite criterion would be a satisfactory option. However, in many cases, performance on any given aptitude is best described in terms of several dimensions, making one dimension insufficient.

Another concern regarding the criterion score is the matter of changes over time: Will the relationships among a group of criterion measurements remain the same as time passes? For example, if selected criterion measures were applied to a group of beginning teachers, would the interrelationships among the measures be the same two years later, or four years later, or six years later for this particular group? The degree of importance of various criteria of good teaching quite possibly might change over the years. Also, if predictions are made from the original set of criteria, and the original interrelations change, the predictions would necessarily be inaccurate. Bereiter (1963) found that a low correlation was obtained for a test given to freshman college students compared with the same test given when these students became seniors, indicating that the test measures different attributes at different stages. In order to take this problem into account, Ghiselli (1960) recommends designing prediction studies so that the period between measurements is short.

Ghiselli also recommends taking into account the dimensionality of the individual when developing a criterion. For example, several teachers at the same school might be considered equally good, yet the nature of their contributions to the school might be quite different. However, these teachers might be evaluated in terms of the same set of criteria, when one teacher actually might contribute most to curriculum development, while another is known for his excellence in teaching. A third might be outstanding in relating to students. According to Ghiselli, the criterion dimensionality of each should be investigated. In an administrative sense there may only be one type of job, but in a psychological sense the jobs are qualitatively different.

The predictor. There is no justification for assuming that a test that logically seems to be a good predictor is so in fact. A high validity coefficient may seem obvious and yet not exist. If the criterion is not quantitatively measurable, predictive validity cannot be determined.

On the other hand, a test might not appear valid, and yet be an excellent predictor. However, even if a high validity coefficient is obtained between the predictors and the criterion, the predictors are still not beyond question. Gulliksen (1950) notes that coaching will destroy test validity if that validity is indirect. If coaching improves the predictor but not the criterion, the validity is indirect. When a predictor test has *intrinsic validity,* improvement on the predictor measure automatically results in improvement on the criterion test. For example, if an investigator suggested that attitudes toward physical education would predict success in physical education classes, then improvement in attitudes should result in improvement in physical education grades, assuming success is measured by grades.

If a track coach suggested that the headstand is a good predictor of sprinting ability, his colleagues would probably look at him in disbelief. The track coach might add that he has been studying this relationship and has figures to prove his point. He produces data yielding a correlation coefficient of 0.82 between the ability to perform a headstand and sprinting ability. Other coaches might respond with a key question: Would improving headstand ability increase sprinting ability? (This question would have to be tested by another method.) If not, the headstand as a predictor lacks intrinsic validity. However, if the coach could establish that, after training individuals on the headstand, their sprinting ability increased, the headstand would, in fact, be a good predictor having intrinsic validity.

Any correlational method yields a coefficient that is a measure of the relationship between or among variables. The relationship is the degree to which the variables are measures of a common element. The correlation coefficient does *not* yield information on the degree to which performance on one variable *causes* performance on another. For example, weight correlates highly with height, because taller people tend to be heavier; but, increasing weight is not necessarily accompanied by an increase in height. Thus, the variables have a *functional* relationship rather than a *causal* one.

Cross-validation. Cross-validation is a technique in which weights determined on one sample are tested for effectiveness on a second, similarly drawn sample (Mosier, 1951). Two random samples are drawn from the same population. The predictor and criterion measures are administered to both samples, although at different points in time. Using the first sample, the best weights for the predictors are computed, based on the criterion data. The weights from Sample 1 are then applied to Sample 2 to compute the multiple correlation coefficient for the predictors of the criterion.

The weights should not be applied to a sample drawn from another population, because the relationships between predictors might differ for the second population. For example, the weights of predictors for ten-year-old boys might differ from the weights for twelve-year-old boys; therefore the multiple correlation coefficient for the twelve-year-olds should not be computed from the weights of predictors for the ten-year-olds.

There are two reasons for using cross-validation procedures. First, if criterion scores are available for a sample, it is unnecessary to predict them. The main value of the sample data is to determine beta weights (used to maximize the correlation) and a multiple correlation "as values which will most likely apply in other samples for which the criterion measures are not and will not be available." (Mosier, 1951, p. 8) Secondly, a multiple correlation coefficient obtained for the first sample is a biased estimate of predictive effectiveness since it capitalizes on the idiosyncrasies of the sample (Cureton, 1950 and 1951; Mosier, 1951). The second sample must be used to get an unbiased (not spuriously high, in this case) estimate.

Mosier (1951) recommends the technique of double cross-validation to avoid wasting data. Briefly, this procedure involves computing beta weights on both samples and then determining a multiple correlation for each sample based on the weights of the other sample.

Cross-validation in physical education research. A great deal of research labeled cross-validation really involves the validation of a test for a sample which differs in some way from the sample on which it was originally validated. An article by Kroll and Petersen (1966) provides an example of this type of validation. Their study was conducted to cross-validate the Booth scale as a measure of competitive spirit. The Booth scale was constructed to discriminate between good and poor competitors in athletics. Booth had suggested that the test had predictive power. Kroll and Petersen administered the Booth scale to six football teams, three with winning seasons and three with losing seasons, and one nonathlete group. The Booth scale failed to distinguish among the groups studied. As a further check on the validity of the Booth scale, good versus poor competitors on the six football teams were studied. Again, no differences were found. In short, the results did not support the earlier results of Booth.

Whenever an investigator attempts to validate a test using a sample that differs from the original sample, the results of his study add to the evidence on the validity of the test. Technically, cross-validation is an inappropriate label for this procedure. When cross-validation procedures are used, the beta weights from the orginal sample are applied to the predictor scores of another sample drawn from the *same population*. The multiple correlation coefficient, obtained by comparing the weighted predictors with the criterion, is computed from the data of the second sample.

Technical aspects of predictive validity. In the case of one predictor and one criterion, the validity coefficient is a simple correlation coefficient. (If both sets of scores are interval or ratio data, the Pearson product-moment correlation coefficient is appropriate. For other types of scales, see the section on correlation in Chapter 4.) For cases of one criterion measure and more than one predictor, multivariate statistics are appropriate, as indicated in Table 5-2. Multiple correlation techniques assess the effectiveness of a composite predictor in predicting a single criterion. Canonical correlation is used to determine the effectiveness of a composite predictor in predicting a composite criterion.

TABLE 5-2 • Types of Predictive Validity Coefficients

Type of Correlation Coefficient	Number of Predictors	Number of Criterion Measures
Simple	One	One
Multiple	Two or More	One
Canonical	Two or More	Two or More

With a composite predictor and a single criterion, it is desirable to have low intercorrelations among the predictors and a high correlation between the predictors and the criterion, although one predictor may correlate zero or even negatively with the criterion. In the latter case, the predictor is a *suppression* variable (Guilford, 1965). If three predictors are used, the suppressor variable may have variance in common with one predictor, but not with the other. This variable may acquire a negative regression weight (that is, a beta weight with a negative value), even though it may correlate only zero, and not negatively, with the criterion.

> [The] . . . function . . . [of the suppression variable] in a regression equation is to suppress in other independent variables whatever variance is not represented in the criterion but which may be in some variable that does otherwise correlate with the criterion (Guilford, 1965, p. 406).

Example of predictive validity study in physical education research. Predictive validity is concerned with future behavior or performance. A study by Vincent (1967) dealt with the prediction of success in physical education activities from attitude, strength, and efficiency measures. The subjects were thirty-seven freshman and sophomore college women. Three predictors were selected for the study: the Wear attitude inventory, selected strength measures, and a physiological efficiency measure. Vincent hypothesized that these measures would predict success in physical education activities. The criterion, success in physical education, was measured by the grade given in a required physical education course. Regression equations were used to determine the appropriate formulas for predicting the criterion measure.

The highest multiple correlation coefficient, $R = 0.56$, was obtained by using all three predictors. However, eliminating the efficiency predictor from the formula only reduced the multiple correlation coefficient to 0.53. Using the attitude predictor alone, a multiple correlation coefficient of 0.49 was obtained. In the latter case, the regression equation equalled 0.370 attitude $+ 31.50$, where 0.370 is the beta value.

In general the sizes of multiple correlation coefficients may be low, but the test user must make his own judgments about the adequacy of the sizes depending upon the kind of predictions to be made. Certainly, a correlation coefficient that is obtained through cross-validation procedures would not reflect the idiosyncracies of the original sample. Since cross-validation procedures were not utilized in the Vincent study, the degree to which the results can be generalized to the population of freshman and sophomore college women is greatly reduced.

There are other logical questions the test user may wish to ask about this study. For example, is a grade in a required physical education course an adequate criterion for success in physical education activities? Perhaps the grade is based in part on attendance or other factors not related to the skill and ability of the student.

Criterion-Related Validity (Concurrent)

Concurrent validity is useful when a test is proposed as a substitute for some other test with established validity. The proven test is then the criterion. Concurrent validity might also be employed for predictive purposes before predictive validity can be established. The predictive tests may be administered to persons whose criterion performance can be observed immediately. This procedure is useful when the true predictive validity cannot be ascertained in the near future.

In a study by Kurucz, Fox and Mathews (1969), cardiorespiratory fitness within safe exercise tolerance limits was appraised. The existing measurements were valid, but were exhausting for the subjects and required expensive equipment and trained technicians. A submaximal cardiovascular step test, referred to as the OSU test, was designed as a simplified measure of cardiorespiratory fitness. If this test correlated highly with existing measures, validation claims would be made on the basis of concurrent validity.

The criterion measure was the Balke Treadmill Test. This test required maximal effort and was applicable to a wide age range.

> Validity for the Balke Test is claimed on the basis that a number of discernible physiological changes occur during a given exercise when the heart rate reaches 180 beats/minute. At this point, the R exceeds 1, pulse pressure and oxygen pulse become maximal, and there is a sharp rise in the respiratory frequency and minute volume, together with a sudden drop in alveolar carbon dioxide tension. At about this time, blood lactate levels begin to rise sharply, indicating the inability of the physiological reserves to keep pace with the increased metabolic needs resulting from exercise (Kurucz, Fox and Mathews, 1969, p. 118).

In the submaximal cardiovascular step test (the OSU Test), for which concurrent validity was established, the subject was required to step on a bench in cadence with a metronome until a heart rate of 150 beats/minute was reached. The test consisted of three phases:

> Phase I consists of 6 innings at 24-step/min cadence on the 15-in. bench.
> Phase II consists of 6 innings at 30-step/min cadence on the 15-in. bench.
> Phase III consists of 6 innings at 30-step/min cadence on the 20-in. bench
> (Kurucz, Fox and Mathews, 1969, p. 116).

Each inning was divided into a 30–second work period and a 20-second rest period. During the rest period, the subject took his pulse for a given ten seconds. The test was completed when the pulse rate reached 25 beats (150 beats/minute) and/or when the subject completed the entire 18 minutes. The score was the inning in which the heart rate reached 150 beats/minute.

Thirty males, ranging in age from 19 to 56, took both the Balke Test and the modified OSU Test. The validity coefficient was 0.94. Thus it appears that the OSU Test is a valid submaximal test of cardiorespiratory fitness. The test is simple to administer, utilizes inexpensive equipment, and an all-out effort is not required of the subjects.

As a note of caution, the OSU Test cannot be substituted for the Balke Test if one is interested in detecting coronary pathology (electrocardiogram changes under exercise stress). It is not until the organism experiences stress (near maximal work) that abnormalities in the presumably normal ECG appear. Since the OSU Test is submaximal, it cannot accomplish the total purpose of the Balke Test. However, as a measure of general cardiorespiratory fitness, the OSU Test is clearly more economical than the Balke Test.

Construct Validity

Construct validity is appropriate when a test purports to measure an attribute or quality which is too complex to be measured precisely. No available criterion is fully valid, and no universe of content is adequate. A construct is "some postulated attribute of people, assumed to be reflected in test performance" (Cronbach and Meehl, 1955, p. 283). Such traits as anxiety, sportsmanship, and athletic ability are examples of constructs. Construct validation deals with defending a proposed interpretation of a test, not with recommending any one type of interpretation. Anastasi (1966) has noted that the idea of construct validity is not new, but that it serves to focus attention on the scientific approach which must be taken in theory development. For fuller discussions of this type of validity, see the articles by Bechtoldt (1959), Campbell (1960), and Cronbach and Meehl (1955) listed in the bibliography.

Once an investigator makes the claim that a given test measures a certain construct, the construct must be amplified from a label into a set of sentences. These sentences form a "complete theory surrounding the construct, every link of which is systematically tested in construct validation" (Cronbach, 1971, p. 465). The most profitable approach toward developing the theory is usually through counterinterpretations of results that yield counterhypotheses, rather than verifying each sentence.

Some meaningful ways to investigate construct validity are through group differences, factor analysis, and studies of internal structure, change over occasions, and process. Group differences can be studied by testing the expectation that two groups will differ on the test. Factor analysis divides the construct into more meaningful parts. Studies of internal consistency allow for an evaluation of the item in terms of the underlying theory of the trait. Studies of change over occasions might indicate the stability of the test scores or the effect of experimental intervention. Studies of process involve observations of the performance process.

The following example of processes involved in devising a test of the construct, "Creativity," is presented in the 1966 *Standards:*

> If the author proposes to interpret the test as a measure of a theoretical variable (ability, trait, or attitude), the proposed interpretation should be fully stated. The interpretation of the theoretical construct should be distinguished from interpretations arising under other theories. . . . The description of a construct may be as simple as the identification of "creativity" with "making many original contributions." Even this definition provides some basis for judging whether or not various pieces of empirical evidence support the proposed interpretation. Ordinarily, however, the test author will have a more elaborate conception. He may wish to rule out such originality as derives only from a large and varied store of information. He may propose explicitly to identify the creative person as one who produces numerous ideas, whether of high or low quality. He may propose to distinguish the ability to criticize ideas from the ability to be "creative." He may go on to hypothesize that the person who shows originality in identifying or describing pictures will also have unconventional preferences in food and clothing. All such characterizations for hypotheses are part of the author's concept of "what the test measures" and are needed in designing and in drawing conclusions for empirical investigations of the psychological interpretation of the construct (American Psychological Association, 1966, p. 23).

Construct validity cannot be summed up in a single measure as a correlation between test scores and criterion scores. "Validity is determined by showing that the consequences which can be predicted on the basis of the theory with respect to the data from the test can, in the main, be confirmed by a series of testings" (Magnusson, 1966, p. 13).

The logic of construct validity is based on an interlocking system of laws which constitutes a theory. These laws may relate observable properties to each other, theoretical constructs to observable properties, or different theoretical constructs to one another. A construct must occur in a nomological, or lawlike network, in which some of the laws involve observable properties that permit prediction about events. This does not mean the construct is reduced to observable parts, but rather is combined with other constructs in the network to make predictions about observables.

Learning more about the theory consists of elaborating the network in which it exists. The network can be enriched by generating hypotheses that are confirmed by observation. Operations which are qualitatively very different measure the same thing when their positions in the network tie them to the same construct variable. For public validation, the same network must be accepted by several users.

If, after experimentation, the hypotheses and the data are discordant, one of three reasons is probably contributory. One, *the test does not measure the construct variable.* Two, *the theoretical network which generated the hypothesis is incorrect.* Three, *the experimental design failed to test the hypothesis adequately.*

The construct can be described as the network of the associations in which it occurs. Investigation of a test's construct validity is not essentially different from the general scientific procedures for developing and confirming theories. For a formal description of construct validity refer to Hempel's (1966) discussion of the philosophy of science.

Theoretical Example of Construct Validation in Physical Education Research

Understanding of the concept of construct validity might be enhanced by noting several possible approaches to this type of validation in physical education. An attitude scale might be developed to measure attitudes toward physical fitness. The construct, then, would be attitudes toward physical fitness. Using the scale, those who have positive and negative attitudes may be identified. They can then be measured on other attributes, thereby developing a theory about the construct determined by obtaining information on how those with positive attitudes toward physical fitness differ from those with negative attitudes.

Another construct that has received limited study in the area of physical education is game sense, which can be considered a component of playing ability. Game sense might include the ability to adjust to novel situations, utilize strategies, and cope with stressful situations in the game. As an example, a game sense test for badminton has been developed by Thorpe and West (1969). A theory about the construct of game sense can be developed by exploring ways in which people with a high level of game sense differ from those with a low level, as measured by the Thorpe and West test. Possible avenues of exploration are success in tournament play, anxiety level (Spielberger, 1969), tension level (Spielberger, 1969), experience, and amount of competition in other sports. Research on these variables might reveal that individuals with a high level of game sense would have the following characteristics: successful tournament player, moderate anxiety level, low to medium tension level, more than four years of experience, and competition in at least one other sport.

These examples typify the deductive method of research. The procedure is initiated by developing a theory about a construct. In the above example, game sense was classified as a construct, and considered one aspect of playing ability. The second step is to make deductions about the characteristics of individuals exhibiting different levels of the construct. In the third step, hypotheses are generated from the deductions. Experimental testing of each hypothesis constitutes the fourth step. In the final step, the results either verify or refute the hypothesis. If the latter occurs, the fault could lie with the theory, the measurement instrument, or the hypothesis.

Controversial Aspects of Construct Validity

Not all measurement and evaluation specialists accept the concept of construct validity. Bechtoldt (1959), for instance, feels that there is no place for the notion of construct validity in methodological thinking. He suggests that the term merely renames the process of building a theory of behavior. Part of the controversy stems from a statement by Cronbach and Meehl (1955) that a construct cannot be operationally defined. While this may be impossible for the construct as a whole, the different aspects that are taken into account in the measuring instrument must be operationally defined.

Cronbach (1971) classifies those who object to the term construct validity as ultraoperationalists. He summarizes the controversial view as follows:

> A construct has scientific status only when it is equated with one particular measuring operation. Then, since no construct has more than one indicator, the nomological net is no more than a list of the empirical relationships of the defining indicator. There is a new list—a new network—for each indicator (Cronbach, 1971, p. 480).

Cronbach suggests that writers on curriculum and evaluation who believe that objectives must be defined in terms of behavior are taking the ultraoperationalist position. If one insists on behavioral objectives, one denies the appropriateness and usefulness of constructs.

> The educator who states objectives in terms of constructs (e.g., self-confidence, scientific attitude, the habit of suiting one's writing style to his purpose) regards observables as indicators from which the presence of the characteristics described by the construct can be inferred. But he will not, for example, substitute "volunteer ideas and answers in class" for "self-confidence." From the construct point of view, behavior such as this is an indicator but not a definer. Indeed no list of specific responses-to-situations, however lengthy, can define the construct since the construct is intended to apply to situations that will arise in the future and cannot be specified now. (Cronbach, 1971, p. 481).

Possibly the issue raised by the ultraoperationalists is one of terminology, since there is universal agreement that operational definitions for all procedures must exist so that experimental work can be verified.

Cronbach further recommends that investigators seek the right breadth for concepts. For example, using citizenship as a concept is perhaps too broad and inclusive. Ego strength, which leads one to anticipate different behavior in situations, all of which might be thought of as calling for citizenship, might be better. On the other hand, such specifics as participation in elections and obedience to speed laws are probably too narrow (Cronbach, 1971).

Construct Validation by the Multitrait-Multimethod Matrix

Campbell and Fiske (1959) have indicated that to demonstrate construct validity, one needs to show that a test not only correlates highly with those variables with which it should (convergent validation), but also that it does not correlate with variables from which it should differ (discriminant validation). The multitrait-multimethod matrix is a systematic experimental design for this type of validation. The design involves assessing two or more traits by two or more methods. Correlations of the *same* trait assessed by *different* methods represent a measure of convergent validity. In this case the correlations should be high. Correlations of *different* traits assessed by the *same* or *similar* methods provide a measure of discriminant validity. In this case the correlation should be low or negligible.

In a hypothetical example of the multitrait-multimethod matrix in physical education two traits, ability in wrestling and ability in fencing, are assessed for the same group of individuals by the same methods, judges' ratings and tests simulating game conditions. For *each* trait, the correlation between the two methods is expected to be high (convergent validity). However, if a given method for the two traits is correlated, the correlation coefficient is expected to be low (discriminant validity). For example, if judges' ratings for wrestling ability and fencing ability were correlated, the correlation coefficient should be low.

Construct Validity and Playing Ability in Athletics

The ability of an athlete to perform in a given sport can be called a construct. Because of the complexities of the playing ability construct, one or two tests probably would never be adequate measures. To date, measures of playing ability reported in the literature consist of batteries of skill tests. It seems certain that there are some personal attributes that are related to taking skill tests that are not relevant to playing ability in a game situation, and vice versa. This concept needs a great deal of exploration and experimentation by measurement specialists.

It would be pertinent to examine an example of a test of playing ability, a battery of ice hockey skill tests designed to measure general ability in ice hockey (Merifield and Walford, 1969). The battery was comprised of six tests: forward skating speed, backward skating speed, skating agility, puck carry, shooting, and passing. The tests were administered to 15 male college students, members of a college hockey club, but of varying levels of ability. The students were rated by the hockey coach who ranked them on overall ability prior to the first day of testing. When the test items were correlated with the coach's ratings, the following validity coefficients were obtained:

Forward skating speed	0.83
Backward skating speed	0.79
Skating ability	0.75
Puck carry	0.96

The intercorrelations among the six tests were examined. The shooting and passing items were dropped due to low validity coefficients. The puck carrying test had the highest correlation of the remaining test items, and therefore, was considered to be the best single measure of overall ice hockey ability .

Several points must be considered here. Construct validity usually involves content validity and criterion-related validity. As test items are developed, each individual test should be validated using logical or content validity whereby good performance is described for each test. A statement regarding the validation of each test should be made.

The criterion score of playing ability was obtained by the coach's ratings. When ratings are utilized, the test constructor should carefully describe the specific characteristics to be rated. Unless the judges are asked to weight the same specific points equally for a hockey pass, one judge might pay more attention to the accuracy of the pass than another, who might emphasize the speed of the pass.

Finally, multiple correlation and regression procedures are appropriate to use in order to examine the contribution of each test to the criterion. Examining the intercorrelations among test items is helpful; however, the overlap among items is not taken into account.

The problem of measuring playing ability has frequently been treated as one of concurrent, rather than construct, validation. Only when interpretations are made about the characteristics of individuals taking a test is construct validation appropriately used.

Other Classifications of Validity

Two different classifications of validity are described by Anastasi (1966). One type is *empirical validity* which refers to "the relation between a test score and a criterion, the latter being an independent and direct measure of that which the test is designed to predict" (Anastasi, 1966, p. 123). This could be considered a criterion-related validity, as defined in the 1966 *Standards* (American Psychological Association). The second type is *factorial validity*, which is "the correlation between the test and a factor common to a group of tests or other measures of behavior —[and] such validity is based on factor analysis" (Anastasi, 1966, p. 123).

Mosier (1957) uses the term *validation by definition,* which assumes that the sample of items adequately represents the total universe of appropriate questions. It is used when the only available measure of the criterion is directly related to the test questions themselves.

Cureton's (1951) definition of *curricular validity* places it as a special case of validity by definition. In a test with curricular validity, the test requirements parallel the content and behaviors that *should* be taught in the course. Curricular relevance differs from logical relevance, in which the test reflects the content and behavior *actually taught* in the course. The content and processes actually taught (logical relevance) may not be those that an expert would judge necessary (curricular relevance).

Validity by hypothesis assumes validity based on similar tests until empirical verification by fact can be accomplished (Mosier, 1957). One can assume validity with varying degrees of confidence depending upon the amount, quality, and pertinence of evidence from previous situations. This type of validity is only appropriate where a quantitative criterion score is ultimately available.

Size of the Validity Coefficient

How high should a criterion-related validity coefficient be? In the case of concurrent validity, the coefficient should be relatively high. If Test A compared with Test B yields a correlation coefficient of 0.50, only 25 percent of the variance of the two tests is common to both. There is no justification for substituting one test for another. As the validity coefficient increases, the two tests are assumed to measure increasingly similar qualities.

When a test is constructed for predictive purposes, a low validity may be acceptable in some cases. If the validity coefficient is higher than the coefficient for other similar predictive measures, a test with a coefficient of 0.50 or 0.60 may be retained (Gronlund, 1965). However, the accuracy of prediction increases as the size of the correlation coefficient increases.

Validity coefficients can be expected to be lower when good criteria are hard to find. A test with a relevant criterion may be more valuable than a test with a higher validity coefficient if the criterion for the latter is less relevant (Lyman, 1971).

Guilford (1956) recommends the use of the index of forecasting efficiency (percent of improvement over chance) which is $100(1 - \sqrt{1-r^2})$, where r is the validity coefficient. However, the precision of prediction is much finer than is often needed in practical situations. If an educator is interested in which general category a student will fall—high, middle, or low—he is justified in using a test with a lower validity coefficient than if he were interested in predicting a student's exact score (Wesman, 1953). Validity coefficients of 0.60, 0.50, 0.40 and even 0.30 are far from useless.

Summary

Validity is the degree to which a test measures that which it is intended to measure. In an attempt to clarify the concept of validity, three types of validity have been identified. These are content validity, criterion-related validity, and construct validity.

Content validity is demonstrated by showing how well the content and behavior of the test sample the universe of content and behavior. When a written test is constructed, the content and behavior universe can be presented in the form of a table of specifications. The relative importance of each aspect must be described in detail. Content validity is then assessed by examining the degree to which the test items are constructed so that all of the elements in the universe are included, with the more important elements receiving greater emphasis. If the test user objects to the universe as described, the issue is no longer one of *content validity* but rather one of *educational importance*.

Three basic assumptions underlie the use of content validity. One, the area of concern to the tester can be conceived as a meaningful, definable universe of responses. Two, a sample can be drawn from the universe in some meaningful, nonrandom fashion. Three, the sample and the sampling process can be defined with sufficient precision to enable the user to judge the adequacy with which the sample performance typifies performance of the universe of responses.

Since the measurement of content validity is not quantitative, there is no scale for determining the representativeness of a sample. Therefore, detailed descriptive evidence of content validity should be given. Factor analysis techniques, expert judgments, or behavioral objectives designed for selected content and behaviors may be used to describe the universe.

When a test of motor skill incorporates and directly measures the important components of the skill being evaluated, logical validity, which can be considered a special case of content validity, may be claimed. In testing a specific skill it is possible to define the aspects of good performance precisely, and to measure these aspects with great accuracy. Logical validity is claimed because the test is designed to measure those elements of good performance which are important components of the skill.

Criterion-related validity is demonstrated by comparing the test scores with one or more external variables that are considered to provide a direct measure of the characteristic or behavior in question. One type of criterion-related validity is predictive validity, dealing with the prediction of future behavior. The other type is concurrent validity, which involves the comparison of a given test with another test of established validity. The latter test is usually excessively time-consuming or costly to administer.

Predictive validity is the degree to which a criterion behavior is predicted from predictor scores. A person's expected future performance can be predicted from a test or a group of tests. Of primary interest is the criterion behavior, the standard against which the usefulness of the test score is judged. Predictors are tests or variables that predict such behavior.

The validity of the criterion must be judged in a logical sense. The criterion is considered the best possible measure of the behavior in question. In order to establish the validity of the criterion through statistical methods, it would have to be compared with an even better measure of criterion behavior. If the test constructor has already developed the best possible measure, references to an "even better measure" are pointless. Thus, logical validity is claimed for the criterion measure.

Four classes of criterion bias can be described. When the criterion test does not adequately measure the criterion behavior, a criterion bias exists. *Criterion deficiency* is the omission of pertinent elements from the criterion. For example, a criterion measure of playing ability in tennis might not include a measure of serving skill. Clearly, the tennis serve is an important element of the game of tennis, and therefore the criterion measure can be described as *deficient* in this respect. *Criterion contamination* introduces extraneous elements into the criterion. If, for instance, final grades in tennis are used as the criterion measure of playing ability, the grade should be based solely on the student's ability in tennis. If attendance affects the grade, an irrelevant element is introduced into the criterion measure, and becomes a contaminating element. *Criterion scale unit bias* is the inequality of scale units in the criterion. If a judge tends to use the middle scores on a scale and exclude the extreme scores, a bias is operating in favor of the middle scores and against the extremes. In this case, *criterion distortion,* which refers to improper weighting in combining criterion elements, occurs because the middle scores are weighted more heavily than the extremes.

The establishment of predictive validity generally follows a standard experimental design. Predictive measures are given to a group before any prediction is actually made. At some future point in time, criterion measures are obtained for all who took the predictive tests. Only when predictor scores are then correlated with the criterion scores can statements legitimately be made about how well the predictors predict the criterion. In order to apply cross-validation techniques, the predictor measures must be administered to two random samples from the same population. The weights (for the predictors based on the criterion) computed for one sample are tested for effectiveness on the second sample by applying them to the predictor scores of the second sample, and a multiple correlation coefficient is computed between the weighted predictors and the criterion. The resulting multiple correlation coefficient reflects the relationship between the predictors and the criterion.

Construct validity is appropriate when a test purports to measure an attribute or quality that is too complex to be measured precisely, making no available criterion fully valid, and no universe of content adequate. A construct is a hypothesized trait that is assumed to be reflected in test performance. The logic of construct validity is based on an interlocking system of laws which constitutes a theory. These laws may relate observable properties to one another, theoretical constructs to observable properties, or different theoretical constructs to one another. Learning more about the theory consists of elaborating the network in which it exists.

The process of construct validation typifies the deductive method of research. The procedure is initiated by developing a theory about a construct. The second step is to make deductions about the characteristics of individuals exhibiting different levels of the construct. In the third step, hypotheses are generated from the deduction. Experimental testing of each hypothesis constitutes the fourth step. In the final step, the results either verify or refute the hypothesis. If the hypothesis is not verified, the fault could lie with the theory, the measurement instrument, or the hypothesis.

When validity is determined statistically, the size of the validity coefficient must be examined. If the validation is concurrent, the coefficient should be relatively high in order to justify substituting one test for another. When a test is constructed for predictive purposes, a low validity may be acceptable in some cases. If the test predicts criterion behavior better than any other available measure, a low validity coefficient should not discourage the test user from using the test. However, the accuracy of prediction increases as the correlation coefficient becomes larger.

Bibliography

American Psychological Association, et al. *Standards for Educational and Psychological Tests and Manuals.* Washington, D.C.: American Psychological Association, Inc., 1966.

ANASTASI, A. "The Concept of Validity in the Interpretation of Test Scores," *Educational and Psychological Measurement,* X (1950), pp. 67–77.

ANASTASI, A. "Some Current Developments in the Measurement and Interpretation of Test Validity," in *Testing Problems in Perspective,* ed. A. Anastasi. Washington, D. C.: American Council on Education, 1966, pp. 307–17.

BECHTOLDT, H. E. "Construct Validity: A Critique," *American Psychologist,* XIV (1959), pp. 619–29.

BEREITER, C. "Some Persisting Dilemmas in the Measurement of Change," in *Problems in Measuring Change,* ed. C. W. Harris. Madison: The University of Wisconsin Press, 1963 pp. 3–20.

BOOTH, E, G. "Personality Traits As Measured by the MMPI," *Research Quarterly,* XXIX (1962), pp. 127–38.

BROGDEN, H. E. "On the Interpretation of the Correlation Coefficient as a Measure of Predictive Efficiency," *Journal of Educational Psychology,* XXXVII (1946), pp. 65–76.

BROGDEN, H. E. and E. K. TAYLOR. "The Theory and Classification of Criterion Bias," *Educational and Psychological Measurement,* X (1950), pp. 159–85.

CAMPBELL, D. T. "Recommendations for APA Test Standard Regarding Construct, Trait, or Discriminant Validity," *American Psychologist,* XV (1960), pp. 546–53.

CAMPBELL, D. T. and D. W. FISKE. "Convergent and Discriminant Validation by the Multitrait-Multimethod Matrix," *Psychological Bulletin,* LVI, (1959), pp. 81–105.

CATTELL, R.B. "Validity and Reliability: A Proposed More Basic Set of Concepts, " *Journal of Educational Psychology,* LV (1964), pp. 1–22.

COOPERATIVE TESTS and SERVICES. *AAHPER Cooperative Physical Education Tests.* Princeton, N. J.: Educational Testing Service, 1970.

CRONBACH, L. J. *Essentials of Psychological Testing.* New York: Harper and Row, Publishers, Inc., 1970.

CRONBACH, L. J. "Test Validation," in *Educational Measurement,* ed. R. L. Thorndike. Washington, D. C.: American Council on Education, 1971, pp. 443–507.

CRONBACH, L. J. and P. E. MEEHL. "Construct Validity in Psychological Tests," *Psychological Bulletin,* LII (1955), pp. 281–302.

CUMBEE, F. Z. and C. W. HARRIS. "The Composite Criterion and Its Relation to Factor Analysis," *Research Quarterly,* XXIV, No. 2 (1953), pp. 127–34.

CURETON, E. E. "Validity, Reliability and Baloney," *Educational and Psychological Measurement,* X (1950), pp. 94–96.

CURETON, E. E. "Validity," in *Educational Measurement,* ed., E. F. Lindquist. Washington, D. C.: American Council on Education, 1951, pp. 621–94.

EBEL, R. L. "Obtaining and Reporting Evidence on Content Validity," *Educational and Psychological Measurement,* XVI (1956), pp. 269–82.

EBEL, R. L. "Must All Tests Be Valid?" *American Psychologist,* XVI (1961), pp. 640–47.

EBEL, R. L. "Content Standard Test Scores," *Educational and Psychological Measurement,* XXII (1962), pp. 15–25.

FLEISHMAN, E. A. *The Structure and Measurement of Physical Fitness.* Englewood Cliffs, N. J. Prentice-Hall, Inc., 1964.

GHISELLI, E. E. "The Validation of Selection Tests in the Light of the Dynamic Character of Criteria," *Personnel Psychology,* XIII (1960), pp. 225–31.

GRONLUND, N. E. *Measurement and Evaluation in Teaching.* New York: The Macmillan Company, 1965.

GUILFORD, J. P. *Psychometric Methods.* New York: McGraw-Hill Book Company, 1956.

GUILFORD, J. P. *Fundamental Statistics in Psychology and Education.* St. Louis: McGraw-Hill Book Company, 1965.

GULLIKSEN, H. "Intrinsic Validity," *American Psychologist,* V (1950), pp. 511–17.

HEMPEL, C. G. *Philosophy of the Natural Sciences.* Englewood Cliffs, N. J.: Prentice-Hall, Inc., 1966.

HUDDLESTON, E. M. "Test Development on the Basis of Content Validity," *Educational and Psychological Measurement,* XVI, No. 3 (1956), pp. 283–93.

KROLL, W. and K. PETERSEN. "Cross-Validation of the Booth Scale," *Research Quarterly,* XXXVII, No. 1 (1966), pp. 66–70.

KROPP, R. P., H. W. STOKER and W. L. BASHAW. "The Validation of the Taxonomy of Educational Objectives, *Journal of Experimental Education,* XXXIV, No. 3 (1966), pp. 69–76.

KURUCZ, R. L., E. L. FOX and D. K. MATHEW. "Construction of Submaximal Cardiovascular Step Test," *Research Quarterly,* XL, No. 1 (1969), pp. 115–22.

LENNON, R. T. "Assumptions Underlying the Use of Content Validity," *Educational and Psychological Measurement,* XVI (1956), pp. 294–304.

LIBA, M. R. and M. STAUFF. "A Test for the Volleyball Pass," *Research Quarterly,* XXXIV, No. 1 (1963), pp. 56–63.

LYMAN, H. B. *Test Scores and What They Mean.* Englewood Cliffs, N. J.: Prentice-Hall, Inc., 1971.

MAGNUSSON, D. *Test Theory.* Palo Alto: Addison-Wesley Publishing Company, Inc., 1966.

MELTON, A. W. "Individual Differences and Theoretical Process Variables," in *Learning and Individual Differences,* ed. R. M. Gagne. Cleveland: Charles E. Merrill Publishing Co., 1966, pp. 238–52.

MERIFIELD, H. H. and G. A. WALFORD. "Battery of Ice Hockey Skill Tests," *Research Quarterly,* XL, No. 1 (1969), pp. 146–52.

MOSIER, C. I. "Problems and Design of Cross Validation," *Educational and Psychological Measurement,* XI (1951), pp. 5–11.

MOSIER, C. I. "A Critical Examination of the Concepts of Face Validity," *Educational and Psychological Measurement,* VII (1957), pp. 191–205.

PEAK, H. "Problems of Objective Observation," in *Research Methods in the Behavioral Sciences,* eds. N. Festinger and D. Katz. New York: Dryden Press, Inc., 1953, pp. 243–300.

SPIELBERGER, C. D., R. L. GORSUCH, and R. E. LUSHENE. *The State-Trait Anxiety Inventory: Test Manual for Form X.* Palo Alto, Calif.: Consulting Psychologists Press, 1969.

THORPE, J. and C. WEST. "A Test of Game Sense in Badminton," *Perceptual and Motor Skills,* XXVIII (1969), pp. 159–69.

VINCENT, M. F. "Prediction of Success in Physical Education Activities from Attitude, Strength, and Efficiency Measurements," *Research Quarterly,* XXXVIII, No. 3 (1967), pp. 502–6.

Webster's New Collegiate Dictionary. Springfield, Mass.: G. & C. Merriam Co., Publishers, 1956.

WESMAN, A. G. "Better than Chance," *Test Service Bulletin No. 45.* The Psychological Corporation, May 1953.

WEST, C. and J. THORPE. "Construction and Validation of Eight-Iron Approach Test," *Research Quarterly,* XXXIX, No. 4 (1968), pp. 1115–20.

6

reliability

One important quality to consider in the evaluation of a test is its reliability. The purpose of this chapter is to examine this concept. Although this material is intended primarily for undergraduate students of measurement, there are sections which deal in depth with certain aspects of reliability. These sections are identified as technical sections, and are appropriate for advanced undergraduate and graduate students.

Reliability theory will be emphasized as it applies to tests of motor performance, although some material on the reliability of written tests is also included. The reader should note from the outset that written test reliability theory is not always applicable to tests of motor performance. A written test consists of items that are similar but never identical to one another, whereas a test of motor performance usually includes more than one trial of the *same* measure.

Some physical education teachers may use tests of motor performance without examining their reliability, especially when the tests have been used from year to year within a school system. Yet, because the results of these tests may be used as a basis for making important decisions about students, it is important that a test yield reasonably precise, or reliable, measures of student performance. The teacher must have a basic understanding of the concept of reliability so that he can select appropriate tests.

Definition of Reliability

The reliability of a test refers to the dependability of scores, their relative freedom from errors. It is the tendency toward consistency exhibited by a given individual's repeated performance of one behavior. Stallings and Gilmore (1971) carefully distinguish precision from accuracy in defining reliability, referring to the following definitions by Eisenhart (1968): The precision of measurement is ". . . the typical closeness together of successive independent measurements of a single magnitude generated by repeated applications of the process under specified conditions . . ." (Eisenhart, 1968, p. 1201). Accuracy is "the closeness to the true value characteristic of such measurements" (Eisenhart, 1968, p. 1201). This definition of accuracy closely parallels the definition of validity. Precision, rather than accuracy, is the appropriate term to use in describing reliability.

Reliability and Validity

A test can be reliable without being valid, whereas a valid test must also be reliable. Reliability, then, refers to the consistency, not the general worthiness or the validity, of the test. For example,

> . . . some English teachers who are distressed by the unreliability of essay grades on writing ability resort to counting the number of errors per one hundred words in usage, punctuation, and spelling. This yields a much more stable reliable measure of writing ability than ratings on general merit, but it does not follow that it is a better measure of writing ability than such ratings. On the contrary, it restricts the attention of both the teacher and the student to mechanics and leaves out far more important elements of good writing such as ideas, organization, wording, and flavor (Diederich, 1967, p. 265).

In a physical education class, wall volley tests are sometimes administered as tests of volleying skill. In most cases, the test score is the number of times the ball hits the wall, with certain height and distance restrictions. Some of these tests have satisfactory reliability estimates for certain groups. However, a student might be able to perform reliably on the test, yet use poor form, executing the skill poorly and, perhaps, illegally by game rules. Reliability does not insure validity. (The concept of validity is discussed in detail in Chapter 5.)

Classifications of Reliability Coefficients

Prior to 1966, three classes of reliability coefficients were recommended by national organizations of educators, psychologists, and measurement personnel. These classes were: coefficient of equivalence, coefficient of stability, and coefficient of internal consistency (APA, 1954). The *coefficient of equivalence* was an estimate of reliability based on the comparison of two equivalent forms of a written test given on the same day. The *coefficient of stability,* or test-retest reliability, involved the repetition of the same test after a specified interval of time, usually in tests of motor behavior. The *coefficient of internal consistency* was obtained by subdividing the total number of items or trials making up a single test and comparing the two subdivisions.

In the 1966 *Standards* (APA), the classification of coefficients into these three categories was no longer recommended.

> Such a terminological system breaks down as more adequate statistical analyses are applied and methods are more adequately described. Hence, it is recommended that test authors work out suitable phrases to convey the meaning of whatever coefficients they report; as an example, the expression, "the stability of measurements by different test forms as determined over a seven-day period" although lengthy, will be reasonably free from ambiguity (APA, 1966, pp. 26–27).

Sources of Variability

When a test is given, factors contributing to the variability of a performer's test score can prevent the test from being a reliable, or precise, measure of an attribute. For instance, if a student ran three trials of the 50-yard dash, his scores would probably not be identical but would vary somewhat from trial to trial. This variation in performance might arise from one or more sources, such as the psychological factor of motivation, or the physiological factor of fatigue. Inaccuracies in timing the dash might provide another source of variability.

Two general categories of variability can be described: systematic variation and error variation. *Systematic variation* is variation in behavior that is biological in nature. Henry (1959) refers to it as intraindividual variability. In general, an individual is unable to execute a motor skill with absolute precision from trial to trial or from day to day. This inconsistency in performance is not due to error in the measurement process, but rather to man's behavioral state. Factors such as level of skill and physical fitness are two examples of systematic variance. *Error variability* is variation due to measurement error, including equipment, scorer, and administrator variability. Both systematic variance and error variance affect the reliability of an individual's performance.

When a student takes a test of motor performance, his score should reflect only his ability in the attribute being measured. The score should not be confounded by the influence of a test administrator who is not consistent in the directions he gives to the students, nor should the score lack precision due to inaccuracies in scoring. Even the choice of the number of trials or days on which the test will be given may unfairly sample the student's performance, and thus affect the precision of the score. The ability to identify sources of variability is essential to an adequate understanding of reliability theory because it is useful in the estimation of reliability. With it, the test constructor is able to plan a measurement situation that can, where possible, provide an estimate of the magnitude of each source of variability relative to the total (observed) variability. The variance estimates are then used to determine ratios that express estimated reliabilities of interest to the test constructor. At the same time, the investigator is equipped with evidence that he can use to improve the test and possibly reduce the variance from undesired sources. The determination of reliability, then, is as much a *logical* as a *statistical* problem.

Several sources of variability are described in the APA *Standards:*

> . . . (1) response variation by the subject (due to changes in physiological efficiency) or in such psychological factors as motivation, effort, or mood, (2) variations in test content or test situation, (3) variations in administration, either through variations in physical factors, such as temperature, noise, or apparatus functioning, or in psychological factors, such as variation in the technique or skill of different test administrators or raters, and (4) variations in the process of observations. In addition to these errors of observation, scoring error variance in test scores reflects variations in the process of scoring responses as well as mistakes in recording, transferring, or reading of scores (APA, p. 26).

The most informative approach to the estimation of reliability is to obtain statistical estimates of clearly labeled components of variance. The way in which the test constructor chooses to estimate reliability is determined by the sources of variability he takes into account. An analysis is possible because the variance of a set of test scores can be broken down into separate parts which combine to give the total variance.

Response Variation by the Subject

Response variation by the subject can occur from trial to trial or from day to day. It is systematic, and can be attributed to numerous potential sources. Lasting and general sources of variability are factors that tend to affect an individual's performance *in the same way* on any type of test no matter when it is taken. Examples of this are general health status, physical fitness, and general attitude toward taking tests. Lasting and specific sources of variability refer to factors that are peculiar to a specific type of test, and that affect performance in the same way whenever that type of test is given. These factors include motivation, attitude toward a particular type of motor performance test, and the level of skill in the attribute being tested.

Temporary and general sources are factors that affect the individual in any testing situation at a given time. Such factors might be acute health status, amount of warm-up preceding testing, hot or cold days, fatigue, and environment. Temporary and specific sources of variability are similar to the temporary and general sources, but are specific to a particular type of test. For example, fatigue might affect the students' performance on a motor skill, but not on a written test. A student may be "hot" on a motor skill test and "cold" on a written test.

Between-days source of variability. If a physical education teacher is interested in assessing achievement on a skill at the end of a unit, he would like to obtain a test score that reflects a student's skill level with precision. The teacher's assessment would be inaccurate if some students obtained high scores on one day and low on another, and vice versa. In this case, a teacher may seek a test for which reliability has been estimated over two or more days. This type of reliability is commonly referred to as test-retest reliability.

If the variability of performance from day to day is sizeable, and the test is given only on one day, the resulting reliability coefficient is likely to be an overestimate, reflecting the individual's fluctuations only within one day. On the other hand, if reliability is estimated for scores collected on two or more days, the precision of the test at a given period of time would be underestimated, but the stability of performance would be precisely estimated. If a test is given twice with the intent of establishing a reliability estimate, and learning takes place between testing sessions, the reliability coefficient will not be a precise estimate. For accurate reliability estimation, the assumption is that no change has taken place in the individual during the time interval between testing sessions.

In the West and Thorpe (1968) eight-iron golf test, reliability was estimated for different combinations of days and trials. Upon examining the reliability coefficients in Table 6–1, the size of a coefficient for testing on one day as opposed to one for testing on two days can be compared. Testing over two days yielded a more reliable estimate regardless of the number of trials administered. This finding was substantiated in another study by West (1969). In tests of motor skills, testing on two days often reflects a more precise representation of the individual's actual performance level than testing on one day.

The type of attribute being measured determines, in part, the way in which reliability coefficients are determined. In tests of physical performance, repeated trials of a skill test are often given. Since the skills are motor skills, it is possible to repeat the same set of measures on another day in order to estimate the consistency of performance over testing sessions. This procedure cannot be used with written tests because a student may remember questions from the first testing session if the same test is given again. Therefore, equivalent tests must be constructed when aspects of mental achievement are being assessed.

TABLE 6–1 • Reliability Estimates Computed by Analysis of Variance for the West and Thorpe Golf Test*

Days	Trials	Reliability Estimates
1	20	.65
1	30	.69
2	12	.75
2	15	.77
2	20	.79
3	10	.80
3	12	.82
3	20	.85
4	12	.86
4	20	.88

*Reprinted from Table 1 of C. West and J. Thorpe, "Construction and Validation of an Eight-Iron Approach Test," *Research Quarterly*, XXXIX, (1968), 1115–1120, published by the American Association for Health, Physical Education, and Recreation, Washington, D.C., by permission of the authors and publisher.

Within-day source of variability. When a test consists of repeated trials, fluctuations from trial to trial may occur. If there is a systematic increase or decrease in performance from trial to trial, a factor is represented which is unrelated to reliability. It is best to have a testing situation in which the fluctuations from trial to trial are random. Two classifications of variability can be described for trial-to-trial score variation. In one case, the variability is due to random fluctuations, and may be described as error. In the second case, the scores increase or decrease from trial to trial. This variability is systematic, and should not be taken into account when estimating reliability.

Possible sources of variability due to random fluctuations from trial to trial are temporary distractions, fluctuations in level of motivation, and natural behavioral variations. They should be taken into account when estimating the reliability of the test. When there is a systematic score increase or decrease from trial to trial, the sources of variability might be the effect of learning, fatigue, boredom, increased familiarity with equipment, or increased or decreased motivation.

A brief discussion of *intraindividual variability* is appropriate at this point since this type of variability is comparable to that being discussed in this section. Intraindividual variability is defined as the variation of an individual's scores around his own mean score (Henry, 1970). Henry (1959) has noted that

$$\text{reliability} = \frac{\text{true score variance}}{\text{obtained score variance}} \qquad \textbf{(Formula 6–1)}$$

or

$$\text{reliability} = \frac{\text{obtained variance} - \text{error variance}}{\text{obtained variance}} \qquad \textbf{(Formula 6–2)}$$

An equivalent statement is

(Formula 6–3)

$$\text{reliability} = \frac{\text{interindividual variance} - \text{intraindividual variance} - \text{measurement error}}{\text{interindividual variance}}$$

where intraindividual and measurement error variance make up the "within" source in an analysis of variance table.

Even though intraindividual variability does contribute to the unreliability of a measure, Henry and others (Fiske and Rice, 1955; Lersten, 1968) do not consider this as error. In this sense, the only existing error is measurement error obtained in conjunction with the process of measuring the trait in question. Intraindividual variability, then, is variation in behavior that is biological in nature. Henry (1959) has shown that measurement error accounts for only a small proportion of the unreliability. For example, he reported a reliability coefficient of 0.962 which took both measurement error and intraindividual variability into account. In computing the reliability coefficient without accounting for measurement error, the coefficient obtained was 0.964, indicating that measurement error only decreased the reliability coefficient by 0.002.

The nature of intraindividual variability has been shown to differ between individuals and to be task specific (Marteniuk, 1969). Lersten (1968) found that intraindividual differences increase in the early stages of learning, although by a smaller magnitude and with less consistency than *inter*individual differences (between individuals). In later stages of practice, no meaningful increases were observed. For a complete review of this topic, see articles by Fiske and Rice (1955), Henry (1970), and Schmidt (1970) listed in the bibliography.

Administrator Source of Variability

Whether or not administrator variability is an important source of variance depends on the nature of the test. If the test administrator merely hands out a paper and pencil test, then collects the test when the students are finished, administrator variability will be practically nonexistent. If the test administrator must give directions or must time the various parts of the test, a greater possibility for variability exists. In tests of motor skills where the administrator must be certain that the students perform the test properly, there is an even greater chance that it will affect the test scores.

Administrator variability should be differentiated from scorer variability. The latter is a result of variability due to inconsistencies in making judgments about the scores of a test. The former refers to the use of inaccurate or inadequate test directions or to the failure to see that the test is executed properly and is difficult to isolate. Possibly administrator variability could be examined by randomly drawing two subgroups from a homogeneous group and assigning a different administrator to each one.

Scorer Source of Variability

The agreement among scorers, raters, or judges is often referred to as the objectivity of the test. However, since a test must be objective to be reliable, objectivity can be included as a source of variability in discussing reliability.

Objective tests are so named because there is little error in scoring these tests. Many individuals could grade the test and obtain the same score. Variability among scorers increases if the scorer is required to make judgments that are more subjective, as in rating playing ability in a sport or using projective techniques in certain psychological tests.

Two types of scorer variability can be identified. One type is *intrajudge error,* which is the amount of variability that occurs when one scorer rates the same test performance two or more times. If the test in question is a written test, intrajudge error can be readily determined. For example, a teacher might grade a set of essay tests once and, at a later date, grade the same set again. Comparison of the two sets of scores would yield an estimate of intrajudge objectivity. In tests of motor skills, estimates of intrajudge objectivity are difficult to obtain because the same performance must be seen twice. By recording the motor performance on film or video tape, it is possible to estimate the magnitude of this type of variability.

The second type of scorer variability is *interjudge variability*, which is the variability existing between two or more independent judgments of the same performance. It is commonly taken into account in gymnastics, diving, and figure skating, where several judges rate each performance. The extent to which the judges agree can be referred to as the interjudge objectivity coefficient. This type of scorer variability may be often computed separately from the remaining sources of variability since the test scores are not meaningful if reasonable agreement among judges cannnot be attained. However, if the sources of variability are examined through interclass correlational methods, each source *must* be examined separately. (There are other disadvantages to using the interclass correlation method for estimating reliability. These disadvantages will be discussed in a later section.) When analysis of variance techniques are used, the scorer variability can be taken into account when estimating the overall reliability of the test. In cases where the variable being judged does not lend itself to direct physical measurement (for example, when assigning grades of A, B, C, D, F), a special analysis of variance model has been developed to determine the degree of accord among observers (Lu, 1971).

Equipment Source of Variability

Variability due to equipment is pure measurement error. Measurement error can occur with such physical education equipment as stopwatches, chronoscopes, cable tensiometers, polygraphs, and gas analyzers. Timing equipment should be calibrated at regular time intervals and other equipment should receive regular maintenance.

Expression of the Reliability of a Test

When two or more sources of variability may be identified for a given test, no one reliability estimate is adequate. That is, if more than one source of variability exists, more than one reliability estimate may be useful. In a study by West (1969), five sources of variability were identified, and the score variance attributable to each source was examined. The five sources of variability were within-day, between-day, timers, readers, and scorers. Examination of the within-day source of variability was possible because more than one trial was administered. Since the test was given over two days, the between-days source could also be studied. Timer source of variability represented the precision with which two or more individuals could time the flight of a ball. Reader source of variability reflected the agreement among individuals who estimated distances on targets. The precision with which individuals observed landing points on targets was referred to as scorer variability.

Given these five sources of variability, it is possible to discuss the significance of each one. West (1969), for example, found a sizeable score variance attributable to between-days source of variability. On this basis, West recommended that the selected projectile skills studied be administered on more than one day. In one test, the timer source of variability provided interesting information. The timers observed the same differences among performers, but the mean scores between timers differed significantly. Either one timer was overestimating the time score, or the other timer underestimated the score. On this basis, West recommended using one timer when the investigator is interested in the *relative* differences among the individuals, although the scores will not necessarily be *accurate*. (Accuracy refers to the closeness of an individual's obtained score value to his true score value.) In essence, there is no single all-encompassing reliability estimate for a test. A reliability estimate describes the influence of a certain source of variability in the test, and is relevant to a specific group of individuals at a specified level of ability.

Statistical Procedures for Estimating the Reliability of Tests of Motor Performance

There are many statistical techniques for estimating test reliability, such as the Pearson product-moment correlation, the Spearman-Brown prophecy formula, the standard error of measurement, and analysis of variance. Because of the nature of tests of motor performance, that is, two or more trials of the same test are given, analysis of variance procedures are appropriate for estimating the reliability of this type of test. The standard error of measurement also provides useful information as an absolute estimate of precision. The Pearson product-moment correlation, although widely applied to tests of motor performance, is not really the most appropriate procedure to use for tests of this type. Correlational techniques that have been used for estimating the reliability of written tests are described in a later section.

Analysis of Variance

The most familiar symbol for the reliability coefficient is r, representing the Pearson product-moment correlation coefficient which is an *interclass* correlation coefficient. When analysis of variance is used to estimate reliability, the appropriate symbol for the reliability coefficient is R, representing the *intraclass* correlation coefficient. The coefficient R represents a ratio of variance estimates that have been obtained through analysis of variance procedures through which it is possible to determine the amount of variance attributable to all measurable sources of variability. Kroll (1962, 1967) and Feldt and McKee (1958) have noted the advantages of the intraclass over the interclass correlation coefficient. The product-moment correlation coefficient does not differentiate from among several possible sources of variability which may be involved in the measurement. By using analysis of variance procedures, however, it is possible to identify specific components of score variation and obtain separate estimates of the relative magnitude of each one.

For example, if a test consists of three trials given on each of two days, computation of the Pearson product-moment coefficient of interclass correlation would necessitate taking the average of three trials for each day and correlate the Day 1 average score with the Day 2 average score. However, any changes in student performance from trial to trial are then ignored.

In addition, if the changes that occur from trial to trial are systematic, this information is important to the test constructor. Several researchers in physical education (Baumgartner, 1969[a]and[b]; Kroll, 1967; Liba, 1962) discuss the importance of information on trial-to-trial variability for tests of motor performance.

The coefficients R and r, if obtained from two sets of scores which have equal means and variances, can have the same numerical value. This does not mean that the two statistics are logically identical or will yield the same numerical estimate in the majority of instances. If the coefficients R and r are not numerically equivalent, R is expected to be more accurate than r, and is never expected to be less accurate (Kroll, 1962). As noted previously, reliability estimates for tests of motor performance are generally based on several trials of the test. Therefore, more than two sets of scores must be taken into account. Although all possible intertrial correlations (r's) could be averaged to obtain a reliability coefficient, use of analysis of variance is more appropriate because a systematic increase or decrease from trial to trial is identified as variability. If the interclass correlation coefficient is used to estimate reliability, systematic increases or decreases from one set of scores to another are treated as reliability, when in reality systematic increases probably reflect the effects of practice or learning while systematic decreases probably reflect the effects of boredom or fatigue.

Technical Aspects of the Intraclass Correlation Coefficient

In 1901, Pearson described the computation of a product-moment correlation coefficient from a symmetrical correlation table when two interchangeable scores are to be correlated (Haggard, 1958). However, the number of entries in a symmetrical table rises very rapidly as class membership increases. Harris (1913) developed a technique which estimated the intraclass correlation coefficient, or R, as a ratio of the variances of the class means to the total variance of all scores in the table. The coefficient R, as well as r, was biased in a negative direction, and a correction factor was needed. This bias was pointed out by Fisher (1959), who developed the concept of achieving an unbiased estimate of the intraclass correlation coefficient through the use of the mean squares in an analysis of variance table.

The coefficient R is a univariate statistic. It is the measure of the relative homogeneity of the scores within the classes in relation to the total variation among all of the scores in the table. Thus, maximal positive correlation exists when all intraclass scores are identical and the scores differ only from class to class. As the relative heterogeneity of the intraclass scores increases, the computed value of R will decrease. Maximal negative correlation exists when the heterogeneity of the intraclass scores is maximal and all the class means are the same (Haggard, 1958).

Test for Trend

Trend is the "fluctuation of the sample mean from trial to trial that is too large to be attributed to the error of measurement" (Alexander, 1947, p. 81). Pictorially, trial means that do not vary markedly from one another represent no trend, as shown in Figure 6–1. Trial means that steadily increase or decrease suggest a linear trend. Those that gradually increase and then gradually decrease (with essentially one bend) suggest a quadratic curve and, depending upon the slope, may represent linear trend as well. Examples of these aspects of curvilinearity are given in Figure 6–1.

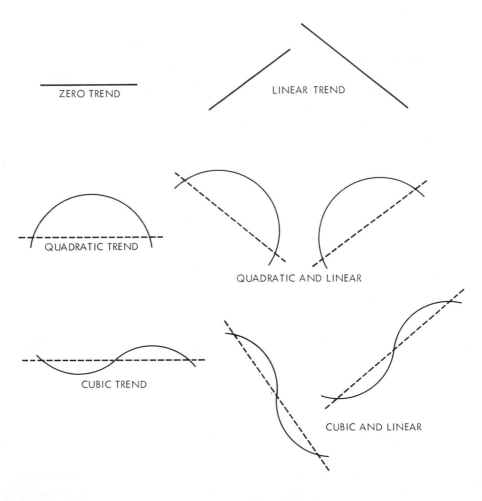

FIG. 6–1   Examples of Trends

The estimation of an intraclass correlation coefficient is obtained through simple analysis of variance procedures. The presence of a trend violates one of the assumptions underlying these procedures, that of randomness of scores. The choice of a suitable measure of reliability is dependent upon the presence or absence of trend. For example, a two-dimensional analysis of variance model is appropriate for estimating the reliability of a test with two identifiable sources of variability if the assumption of random variation for a series of trials is tenable. (Use of this model for tests of motor performance has been described by Feldt and McKee, 1958.) When there is evidence of systematic variation from trial to trial, an adjustment of the model would be necessary.

Although one does not expect the mean scores for a group of trials to be identical, the fluctuations from one mean to another are expected to be random. In other words, some trial score means will be higher than the mean scores for all trials, and some will be lower, but none will differ significantly from other trial scores. If, in fact, some trials do differ significantly from others, a trend analysis should be applied to the data. A selection of test scores can be made that eliminates the trend effect, and the standard intraclass correlation formula can be used to obtain a reliability estimate. Under certain circumstances, the investigator may wish to retain trials causing the trend effect, and use an intraclass correlation formula that is adjusted for trend.

Technical Aspects of Test for Trend

A formula described by Alexander (1949) tests whether the trial means are significantly different. The formula is

$$F_t = \frac{V_t}{V_{it}} \qquad \text{(Formula 6–4)}$$

where V_t = variance between trials

           V_{it} = interaction between individuals and trials.

In the case of two trials, a t test could be used as a test of trend, although Alexander suggests that more information can be obtained from an analysis of variance. If a test consists of more than two trials, the investigator must go beyond both the t test and the F test, and use tests for higher order polynomial trends. Since the Alexander formula is only a test for linear trend, tests for higher order polynomial trends must be made using other procedures, such as those developed by Grant (1956).

Trend tests have not been widely used in the estimation of reliability for motor performance tests. Liba (1962) applied tests of overall and relevant components of trend to bowling and softball velocity data. (The number of "relevant" components of trend is determined by the number of trials for the test. If two trials are used, the only possible trend is a linear one. With three trials, the trend may either be quadratic, a combination of linear and quadratic, or linear. With four trials, a cubic polynomial is possible, and so on.) When the velocity trial means were plotted, the bowling data gave the appearance of linearity, and the softball data gave the appearance of curvilinearity. The overall trend was not significant. The test for relevant components of trend showed that the bowling data represented a linear trend. No other polynomial was significant. Because of the presence of a linear trend, the standard two-dimensional analysis of variance model was not appropriate for estimating the reliability of the bowling velocity data.

Formula for Intraclass Correlation Coefficient

If the F value obtained in the trend test is not significant, and the variance between trials $(s_t{}^2)$ is zero, the variance assoicated with trials and the variance associated with individuals and trials should be replaced by a pooled estimate known as the within-individuals mean square, as shown in Formula 6–5. The *sums of squares* of both V_t and V_{it} are used in Formula 6–5 rather than the mean squares.

$$V_{wi} = \frac{V_t + V_{it}}{df_t + d_{it}}$$ (Formula 6–5)

where df_t = degrees of freedom for trials
df_{it} = degrees of freedom for interaction
between individuals and trials
V_{wi} = variance within individuals.

The pooled estimate, V_{wi}, obtained in Formula 6–5 is then used in Formula 6–6 which yields an estimate of reliability that is appropriate when no trend is present.

$$R = \frac{V_i - V_{wi}}{V_i + (\frac{k}{k'} - 1) V_{wi}}$$ (Formula 6–6)

where k = number of trials administered
k' = number of trials for which estimated reliability coefficient
is determined.

The *mean squares* of V_i and V_{wi} are used in Formula 6–6. This is the intraclass correlation proposed by Fisher, using the symmetrical table estimate. The presence of trend would lower the value of R.

If the test for trend *is* significant, the investigator may proceed in one of two possible directions. One choice would be to use an intraclass correlation formula adjusted for trend (Alexander, 1946). This is done in Formula 6–7, where the variation apart from trials is considered. In other words, the trials source of variability is omitted from the computation of the reliability estimate as described in Formual 6–7.

$$R = \frac{V_i - V_{it}}{V_i + (\frac{k}{k'} - 1) V_{it}}$$ **(Formula 6–7)**

Here again, the mean squares of the variance estimates are used in the formula. The coefficient R is an estimate of the value that would have been obtained if the trial fluctuations had been avoided, that is, if no trend existed. The coefficient R provides a fair estimate of the reliability coefficient, and is independent of the presence of trend.

The other choice would be to use a measure that is free of systematic trend. If achievement is being measured at the end of a unit in physical education, the teacher would like to use a test that does *not* reflect systematic variation such as learning or practice. The researcher, while expecting normal human variation, would like to avoid systematic increases or decreases in performance. If Formula 6 7 is used, we do not solve the problem of how, if at all, it is possible to avoid obtaining the trend over trials the next time the test is administered. Kroll (1967) has suggested that, rather than computing the reliability estimate by Formula 6–7, the trials affected by trend be omitted, and a reliability estimate using Formula 6 6 be computed for the remaining trials. If the reliability estimate is satisfactory under these conditions, the trials not affected by trend may be used as the criterion score. If reducing the number of trials yields an unsatisfactory reliability coefficient, the investigator must attempt to find another measure that is free of the trend effect and yet yields a satisfactory reliability coefficient.

Baumgartner and Jackson (1970) have studied the effect of trend on numerous measures of motor performance. They found that the trend effect can operate differently for the same test administered to different age groups. For example, a trend effect occurred on the *first* three of six trials of the standing broad jump when senior high school boys were measured. For junior high school boys, the trend effect occurred during the *last* three of six trials of the jump. These results indicate that six trials of the standing broad jump should be administered to senior high school boys, but only the last three trials should be utilized. Conversely, only three trials of the jump are necessary for junior high school boys, and all three of these trials should be used. Knowledge of trend effects, then, provides useful information for physical education teachers.

To summarize, the first step in the estimation of reliability for repeated measures is to test for trend. If no trend of any kind is present, then Formula 6–6 should be used. If a trend is present, the investigator may drop the trials which appear to show the trend effect, and compute the reliability coefficient again on the remaining trials. As an alternative the investigator can compute the reliability estimate using Formula 6–7, in which the trials source of variance is removed.

Example of a Simple Case of Analysis of Variance with No Trend

The simple case of the analysis of variance for the estimation of reliability has been described in the preceding sections. Formulas 6–6 and 6–7 are appropriate when only one undesirable * source of variability can be measured. (Variability among individuals is usually expected, and thus would not be considered an "undesirable" source of variability.) Any source of variability could be handled in these formulas in place of the trial-to-trial source of variability that occurs in this example.

In this section, a computational example of the simple case will be presented. The data include two trials for each of five individuals, and are artificially produced for purposes of simplicity. The raw scores and several of the basic computations are presented in Table 6–2.

TABLE 6–2 • Data for Reliability Estimation Using Analysis of Variance Procedures

Individuals	Trial 1	Trial 2	$T_r.$*	$T_r.^2$
1	10	6	16	256
2	8	9	17	289
3	7	5	12	144
4	4	7	11	121
5	2	3	5	25
$T._c$**	31	30	61	835
$T._c^2$	991	900	= 1891	

*$T_r.$ = sum of rows
**$T._c$ = sum of columns

*The question of an *undesirable* source of variability requires further clarification. In the simple case of the analysis of variance, three sources of variability may be identified. These sources are individuals, trials (following our example), and individuals by trials. The individuals source of variability is expected (and desirable) and the interaction variance serves as the error term. If an investigator wishes to obtain very precise measures, he may

The computation of variance components follows:

$$V_i = \frac{\sum T_r.^2}{k} - \frac{(T_r.)^2}{nk}$$

where n = individuals (5)
k = trials (2)

$$= \frac{835}{2} - \frac{(61)^2}{10} = 45.4$$

$$V_t = \frac{\sum T_c.^2}{n} - \frac{(T_r.)^2}{nk}$$

$$= \frac{1891}{5} - \frac{(61)^2}{10} = 6.1$$

$$V_{total} = \sum\sum X_{rc}^2 - \frac{(T_r.)^2}{nk}$$

where $\sum\sum X_{rc}^2 = (10^2 + 8^2 + \ldots + 7^2 + 3^2)$
$$= 433 - 372.1 = 60.9$$
$$V_{it} = \text{Total} - (V_i + V_t)$$
$$= 60.9 - (6.1 + 45.4) = 9.4$$

A summary of the sums of squares, the degrees of freedom, and the mean squares for the three variance components is given in Table 6–3.

TABLE 6–3 · Analysis of Variance Summary Table

Sources of Variance	Sums of Squares	Degrees of Freedom	Mean Square
V_i	45.4	4	11.35
V_t	6.1	1	6.10
V_{it}	9.4	4	2.35
Total	60.9	9	

The first step in the estimation of reliability is to test for trend using Formula 6–4.

$$F = \frac{V_t}{V_{it}} = \frac{6.10}{2.35} = 2.59$$

consider "trials" variability as undesirable. This variability is measurable, and can, to some extent, be controlled by the investigator. The investigator may strive to reduce measurement error in an attempt to reduce trial-to-trial variability, but may consider individual fluctuations from trial to trial as normal biological variations. Thus, different investigators might have different views of *undesirable* variability.

According to the table of F values, an F value of 7.71 is necessary to reflect a significant difference between the two trials at the 0.05 level. A table of F values can be found in the appendix of this text. The value of 7.71 is determined using the degrees of freedom for the greater mean square and the lesser mean square. In this case, the greater mean square is associated with the trials source of variability, and the degrees of freedom are $k-1$, where k equals the number of trials. The lesser mean square is the interaction source of variance or V_{it}, and the degrees of freedom are determined by multiplying the V_i degrees of freedom times the V_t degrees of freedom. (See Table 6–3.) Since the F value of 2.59 is not significant, the difference between the two trials is not systematic.

Since there is no evidence of trend, the interaction and trial sources of variance may be combined using Formula 6–5.

$$V_{wi} = \frac{V_t \text{ sum of squares} + V_{it} \text{ sum of squares}}{df \text{ for } V_t + df \text{ for } V_{it}} = \frac{6.1 + 9.4}{1 + 4} = 3.1$$

Note that the *mean square* variances are used in the trend test, while the *sum of squares* values are used in obtaining the within-individuals variance estimate. In the latter case, the variance estimates must be added, and only the sum of squares values are additive. The fact that these components are additive is, of course, one of the advantages of using the analysis of variance technique to estimate reliability.

The reliability coefficient can now be determined using the within-individuals variance as the estimate of error, and Formula 6–6.

$$R = \frac{V_i - V_{wi}}{V_i + (\frac{k}{k'} - 1) V_{wi}}$$

$$= \frac{11.35 - 3.1}{11.35 + (\frac{2}{2} - 1) 3.1} = 0.727 \text{ (mean of 2 trials)}$$

This estimate reflects the reliability of the test as given, which consisted of two trials. The test user may wish to know the degree to which the reliability coefficient will be altered if the number of trials is changed. Any number of trials may be inserted for k'. For example, if one wishes to estimate the reliability for one trial, k' would equal 1.

$$R = \frac{11.35 - 3.1}{11.35 + (\frac{2}{1} - 1) 3.1} = 0.571 \text{ (1 trial)}$$

Or, if the estimate for four trials is desired, $k' = 4$.

$$R = \frac{11.35 - 3.1}{11.35 + (\frac{2}{4} - 1)\, 3.1} = 0.764 \text{ (mean of 4 trials)}$$

In a test consisting of only two trials that are not affected by trend, the Pearson product-moment correlation method yields similar results for one and two trials, as shown in Table 6–4. Note that the interclass correlation coefficient for four trials is inflated compared to the intraclass correlation coefficient. The tendency for the Spearman-Brown formula to yield spuriously high estimates has been noted for several tests of motor performance (Baumgartner, 1968).

TABLE 6–4 • **Comparison of Intraclass (R) and Interclass (r) Correlation Coefficients in Simple Case of Two Trials**

Number of Trials	r	R
1	0.569	0.571
2	0.725*	0.727
4	0.841*	0.764

*Estimated using Spearman-Brown prophecy formula.

When more than two trials are used, the analysis of variance technique has computational advantages over the product-moment correlation coefficient, even though the average of all possible product-moment intercorrelations will yield similar results to the intraclass method. When two sources of undesirable variability can be isolated, such as individuals, trials and scorers, a two-dimensional analysis of variance model must be used (Lindquist, 1958; Feldt and McKee, 1958). When more than two sources of undesirable variability can be measured, multivariate analysis of variance (extension of the Lindquist model) is used.

Standard Error of Measurement

The standard error of measurement (SE_m) is an absolute measure of precision. The estimate of the standard error is presented in the actual score units of the data. The intraclass correlation coefficient, on the other hand, is a relative measure of precision because it describes the consistency with which an individual maintains his position in the total group when the measurement procedure is repeated. One advantage of the standard error of measurement over the correlation coefficient is that it is independent of the exact spread of scores.

If it were possible to administer a test repeatedly to an individual, the standard deviation for the distribution of test scores would be the standard error of measurement for that individual. Since it is not practical (or often reasonable) to administer a test repeatedly, the standard error can be estimated from the scores of a group by using Formula 6–8.

$$SE_m = s\sqrt{1 - r} \qquad\qquad \text{(Formula 6–8)}$$

When the standard error of measurement is estimated using Formula 6–8, it represents the average value of each individual's standard deviation around his own mean. The standard error can also be computed by taking the square root of the error variance term obtained in an analysis of variance. For example, the standard error of measurement in the computational example presented in Table 6–2 (using Formula 6–5 to compute the within-individuals error variance) is

$$SE_m = \sqrt{3.1} = 1.76$$

We must keep in mind that an individual's true score, the score that would be obtained if the measure were absolutely precise, is not known. If we knew the true score and the standard error of measurement, we would know that 68 percent of the scores of the individual (if he took the test repeatedly) would fall within one standard error of measurement above or below his true score. For example, if an individual's true score on the shuttle run was 11.2 seconds and the standard error was 1.4, 68 percent of his scores would fall between one standard error above the true score and one standard error below the true score, or between 9.8 and 12.6 seconds. If we considered the variability encompassed by two standard errors of measurement above and below the score, this area would include 95 percent of the obtained scores, while over 99 percent would be contained within three standard errors of measurement.

Since the true score is unknown, it can only be said with reasonable certainty that 1 SE_m above and below the obtained score will span the true score 68 percent of the time, but it cannot be said with any certainty that the true score will fall within these limits 68 percent of the time. The latter statement implies that the true score is variable. On the contrary, the theoretical true score is fixed, whereas the limits set by the standard error of measurement are variable (Doppelt, 1968; Gronlund, 1965).

In general, the smaller the SE_m the more reliable the test. This is not true automatically, since the standard error of measurement is related to the magnitude of the standard deviation of the test. A test with a standard deviation of 16 may have the same reliability as a test with a standard deviation of 8. However, the standard error of measurement of the first test will be numerically twice that of the second. See Table 6–5 for other examples of this relationship. Lord (1959) in his study of standardized written tests, demonstrated that tests of the same length have the same standard error of measurement. As the test length increases, the standard error of measurement increases, unless the test is unusually easy or excessively difficult.

TABLE 6–5 • Standard Error of Measurement for Given Values of
Reliability Coefficient and Standard Deviation*

SD	Reliability Coefficient					
	0.95	0.90	0.85	0.80	0.75	0.70
30	6.7	9.5	11.6	13.4	15.0	16.4
28	6.3	8.9	10.8	12.5	14.0	15.3
26	5.8	8.2	10.1	11.6	13.0	14.2
24	5.4	7.6	9.3	10.7	12.0	13.1
22	4.9	7.0	8.5	9.8	11.0	12.0
20	4.5	6.3	7.7	8.9	10.0	11.0
18	4.0	5.7	7.0	8.0	9.0	9.9
16	3.6	5.1	6.2	7.2	8.0	8.8
14	3.1	4.4	5.4	6.3	7.0	7.7
12	2.7	3.8	4.6	5.4	6.0	6.6
10	2.2	3.2	3.9	4.5	5.0	5.5
8	1.8	2.5	3.1	3.6	4.0	4.4
6	1.3	1.9	2.3	2.7	3.0	3.3
4	0.9	1.3	1.5	1.8	2.0	2.2
2	0.4	0.6	0.8	0.9	1.0	1.1

*Reprinted from J.E. Doppelt, "How Accurate is a Test Score?," *Test Service Bulletin No. 50* (1956), published by the Psychological Corporation, New York, and by permission of the author and publisher.

To summarize: The smaller the standard error of measurement for a given test, the more reliable the test. When comparing two different tests, the standard error should be evaluated with the magnitude of the standard deviation in mind. For information on different methods of computing the standard error of measurement, see the article by Horn (1971) listed in the bibliography.

Statistical Procedures for Estimating
the Reliability of Written Tests

Four statistical techniques for estimating the reliability of written tests are described in this section. These techniques are the Pearson product-moment correlation, split-half methods, Spearman-Brown prophecy formula, and analysis of variance. Each has been used extensively in estimating the reliability of written tests.

Pearson Product-Moment Correlation

The Pearson product-moment coefficient of interclass correlation compares the relative positions of a group of individuals on two sets of scores. Although analysis of variance techniques are available to estimate the reliability of equivalent forms of written tests, interclass correlation methods have been and are frequently used to estimate reliabilities for such tests. It should be emphasized that interclass correlation techniques are *not* recommended for the estimation of the reliability of motor performance measures.

The product-moment correlation coefficient is a bivariate coefficient of interclass correlation. It can be used when the score units of two tests differ. This coefficient estimates the degree of relationship between pairs of scores on two different variables for the same individuals. However, the correlation between two trials of the *same* test for the same individuals can also be obtained using the product-moment method. Because this type of computation is possible, the Pearson product-moment coefficient has often been incorrectly used to estimate the reliability of tests involving repeated measures, including tests of motor performance.

In order to compute the correlation coefficient for two tests, the scores on each test are converted from raw scores into z scores. This step is essential when the score units of two tests differ. However, when there are two sets of scores for the *same* test, the conversion of raw scores to z scores will mask any systematic increases or decreases from one set of scores to another. Table 6–6 gives an example of a systematic increase in scores from one day to another.

Note that systematic shifts from one trial to another occur in Table 6–6, and that there is a marked difference in the means of the two sets of scores. However, the correlation between the two sets of scores is +1.00, a perfect correlation. Yet the two scores for any given individual do not reflect consistency of performance. Why then does the correlation coefficient indicate a perfect positive relationship? The reason is that the computation of a correlation coefficient involves transforming the raw scores to z scores. When this type of transformation is applied to the data in Table 6–6, the

TABLE 6–6 · Systematic Increase in Scores from Day 1 to Day 11

Student	Test I, Day I	Test I, Day II
A	2	20
B	4	40
C	6	60
D	8	80
E	10	100
	30	300
	$\bar{X} = 6$	$\bar{X} = 60$
	$s = 3.16$	$s = 31.62$

mean of each set of data is converted to a z score of zero and the standard deviation is converted to a z score of one. The two scores for each individual, after transformation, become identical z scores. Thus, the correlation between the two sets of scores is clearly $+1.00$. The correlation coefficient is sensitive to changes in the order of scores, but not to consistent increases or decreases from one set of scores to another. Therefore, the use of the interclass correlation coefficient to estimate the reliability of repeated measures may yield an inaccurate estimate.

To summarize: The interclass correlation coefficient reflects the relative position of paired scores in each of the two z score distributions. This coefficient, then, is independent of any possible differences in the means and variances of the raw data. If the variables are measured in differing units, use of the Pearson product-moment correlation coefficient is appropriate. If this is not the case, and the variables are measured in the same units, differences in the means and the variances are meaningful, especially in the computation of a reliability estimate. The interclass correlation coefficient, then, is insensitive to the presence of trend and inadequate as a reliability estimate where more than one source of random variability is present.

If it is impossible to develop equivalent forms of a written test, the internal consistency of the test can be assessed by assembling half-test scores in one of several ways, and correlating the two half-tests. Four methods of splitting a test are most commonly used. One, sets of items for the two half-tests can be selected on the basis of equivalence in content and difficulty. Two, alternate items, sometimes referred to as odd-even split-halves, can be placed in each half-test. Three, alternate groups of items can be placed in each half-test. Four, the first half of the items can be used as one half-test and the second half as the other half-test.

The use of *split-half methods* for estimating reliability has certain limitations. The application of a split-half method to scores on a timed written test will yield a correlation coefficient that lacks meaning. A timed test is constructed so that the items, although not necessarily difficult, are too numerous to be completed within the given time limit. The purpose of the test is to measure the speed with which the individual can respond to the items. If an odd-even split is used, the reliability coefficient may be misleadingly high. If none of the students have time to answer the latter part of the test, these items will be scored as incorrect answers. The odd and even items on this part of the test will therefore receive the same score, and the resulting correlation coefficient will be inflated. If a first half-second half split is used, the reliability coefficient will be spuriously low. When speed is important in test performance, the reliability coefficient should be determined by test-retest methods. A second limitation of the split-half method is the lack of a time interval between the two halves of the test. Again, the reliability coefficient will tend to be misleadingly high.

The half-tests should be selected so that their content conforms to the specifications for the total test, but within these limits, chance should determine which items go in which half of the test. Lindquist (1952) suggests constructing the two half-tests separately to get a correlation coefficient, and then adding the scores for the total test score.

If alternate, or odd-even, items are used as the basis for estimating the reliability of a power test (in which sufficient time is allowed to complete the test), the errors of measurement in successive administrations of the test are correlated rather than independent. For example, if one item is missed in a half-test, the alternate item in the other half-test is likely to be missed. This is treated as systematic rather than error variance. The odd-even procedure causes fluctuations in individual performance that occur during the testing period to operate together to overestimate the reliability of the test (Thorndike, 1951). If an individual's motivation drops during a portion of the test and affects performance on that part, the individual's inconsistency will be reflected as consistency if an odd-even split is used.

The reliability coefficient of a power test in which the first-half and second-half split is used will reflect individual fluctuations that occur within a given time period. If the test is too long, fatigue or boredom may affect performance during the latter part of the test. Such factors will function to lower the reliability of the test.

Analysis of Variance for Written Tests

An analysis of variance among items can be used to estimate the consistency of a test at a specific time (Hoyt, 1941). The reliability coefficient is estimated from the ratio of the total test variance to the item variance. Reliability computed through analysis of variance and intraclass correlation reflects the consistency of individual performance upon items of a test.

Using the procedures described by Hoyt (1941) for estimating the reliability of a written test by analysis of variance, the appropriate formula is

$$r_{tt} = \frac{V_{\text{items}} - V_{\text{residual}}}{V_{\text{items}}}$$ (Formula 6-9)

where V_{items} = mean square of the among items variance

V_{residual} = sums of squares of among item variance and among individuals variance subtracted from sum of squares for total variance, divided by appropriate degrees of freedom.

The sum of squares for items and the sum of squares for individuals is subtracted from the total sum of squares, leaving the residual sum of squares. The residual sum of squares is used as the basis for estimating the discrepancy between the obtained variance and the true variance. This method is superior to any method based upon an arbitrary division of the test into halves.

The Hoyt method of analysis of variance yields the same results as the Kuder-Richardson Formula No. 20 (Kuder and Richardson, 1937). Formula 6-9 can be extended if two or more equivalent forms of the test are administered so that the between-forms source of variability can be taken into account.

Spearman-Brown Prophecy Formula

When a reliability estimate is obtained by splitting the test in some way, the reliability coefficient is computed for only half of the test. If a written test consists of fifty items given during the same period of time, the fifty items will be split into two sets of twenty-five items each. By comparing the two sets of items, a reliability estimate can be computed, but this will be the estimate for twenty-five items. Since the test actually consists of fifty items, the test user is interested in the reliability of the 50-item test. The reliability for the mean of the 50-item test can be estimated using the Spearman-Brown prophecy formula, which is Formula 6-10.

$$r^* = \frac{nr}{1 + (n - 1)r}$$ (Formula 6-10)

where n = number of times test length is increased

r = reliability of one half with second half

r^* = estimated reliability for desired test length.

Formula 6-10 can be used in the same way with the intraclass correlation coefficient. However, only one source of variability can be considered when the Spearman-Brown prophecy formula is used. The analysis of variance model is appropriate when estimated reliability coefficients are desired for tests with two or more sources of variability, such as a combintaion of between-days variability and within-days variability.

For written tests made up of many items, correlation coefficients estimated using the Spearman-Brown prophecy formula are usually, though not always, higher than those obtained by correlating equivalent forms (Jackson, 1941). Baumgartner (1968) investigated the relationship between split-half reliability coefficients and test-retest coefficients for four physical performance tests: standing broad jump, shuttle run, reaction time, and speed of movement. He found that when all physical performance test scores were collected on the same day, the split-half reliability coefficient tended to be higher than the test-retest coefficient. This was also true when data were collected over two days. Baumgartner recommends using the Spearman-Brown formula only when tests are given on two different days if day-to-day variation is important. Even then, the predicted reliability is considered the upper limit of reliability for the number of trials utilized.

Advantages of the Intraclass Correlation Coefficient

When is the use of the interclass correlation coefficient appropriate? According to Lindquist (1951), when there is only one distinguishable source of undesirable variability, as in a single form of a written test, the product-moment correlation may be used. The use of correlational methods is decidedly inadequate, however, when several sources of undesirable variability can be distinguished.

It is possible to obtain a number of reliability coefficients from one set of data. If a set of data consisted of fifty subjects, four trials, and two observers, reliability coefficients could be computed for subjects over trials, and between observers. These coefficients would have some descriptive value, but they would not lead directly to a quantitative estimate of the relative importance of the various sources of variability.

If no trend is present for a set of two trials, the product-moment correlation coefficient could be used to estimate reliability. With more than two trials, one might compute the correlation for each of the possible pairs of scores and use the average of the coefficients. However, analysis of variance is more convenient because it can be calculated more easily and it leads to the intraclass correlation coefficient that is equivalent to the average of all possible paired-score product-moment correlation coefficients (again assuming no trend exists). In most cases, the use of analysis of variance to estimate reliability is widely preferred and recommended.

Factors Influencing the Reliability of a Test

Numerous factors influence the reliability of a test. Some of these factors are range of ability, level of ability, interval between testing, part-vs-total reliability, length of test, and intrinsic factors.

Range of Ability

The greater the range of ability within the group taking the test, the higher the reliability coefficient, whether or not the measure is accurate (Wesman, 1952; Ebel, 1962). For a simplified example, examine the two samples of scores in Table 6–7.

TABLE 6–7 • Effect of Range of Ability on Reliability

Student Number		Broad Jump 1		Broad Jump 2
1		77		70
2		76		69
3	Sample I	72		73
4		70		70
5		69		75
6		69		66
7		67		67
8		65		67
9		65		64
10		65		61
11		63	Sample II	62
12		61		60
13		60		60
14		60		64
15		59		61
16		57		55
17		54		50
18		50		48
19		49		46
20		47		48

Sample I, containing five students, is embedded in Sample II, containing twenty. Normally, it would be highly undesirable to estimate reliability based on a sample of only five people. However, the effect of range of ability can be seen more easily using small samples.

Note the distribution of scores in the first trial for Sample I in the broad jump. Compare these scores for the five subjects with their scores on the second trial. Student 1 has the best jump in the first trial, but his jump is second best in the second one. Fluctuations like these for a sample of this size operate to reduce the reliability of the test. After all, student 1 can drop down to no less than fifth place and student 5 can rise to no more than first place. However, in a sample of twenty, the same fluctuations by the first five students will no longer reduce the reliability in the same way. Now student 1 could theoretically drop down to the twentieth position. In reality, he is not likely to fluctuate to that extent, so as the range of skill increases, so does the reliability. Thus, when test reliability is reported based on the test scores of a wide range of grades or ages, the teacher should be suspicious of the reliability estimate. If the scores are obtained from grades 3 to 8 or ages 7 to 11, a wide range of ability is obviously represented, and the reliability coefficient will be an overestimate. The appropriate procedure is to select a test which has a reliability estimate for the age or grade for which the test is intended.

The range of scores as well as the reliability estimate should be reported by the test constructor. A reliability coefficient of 0.65 based on a narrow range of talent is as good as a coefficient of 0.90 based on a group with twice that range of scores.

Level of Ability

Closely related to the range of ability is the level of ability and its effect on reliability. In physical education activities, we expect skilled individuals to perform with more consistency than beginners. Therefore, many skill tests will be more reliable when administered to highly skilled players. One should not, however, assume that this is automatically true, but should base test selection on a stated numerical reliability estimate. For example, the charts in Table 6–8 note the differences in reliability coefficients (SE_m) of two written tests at different ability and age levels.

Interval between Testing

As discussed earlier, the reliability estimate derived from testing on one day will be an overestimate if the magnitude of day-to-day variability is relatively large. If one is interested in stability of performance over a specified length of time, the reliability estimate will be more accurate when the same time interval exists between repetitions of the test.

Part vs Total Reliability

Even if a battery of tests has a high reliability estimate, there is no assurance that the individual tests in the battery, when used singly, are

TABLE 6–8 · Effect of Level of Ability on the Reliability Estimate*

Revised Stanford-Binet		Wechsler Intelligence Scale	
IQ Level	Standard error of IQ	Age	SE_M of IQ
130 and over	5.2	$7\frac{1}{2}$	4.2
110–129	4.9	$10\frac{1}{2}$	3.4
90–109	4.5	$13\frac{1}{2}$	3.7
70–89	3.8		
Below 70	2.2		

*From R.L. Thorndike and E. Hagen, *Measurement and Evaluation in Psychology and Education,* 3rd ed. Copyright © 1955, 1961, 1969, by John Wiley & Sons, Inc. Reprinted by permission.

reliable. Only when satisfactory reliability estimates are given for each test in a battery, or each part of a test, should they be used individually (Wesman, 1952).

Length of Test

All else being equal, the longer the test, the higher the reliability. However, after a certain point, increased length will have such a minor effect on the reliability estimate that further increases will not be worthwhile, as shown in Table 6–9. In measures of physical performance, the effect of fatigue or boredom prohibits excessive test length in many cases.

TABLE 6–9 · Relation of Written Test Length to Test Reliability*

Items	Reliability
5	0.20
10	0.33
20	0.50
40	0.67
80	0.80
160	0.89
320	0.94
640	0.97
Infinity	1.00

*Reprinted from Table 10.13 of Ebel, *Measuring Educational Achievement* (Englewood Cliffs, N.J.: Prentice-Hall, Inc., 1965), p. 337, by permission of the publisher.

Range of Difficulty of Items in a Written Test

The narrower the range of difficulty of items of a written test, the greater the reliability (Symonds, 1928). If no one can answer a question or if everyone can, the reliability is not influenced. Such items do not discriminate, and thus are not useful. A maximum reliability coefficient is obtained when the items are of the 50 percent difficulty level (Lindquist, 1952). However, selecting only items at the 50 percent difficulty level is not done in practice.

Individual Variability Affecting Test Reliability

Many individual factors affect the reliability of a test. Some of these are speed and accuracy in taking a test, incentive or effort, obtrusion of competing ideas, distractions, health and cheating (Symonds, 1928).

Size of Reliability Coefficient

Reliability coefficients cannot be expressed as percentages, and thus cannot be evaluated as proportions of total variance. However, the coefficient can be squared to determine the amount of shared variance between the test scores. Shared variance indicates the degree to which the test scores are measuring the same thing. A coefficient of 0.80 when squared equals 0.64, which means that 64 percent of the variance of the test scores is held in common.

The interpretation of the reliability estimate also depends upon the type of skill being measured. In one of the early books on measurement in physical education, Glassow and Broer (1938) indicated that strength measures can be highly reliable when only a few trials are taken. High reliability estimates were also obtained for measures of throwing and jumping for distance; however, lower estimates were obtained for elementary children performing the same skills. Striking and kicking skills yielded lower reliability estimates, and accuracy tests were the least reliable. Basically, these generalizations about the estimates of reliability for tests of motor performance remain appropriate. The greater the force requirements (throw as hard as possible, jump as far as possible, squeeze the dynamometer as hard as possible), the higher the reliability coefficient may be expected to be. As accuracy demands increase, the reliability coefficient can be expected to decrease.

For a stringent evaluation of the size of reliability coefficients, one can refer to Kelley's table (Kelley, 1927). According to Kelley, this type of evaluation should be made in light of the types of decisions the test user will make based on the test results. If the level of group accomplishment is of interest, a reliability as low as 0.50 may be adequate. If the user is concerned with the level of individual accomplishment (such as using the score to determine a grade for a student), a minimal reliability coefficient of 0.94 is recommended.

In general, physical educators have assumed that highly skilled persons perform more reliably than those poorly skilled. However, Kroll (1970) has shown that girls in a low strength category displayed less error variance than girls in a high strength category. The low strength group also had a lower true score variance than the high, and as a result, reflected less reliability. These results indicate that the proportions of variance need to be examined as well as the reliability coefficient.

To summarize, the reliability coefficient can be evaluated in several ways: 1) by squaring the coefficient, 2) by referring to standards in published tables, 3) by using the logical expectation for the type of skill being measured, and 4) by referring to the age and skill level of the students for whom the coefficient was determined.

Summary

Reliability is defined as the precision of an individual's score and is an integral aspect of validity. A test that is not reliable cannot be valid, whereas a test can be reliable without being valid.

The determination of reliability is a logical as well as a statistical procedure. The logical process consists of planning a measurement schedule that will take into account as many measurable sources of variability as possible. Three general sources of variability can be described. Response variation by the subject is variability that can occur from trial to trial or from day to day. This source represents variation in behavior that is biological in nature. Within this category, a between-days source of variability and a within-days source of variability can be identified. The between-days source includes variability that occurs from day to day, whereas the within-days source refers to the variability from trial to trial. Variation in the response of the student may also be called intraindividual variability.

A second general category of sources of variability is administrator variation. Administrator variability is the product of inaccurate or inadequate test directions or the failure to see that a test is executed properly. A third general category, scorer source of variability, is a result of inconsistencies in making judgments about the scores of tests.

When more than one source of variability can be identified for a given test, the variance attributable to each of the sources can be examined. Thus, more than one estimate of reliability may be useful for a given test. It is then possible to plan a measurement schedule in which the variability is reduced as much as possible.

Since most tests of motor performance utilize two or more trials of the same measure, analysis of variance procedures are appropriate statistical techniques for estimating the reliability of this type of test. The reliability coefficient obtained through analysis of variance procedures is called the intraclass correlation coefficient, or R. Use of this technique allows the investigator to identify specific components of score variation and to obtain estimates of the relative magnitude of each variance component. The product-moment correlation method is not an appropriate method for estimating the reliability of a test of repeated measures because the variance associated with the existing sources of variability cannot be estimated. In addition, the correlation method incorrectly treats systematic increases or decreases from one set of scores to another as reliability.

The estimation of an intraclass correlation coefficient should be preceded by a test for trend. A trend is a systematic increase or decrease from trial to trial. If a trend is present, the investigator can omit the trials which show the trend effect, and compute the reliability coefficient again on the remaining trials. As an alternative, the investigator can compute the reliability estimate using the formula adjusted for trend, in which the trials source of variance is removed.

The reliability of tests of motor performance can also be estimated using the standard error of measurement, which is an absolute measure of precision that is given in the actual score units of the data. The smaller the standard error of measurement for a given test, the more reliable the test. When comparing two different tests, the standard error should be evaluated with the magnitude of the standard deviation in mind.

The reliability of written tests is sometimes estimated by correlating two equivalent forms of a test or two half-tests that are equivalent in content and difficulty. However, the split-half reliability adjusted by the Spearman-Brown prophecy formula tends to be spuriously high. The Hoyt analysis of variance procedure is recommended for estimating the reliability of written tests.

The reliability of a test is affected by many factors. The greater the range of ability, the higher the reliability coefficient. Highly skilled individuals tend to perform on motor skills measurements with more consistency than poorly skilled persons. If there is a time interval between testing sessions, the reliability coefficient may be affected. Generally, the longer the time interval, the lower the reliability estimate. When all else is equal, the longer the test, the higher the reliability. Many individual factors affect the reliability of a test, such as effort, motivation, distraction and cheating.

The reliability can be evaluated by squaring the coefficient, by referring to standards in published tables, and by using the logical expectation for the type of skill being measured. The coefficient must also be interpreted in light of the age and skill level of the students for whom it was determined.

Bibliography

ALEXANDER, H. W. "A General Test for Trend," *Psychological Bulletin,* XLIII (1946), pp. 533–57.

ALEXANDER, H. W. "The Estimation of Reliability When Several Trials Are Available," *Psychometrika,* XII (1947), pp. 79–99.

American Psychological Association, et al. *Standards for Educational and Psychological Tests and Manuals.* Washington, D. C.: American Psychological Association, Inc., 1954.

American Psychological Association, et al. *Standards for Educational and Psychological Tests and Manuals.* Washington, D. C.: American Psychological Association, Inc., 1966.

BAUMGARTNER, T. A. "The Applicability of the Spearman-Brown Prophecy Formula When Applied to Physical Performance Tests," *Research Quarterly,* XXXIX, No. 4 (1968), pp. 847–56.

BAUMGARTNER, T. A. "Stability of Physical Performance Test Scores," *Research Quarterly,* XL, No. 2 (1969), pp. 257–61.

BAUMGARTNER, T. A. "Estimating Reliability When All Test Trials Are Administered on the Same Day," *Research Quarterly,* XL, No. 1 (1969), pp. 222–25.

BAUMGARTNER, T. A. and A. S. Jackson. "Measurement Schedules for Tests of Motor Performance," *Research Quarterly,* XLI, No. 1 (1970), pp. 10–14.

BROZEK, J. and H. ALEXANDER. "Components of Variation and the Consistency of Repeated Measurements," *Research Quarterly,* XVIII (1947), pp. 152–66.

CATTELL, R. B. "Suggested Restructuring of the Concept of Reliability," *Journal of Educational Psychology,* LV (1964), pp. 1–22.

CURETON, E. E. "The Stability Coefficient," *Educational and Psychological Measurement,* XXXI (1971), pp. 45–55.

DAVIS, F. B. *Educational Measurements and Their Interpretation.* Belmont, Calif.: Wadsworth Publishing Company, Inc., 1964.

DIEDERICH, P. B. "Pinhead Statistics," *Evaluations as Feedback and Guide.* Association for Supervision and Curriculum Development Yearbook, 1967, pp. 264–69.

DOPPELT, J. E. "How Accurate Is a Test Score?" in *Readings in Measurement and Evaluation,* ed., N. Gronlund. New York: The Macmillan Company, 1968, pp. 203–7.

EBEL, R. L. "Estimation of the Reliability of Ratings" *Psychometrika,* XVI (1951), pp. 407–24.

EBEL, R. L. "Measurement and the Teacher," *Educational Leadership,* XX (1962), pp. 20–24.

EBEL, R. L. *Measuring Educational Achievement.* Englewood Cliffs, N. J.: Prentice-Hall, Inc., 1965.

EISENHART, C. "Expression of the Uncertainties of Final Results," *Science,* CLX (1968), pp. 1201–4.

FELDT, L. S. and M. E. McKEE. "Estimation of the Reliability of Skill Tests," *Research Quarterly,* XXIX (1958), pp. 279–93.

FISHER, R. A. *Statistical Methods for Research Workers.* Edinburgh: Oliver and Boyd Limited, 1925.

FISKE, D. W. and L. RICE. "Intra-Individual Response Variability," *Psychological Bulletin,* LII, No. 3 (1955), pp. 217–50.

GLASSOW, R. B. and M. R. BROER. *Measuring Achievement in Physical Education.* Philadelphia: W. B. Saunders Company, 1938.

GRANT, D. A. "Analysis of Variance Tests in the Analysis and Comparison of Curves," *Psychological Bulletin,* LIII (1956), pp. 141–54.

GRONLUND, N. E. *Measurement and Evaluation in Teaching.* New York: The Macmillan Company, 1965.

HAGGARD, E. A. *Intraclass Correlation and the Analysis of Variance.* New York: The Dryden Press, Inc., 1958.

HARRIS, J. A. "On the Correlation of Intraclass and Interclass Coefficients of Correlation from Class Moments When the Number of Possible Combinations Is Large," *Biometrika,* IX (1913), pp. 446–72.

HENRY, F. M. "Reliability, Measurement Error, and Intra-Individual Difference," *Research Quarterly,* XXX, No. 1 (1959), pp. 21–24.

HENRY, F. M. "Influence of Measurement Error and Intra-Individual Variation on the Reliability of Muscle Strength and Vertical Jump Tests," *Research Quarterly,* XXX, No. 2 (1959), pp. 155–59.

HENRY, F. M. "Individual Differences in Motor Learning and Performance," in *Psychology of Motor Learning,* ed., L. E. Smith. Chicago: The Athletic Institute, 1970, pp. 243–56.

HENRY, F. M. et al. "Errors in Measurement," in *Research Methods Applied to Health, Physical Education and Recreation.* Washington, D. C.: AAHPER, National Education Association, 1949, pp. 459–77.

HORN, J. L. "Integration of Concepts of Reliability and Standard Error of Measurement," *Educational and Psychological Measurement,* XXXI (1971), pp. 57–74.

HOYT, C. J. "Test Reliability Estimated by Analysis of Variance," *Psychometrika,* V (1941), pp. 153–60.

HOYT, C. J. "Reliability," in *Encyclopedia of Educational Research,* ed., C. H. Harris. New York: The Macmillan Company, 1960.

JACKSON, R. W. B. "Studies on the Reliabilities of Tests," Bulletin No. 12, Department of Educational Research, University of Toronto, 1941.

KELLEY, T. L. *Interpretation of Education Measurements.* Yonkers-on-Hudson: World Book Company, 1927.

KROLL, W. "A Note on the Coefficient of Intraclass Correlation as an Estimate of Reliability," *Research Quarterly,* XXXIII (1962), pp. 313–16.

KROLL, W. "Reliability of a Selected Measure of Human Strength," *Research Quarterly,* XXXIII (1962), pp. 410–17.

KROLL, W. "Reliability Variations of Strength in Test-Retest Situations," *Research Quarterly,* XXXIV (1963), pp. 50–55.

Kroll, W. "Reliability Theory and Research Decision in Selection of a Criterion Score," *Research Quarterly,* XXXVIII, No. 3 (1967), pp. 412–19.

KROLL, W. "Test Reliability and Errors of Measurement at Several Levels of Absolute Isometric Strength," *Research Quarterly,* XLI, No. 2 (1970), pp. 155–63.

KUDER, G. F. and M. W. RICHARDSON. "The Theory of the Estimation of Test Reliability," *Psychometrika,* II (1937), pp. 151–60.

LERSTEN, K. C. "Inter-and Intra-Individual Variations during the Progress of Motor Learning," *Research Quarterly,* XXXIX, No. 4 (1968), pp. 1013–19.

LIBA, M. "A Trend Test as a Preliminary to Reliability Estimation," *Research Quarterly,* XXXIII (1962), pp. 245–48.

LINDQUIST, E. F. *Design and Analysis of Experiments.* New York: John C. Wiley and Sons, Inc., 1952.

LINDQUIST, E. F. *Design and Analysis of Experiments in Psychology and Education.* Boston: Houghton Mifflin Company, 1956.

LORD, F. M. "Tests of the Same Length Do Have the Same Standard Error of Measurement," *Educational and Psychological Measurement,* XIX (1959), pp. 233–39.

LU, K. H. "A Measure of Agreement Among Subjective Judgments," *Educational and Psychological Measurement,* XXXI (1971), pp. 75–84.

MARTENIUK, R. G. "Individual Differences in Intra-Individual Variability," *Journal of Motor Behavior,* I, No. 4 (1969), pp. 309–18.

SCHMIDT, R. A. "Critique of Henry's Paper," in *Psychology of Motor Learning,* ed., L.E. Smith. Chicago: The Athletic Institute, 1970, pp. 256–60.

STALLINGS, W. M. and G. M. GILLMORE. "A Note on 'Accuracy' and 'Precision'," *Journal of Educational Measurement,* VIII, No. 2 (1971), pp. 127–29.

STANLEY, J. C. "Reliability," in *Educational Measurement* (2nd ed.), ed., R. L. Thorndike. Washington, D.C.: American Council on Education, 1971.

STANLEY, J. C. "Reliability of Test Scores and Other Measurements," in *Encyclopedia of Education,* ed., L. C. Deighton. New York: The Macmillan Company, 1971.

SYMONDS, P. M. "Factors Influencing Test Reliability," *Journal of Educational Psychology,* XIX (1928), pp. 73–87; in *Educational and Psychological Measurement,* eds., D. PAYNE and R. McMORRIS. Waltham, Mass.: Blaisdell Publishing Company, 1967, pp. 46–54.

THORNDIKE, R. L. "Reliability," in *Educational Measurement,* ed., E. F. Lindquist. Washington, D. C.: American Council on Education, 1951, pp. 560–620.

THORNDIKE, R. L. and E. HAGEN. *Measurement and Evaluation in Psychology and Education.* New York: John Wiley and Sons, Inc., 1955.

WESMAN, A. G. "Reliability and Confidence," in *Readings in Measurement and Evaluation,* ed., N. GRONLUND. New York: The Macmillan Company, 1968, pp. 208–14.

WEST, C. "Estimates of Reliability and Interrelationships among Components of Selected Projectile Skills." Unpublished Doctoral dissertation, University of

Wisconsin, Madison, 1970 (Microcard PE 1170, University of Oregon, Eugene).

WEST, C. and J. THORPE. "Construction and Validation of an Eight-Iron Approach Test." *Research Quarterly,* XXXIX (1968), No. 4, pp. 1115–20.

WIDULE, C. J. "The Application of Trend Analysis to Research in Physical Education." Paper presented to the Midwest Association for Physical Education of College Women Fall Conference, Oglebay Park, W. Va., October 1964.

7

construction of tests
of motor performance

The construction of tests of motor performance varies according to the purpose of the test. A test can be designed to measure a specific skill, a combination of skills, or playing ability; or to contribute to a battery of tests. The type of test that measures a specific skill should be distinguished from the type that measures a combination of skills. For instance, a teacher may wish to select a test of the jump shot in basketball. If so, he would choose a test that measures only the jump shot. If he wishes to measure a combination of basketball skills, such as dribbling and shooting, he would select a test in which the student is required to dribble and shoot. However, he must recognize that two skills—dribbling and shooting—are being measured in this case. When more than one skill is measured by a given test, the diagnostic value of the test is often limited. Do the student's errors occur in dribbling or in shooting? After the skills of dribbling and shooting are mastered separately, the teacher may then wish to test the skills in combination. When selecting a test for a *specific skill*, the teacher should carefully differentiate between tests of specific skills and tests of combinations of skills.

A battery of tests is usually designed to measure some overall ability, such as playing ability. Because certain elements exist in the game situation that do not occur during the administration of a battery of tests, the better measures of playing ability may be determined through the assessment of performance in the game situation. As the student develops skill in an activity, the assessment of the skill can increase in complexity by measuring the skill as it is used in the game. The latter test would be a measure of one component of playing ability, but not playing ability in its entirety.

Aside from the question of the purpose of the test, a second consideration in selecting tests is the proposed use of the test. If the test is to be used in a formative sense, appropriate mastery levels are needed. If the test is to be used for summative purposes, a table of norms should be provided. In the latter situation, the criteria for selection of tests should be strictly applied since lasting decisions are frequently based on summative evaluations.

Development of Tests of a Single Skill

This section will deal with the construction of tests measuring a specific skill, such as the football punt, the baseball throw, or the badminton short serve. This type of test would be appropriate when the students are working on specific skills during a unit. If the major emphasis in a given unit is on skill development, tests of specific skills may be used as summative measures. The distinguishing aspect of this type of test is that a single skill rather than a combination of skills is being measured. There are times when this type of test would be totally inappropriate. For example, using *only* specific skill tests to assess intermediate players at the end of a unit would be insufficient, because the way in which these skills are used in the game is also important at the intermediate level.

Definition of Good Performance

The first stage in constructing a skill test is the specification of the important components of the skill. When these components of the test have been determined, a definition of *good performance* for the skill can be written. This definition provides the basis for developing and validating the test as described in Chapter 5. In the development of the Liba and Stauff Volleyball Pass Test (1963) for example, the two important components of the pass were specified as height of the pass and distance over which the ball travels. The desired height of the pass was described as 15 feet, allowing a teammate adequate time for positioning and receiving the pass. The desired distance of the pass was designated as 20 feet, representing the optimal distance from a back row player to a front row player. (The components of the type of passing skill currently required in power volleyball may be somewhat different from the above description of the pass.) The two components of the volleyball pass then formed the basis for the definition of good performance.

Review of Literature

Once the definition of good performance has been determined, a review of the literature on available tests of the skill is appropriate. If a test is available that meets the criteria stated in the description of good performance, it is not necessary to construct a new test. Even when an appropriate test is not available, useful ideas for test construction may be obtained by examing other tests of the skill.

In addition to reviewing tests of the specified skill, a review of descriptions of the skill by experts may be helpful. Experts include such persons as successful teachers, coaches, and outstanding players. A review of expert opinion is essential unless the test constructor is highly skilled in the sport or very successful in teaching the sport. Regardless of the qualifications of the test constructor, an examination of expert opinions may provide a basis for revising the definition of good performance. For instance, developing a definition of good performance for a swimming stroke without reviewing the work of Counsilman (1968) would be a questionable practice. Once available tests and expert opinions have been reviewed, it may be necessary to rewrite the definition of good performance to include additional information since the development of the test will be based on this definition.

Design of Test

The skill test should be designed for a specific level of ability in a specific learning situation. Economy of administration must also be taken into account. A skill can be measured in several ways, such as time, distance, accuracy, and force. Measures of form (process) can also be included in skill assessment.

Measures of time. When a time measure is used to measure a skill, the product rather than the process of skill execution is measured. The difference between product and process can be described using the example of measuring the speed of an ice hockey puck over a given distance. The *product,* the action of the puck, is being measured. The *process,* the force-producing actions of the player, is of indirect concern but is not directly measured. Time measures have also been used to measure the repeated executions of a skill.

Time measures are appropriate for speed events in such activities as swimming and track, and for skills in which the projectile remains on the ground or floor, such as ice hockey and bowling. (The assumption is that minimal resistance will result from the object contacting the ground or floor.) If the object is projected into the air, a velocity rather than a time measure should be used to measure force.

When a given number of executions of a skill is timed, the use of time as a measure has questionable validity. First, the student is encouraged to hurry at the expense of accuracy. Second, when measuring ball skills in this way, the student is required to rebound the ball off the wall continuously. There are very few sports in which the player is required to receive his own rebound. Thus, handling the rebound may add an unrealistic element of skill to the test. Third, the use of repeated measures of a skill provides little diagnostic information on the skill itself. If throwing is being measured, for example, a ball rebounding off the wall may be poorly caught resulting in a poor score. Measuring a single execution of a skill over several trials is preferable to measuring repeated executions of a skill within one trial.

Measures of distance. Distance measures are frequently used to measure jumps and throws. The distance measure is probably adequate for measuring skill in jumping. However, when measuring skill in throwing, the distance measure is often inappropriate. Skill in throwing requires a combination of force and accuracy. If two objects were thrown, both might land at the same point and yet the trajectories of the two objects could be quite different. In this case, both throws are equally accurate, but the force applied to each differs. Or, conversely, two objects might be projected with the same force and yet the distances of two throws could vary, due to differences in the angle at which the object is thrown. Thus, skill in throwing should be measured by taking both the accuracy and force components of the skill into account. This can best be done by utilizing both velocity and accuracy measures. The concept of measuring both force and accuracy does not apply to competitive situations in field events, where the skill is not a sport skill but rather is a specific skill involving coordination and power. The latter skill requires *maximum* force and *limited* accuracy as opposed to a throw in softball where the accuracy demands are *high* and an *optimal* force is required.

Measures of number of executions in a given time. Another variety of motor skills tests measures the number of executions of a given skill that can be performed in a specified time period. A common example of this type of measure is a test of the number of repeated wall volleys that can be executed in 30 seconds. The problems inherent in this type of measure as a test of a specific skill are similar to those described for measures of time: the student is required to receive his own rebound, the time limit stresses speed rather than a combination of speed and accuracy, and the test has limited diagnostic value for the skill in question.

Measures of velocity. Velocity measures take the speed, angle of projection, and distance components of the projectile skill into account. Thus, the force aspect of the skill is measured with a great degree of precision. Velocity is determined by dividing distance by time, and is recorded in feet per second, and should be used for any skill in which an object is projected into the air. The velocity score reflects the amount of force applied, and should be accompanied by an accuracy measure.

Measures of velocity can be approximated in several ways. One method is to use ropes to measure the height of the trajectory. An early test in which a rope was used to measure force was the Tennis Drive Test developed by Broer and Miller (1950). In this test, a rope was placed four feet above the net, and any drive in which the ball passed between the net and the rope was given a higher score than an equally accurate drive in which the ball passed over the rope. By giving more points for a ball that passes between the rope and the net, the velocity (or force) of the ball is taken into account in a rough sense. However, Glassow (1957) showed that a wide range of velocities could be obtained within any given scoring area for this particular test, and suggested the need for reducing the area between the rope and the net. A refinement of this method was developed by Liba and Stauff (1963) in the Volleyball Pass Test. Three ropes were used instead of one. The top rope was placed so that the trajectory of the volleyball would have a minimum high point of 15 feet in accordance with the definition of good performance. The remaining ropes defined scoring areas at lesser heights. Ropes are useful measures of force as long as their placement is such that the velocity scores within a given target area do not vary to a great extent. A four-foot range in velocities within a given area should be acceptable. However, the use of ropes will provide only an approximation of the force applied to the ball.

Another method of roughly assessing a component of velocity (vertical angle of projection) has been described by West and Thorpe (1968). In measuring the short shot in golf using the eight-iron, the authors used ratings of the vertical angle of projection to categorize the height of the trajectory. If the ball was hit at an angle of 29 degrees or more, three points were given for the flight score. If the angle was judged to be less than 29 degrees, two points were given. A topped ball received one point. Because of the subjectivity involved in making these judgments, the interjudge objectivity should be determined. (Interrater objectivity was satisfactorily established for the West and Thorpe Test.)

The most precise measure of determining velocity is through the use of electronic equipment such as the velocimeter currently in use at the University of Wisconsin. Less accurate but usable velocity scores can be obtained using a stopwatch and a wall target. This procedure has been described by Safrit and Pavis (1969) for a measure of the force of the overarm softball throw. The velocity scores can be computed using the method described in Cooper and Glassow (1972). This process is extremely time-consuming, and the use of velocity tables is recommended as a more expedient method. A velocity table for objects projected from a distance of 30 feet is presented in the appendix of the Cooper and Glassow book. Tables are available at the University of Wisconsin for other distances. Such tables can easily be developed through the use of a simple computer program.

Measures of accuracy. Accuracy is one of the most frequently measured components of a skill, and is generally measured using a target of some sort which can range from the simple to the complex. In beginning badminton, for example, a useful target to aid in measuring the accuracy of the long serve might be a simple division of the long service court into three sections, as shown in Figure 7–1. A major emphasis for beginners is to hit the shuttlecock to the back of the court. Since the student is learning the skill, deviations *beyond* the "3" area might be scored the same as those in front of the "3" area. In fact, since many girls lack strength, a girl who consistently scores in the "2L" area is a step closer to perfecting the skill than a girl who consistently scores in the "2S" area. The first girl needs to control her force, while the second still needs to develop adequate force.

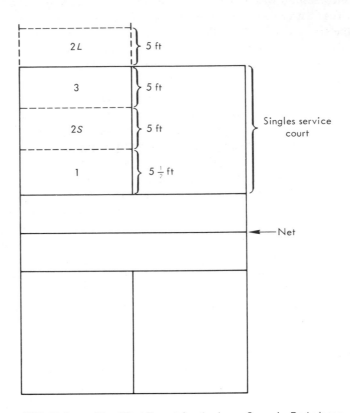

FIG. 7-1   Simplified Target for the Long Serve in Badminton

It is assumed that the height of the trajectory is also being measured, since this is an important component of the badminton serve. Clearly, the measurement of accuracy alone is insufficient for the assessment of a skill. Two shuttlecocks may land on the same section of a target, and yet have different trajectories. Thus, both force and accuracy must be taken into account.

The target for assessing accuracy can be made more discriminating by using a test such as the Wisconsin Badminton Test (1963) where the distances from the one-foot area in front of the baseline are marked off in feet as shown in Figure 7–2. As the student begins to develop his skill, this type of target might be more appropriate than that shown in Figure 7–1.

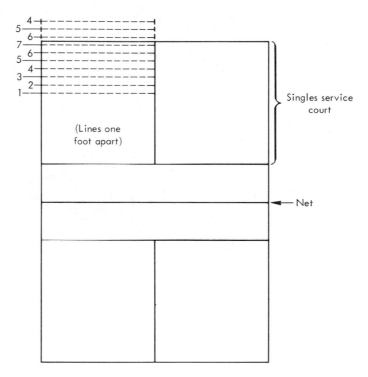

FIG. 7–2   Target for the Wisconsin Long Serve Test (Badminton)

A more complicated target can be designed using arcs and rays. A target designed by Hale (1970) for the long serve is shown in Figure 7–3 and represents a more refined measure of accuracy. Deviations from the area with the greatest point value (10) are given in the upper left hand corner, and distances from the net are presented in the lower right hand corner. It was designed to include the majority of landing points that can result from aiming at the right-hand corner of the left long service court (the area scored 10). The test is diagnostic in that both an accuracy and a deviation score (as well as a height score) are obtained. Almost all of the attempted serves will be scored, which is advantageous, because when many zero scores are obtained, no information is provided about the students' weaknesses.

Measures of form. Very often, physical educators express an interest in the measurement of form, the process by which a skill is executed. Measures of form are frequently carried out by means of a check list or a rating scale. Both of these methods are discussed in a later section.

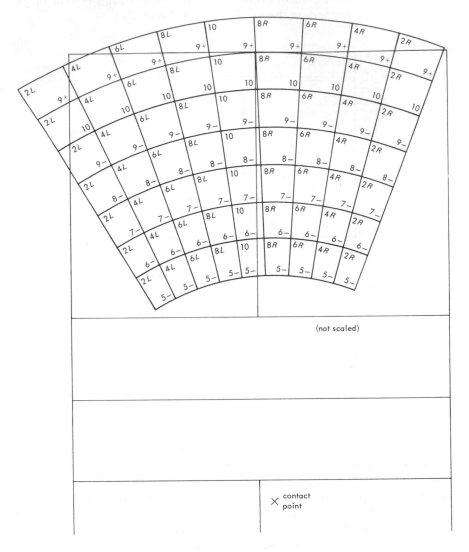

FIG. 7–3   Target for the Hale Long Serve Test (Badminton)

If the product is satisfactory, there is some question regarding the need to measure the process. For example, if a boy can execute a good place-kick in football, does it matter if his form does not fit a "typical" pattern? Certainly a professional football coach would not consider changing a successful soccer-style place-kicker to the more traditional method of kicking off of the toe. However, it may be desirable to measure beginners on some aspects of form, especially when deviations from the typical pattern of form are likely to hinder further development in the skill. However, as the student develops a skill that is consistently satisfactory in terms of product, the teacher should no longer attempt to change idiosyncrasies of style. The measurement of form or process should probably be de-emphasized after the students have advanced beyond the beginner's level in most sports activities, although this may not be true in such areas as movement education, dance, gymnastics, and swimming.

Selection of Subjects

Once the test has been designed, a pilot study should be run utilizing students similar to those for whom the test is intended. For example, if the test is to be used for junior high school girls, the sample selected for initial testing should consist of junior high school girls. Ideally a random sample of at least forty students should be used. However, if a teacher is constructing a test for a group of students in his school, he will probably have to use these students for initial testing. This procedure will limit the degree to which the test can be generalized to other samples, but nonetheless the test will be useful in his school as long as satisfactory standards of validity and reliability are established before decisions are made based on the test results.

Standardization of Directions

The directions for administering the test should be standardized so that each individual will receive the same information prior to being tested. As the instructions vary from student to student, the administrator source of error increases.

Validity and Reliability

The validity of a test of a specific skill can be established through logical validity, which is justified when the test is constucted according to the specifications of the definition of good performance. In the event that a previously developed test is found that is a valid measure of the skill in question but is too expensive or complex to be used in a school setting, this test may be used as a criterion against which a newly developed test can be compared. In this case criterion-related validity, as well as logical validity, would be appropriate.

During the initial testing period, several trials of the test should be administered over more than one day so that the important sources of variance can be examined. Anaylsis of variance procedures should be used to determine the amount of variance attributable to each source and the reliability of the test. The appropriate number of trials is selected according to the size of the intraclass correlation coefficient for trials that are not affected by trend. For greater detail on reliability and validity, see Chapters 5 and 6.

Development of Norms

If the test meets satisfactory criteria for reliability and validity, norms should be developed based on the available test data. If norms are desired that reflect a student's score relative to the scores of other students in the initial testing, either percentile or standard scores are recommended. If the test is formative in nature, mastery levels can be determined using the percentage-correct scores. For details on norms and derived scores, see Chapter 11.

Development of a Battery of Skill Tests

Generally, a battery of skill tests is developed in order to measure playing ability in an activity. One method of developing such a battery is to compare the combined tests with a criterion measure of playing ability using multiple correlation procedures. A regression equation is then written for the combination of tests yielding a satisfactory multiple correlation coefficient. The following is one of the regression equations for the Scott Motor Ability Test (1959):

2.0 basketball throw $+$ 1.4 broad jump $-$ obstacle race $=$ score that is predictor of general motor ability.

Playing ability, like motor ability, is difficult to define. If a satisfactory regression equation can be written as a predictor of playing ability in an activity, the high scoring students, as determined by the results of the regression equation, are those who are predicted to have better playing ability in the game. The primary difficulty in developing a regression equation is to develop an adequate criterion measure with which to compare the battery of tests. For a more complete discussion of prediction, see the section on criterion-related validity in Chapter 5.

A second method of developing a battery of skill tests is to determine a hypothetical structure that includes all of the important components of playing ability. This structure can be tested through factor analytic techniques. In this case, no criterion measure is considered adequate, and therefore no multiple correlation can be computed. See the section on construct validity in Chapter 5 for elaboration of this topic.

Development of Tests of Playing Ability

Very little experimentation has been done on the measurement of playing ability. When a battery of tests has been compared to a criterion measure of playing ability, either tournament rankings or judges' ratings have frequently been used as the criterion measure. Tournament ranking, probably the weaker of the two measures, is a gross measure of playing ability that provides no specific information on the student's strengths and weaknesses. Tournament play may involve elements of competition and chance factors that affect winning or losing, but these may not be the factors with which the teacher is primarily concerned at given stages of learning.

Rating Scales

Judges' ratings can also be weak criterion measures if the rating scale is not well defined. A rating scale should be developed as carefully as a skill test. When assessing playing ability, it is highly unlikely that any one rating scale will suffice as a measure of playing ability. A scale should be developed for *each* component of playing ability that has been identified. For example, one of the important components of badminton playing ability is the ability to use the short serve in the game. The following scale might be used to rate a student on the short serve:

5   Excellent
4   Good
3   Average
2   Fair
1   Poor

This type of scale lacks value because the meaning of "Excellent," "Good," and so on, is not described. Thus, a serve that is rated "Good" by one judge may be rated "Average" by another judge. At the same time, the feedback to the student is poor. A student receiving a score of "2" knows that his serve is rated as fair, but he does not know the reason for the rating.

A better rating scale might be the following:

5   No faults;* serve close to net; serve close to short service line; placement appropriate for opponent's weaknesses or position.
4   No faults;* serve close to net; serve close to short service line; no apparent placement.
3   No faults;* serve *either* close to net *or* close to short service line; no apparent placement.**

2 No faults;* serve *neither* close to net *nor* close to short service line; no apparent placement.**

1 One or more faults; serve neither close to net nor close to short service line; no apparent placement.**

This scale can be used with greater objectivity than the previous one. In addition, the student can attach some meaning to his score. However, some aspects of the scale may still be too vague. For instance, what does "close to the net" mean? Perhaps the specifications should read "within one foot of the net" and "within one foot of the short service line." A one-foot marker could then be placed on the net standards to aid the raters in making judgments about the shuttlecock in relation to the net. Tape could be placed on the floor in order to judge the landing point more accurately. The short serve should be rated on as many occasions as possible, so that the results are representative of the student's skill.

Game Statistics

Rating scales used as measures of playing ability can be supplemented by collecting game statistics. These statistics should not be used as the sole measure of playing ability because of the effect of extraneous factors on such data. However, information collected over several badminton games, such as the number of good serves not returned, the number of good serves returned successfully, and the number of serves that were not good, might be useful to the teacher and the student.

Summary

When a teacher selects a test for a specific purpose, he must distinguish between summative and formative tests, as well as among measures of a single skill, of several skills combined, and of playing ability. The teacher can then proceed with the selection or construction of a test.

If a test of a specific skill is desired, the skill must be defined in terms of good performance. If no test is available that measures the skill according to the prescribed definition, the teacher may wish to construct a suitable one.

A skill test can be designed to use a measure of time, distance, number of executions in a given time, accuracy, velocity, or form, as well as some combination of these measures. While time measures are useful for speed

---

*If one or more faults occur, lower the score by one point.
**If placement is considered satisfactory, raise the score by one point.

events, such measures are not recommended for measuring the amount of time required to execute a skill a given number of times. The measurement of one execution of the skill over several trials is recommended. Distance measures are appropriate for selected field events, but inappropriate for measuring a skill such as throwing, in which time, distance, and angle of projection must be taken into account. Velocity measures are appropriate measures of the force applied in projecting an object. Measures of the number of executions of a skill within a given time period tend to encourage speed over accuracy, and the results provide little feedback to the students. Measures of accuracy in conjunction with measures of force are recommended for object projection skills.

Once the skill test has been designed, it should be administered to a group of students who are similar to those for whom the test is developed. The directions should be standardized, and satisfactory validity and reliability should be established. If the validity and reliability of the test are adequate, norms should be developed for the test.

A battery of tests that is designed to measure playing ability can be developed in two ways. In one, a battery of tests is correlated with a criterion measure, and a regression equation is written in which each test is given an optimal weighting. The weighted tests correlated with the criterion yield the maximal multiple correlation coefficient. In the second method, the important components of playing ability are hypothesized and the hypothesis can be tested through factor analytic techniques.

A highly desirable method of measuring playing ability is through the use of well developed rating scales that can be used during the game. (Individual skills, especially in activities such as gymnastics and swimming, can also be measured by rating scales.) Each category of the scale should be described in such detail that raters can be trained to use the scale objectively and students can receive meaningful feedback about their scores.

Tests of motor performance should be developed in a scientific manner in order to assess students' abilities accurately. The sources for a number of available tests for various aspects of motor performance are given in Appendix A.

Bibliography

BROER, M. R. and D. M. MILLER. "Achievement Tests for Beginning and Intermediate Tennis," *Research Quarterly,* XXI, (1950), pp. 303–13.

COOPER, J. M. and R.B. GLASSOW. *Kinesiology.* St. Louis: The C.V. Mosby Company, 1972.

COUNSILMAN, J. *The Science of Swimming.* Englewood Cliffs, N.J.: Prentice-Hall, Inc., 1968.

GLASSOW, R. B. "Comments on the Miller-Broer Tennis Test." Unpublished paper, The University of Wisconsin, Madison, January 1957.

HALE, P. A. "Construction of a Long Serve Test for Beginning Badminton Players." Unpublished Master's thesis, The University of Wisconsin, Madison, 1970.

LIBA, M. R. and M. STAUFF. "A Test for the Volleyball Pass," *Research Quarterly*, XXXIV, No. 1(1963), pp. 56–63.

SAFRIT, M.J. and A. PAVIS. "Overarm Throw Skill Testing," in *Selected Softball Articles*, eds. J. Felshin and C. O'Brien. Washington, D.C.: American Association of Health, Physical Education and Recreation, 1969.

SCOTT, M. G. and E. FRENCH. *Measurement and Evaluation in Physical Education.* Dubuque, Iowa: Wm. C. Brown Company Publishers, 1959.

University of Wisconsin, Department of Physical Education for Women. "Badminton Report." An unpublished report prepared by the Badminton Committee, 1963.

WEST, C. and J. THORPE. "Construction and Validation of Eight-Iron Approach Test," *Research Quarterly*, XXXIX, No. 4 (1968), pp. 1115–20.

8

written text construction

A basketball player improves his jumping ability through practice. However, any improvement in his performance should be facilitated by an understanding of the mechanical principles, such as the principles of rebounding, that affect jumping ability in various situations. The physical educator is concerned not only with the development of motor skills and abilities, but also with the assimilation of knowledge about movement. Thus, we must be able to develop and utilize written tests as well as skill tests. Even though physical educators may use written tests less frequently than the classroom teacher, such tests should be developed on the basis of sound test construction practices.

This chapter is designed to aid the teacher in the development of various types of written tests. The sections on test construction will be followed by a section on item analysis, including computational methods that can be carried out by hand and typical output of an item analysis obtained through a computer. As more school systems have access to computers, the process of scoring and analyzing written examinations will be greatly facilitated for the individual teacher. The computer can be used to score and analyze essay tests (Page, 1967) as well as objective tests (Baker, 1971), although the major developments using the computer have been in the area of objective testing.

Test Specifications

The process of constructing a written test is a complex one. A teacher may attempt to put together a written test in one or two free periods, whereas an item writer employed by a testing service may be satisfied if he writes 10 to 15 good items a day. The teacher may write down items as they come to mind, with little or no organization. The results of these efforts may be somewhat haphazard. To insure a more systematic approach, Tinkelman (1971) recommends that the teacher develop a test blueprint.

The test blueprint is determined by the purposes of the test. The major purpose is related to the specific area of achievement to be tested. If the test is being constructed for a basketball unit, the teacher must decide the degree to which he is concerned with knowledge of rules, mechanical principles, knowledge of strategies, history of the sport, and so on. Then, are these knowledges to be measured at a low, medium, or high level of cognitive behavior? The content and behaviors should then be noted in a table of specifications, as described in Chapter 2. Such factors must be considered in conjunction with the nature of the group that will be tested, that is, the grade level and ability level of the group.

Another consideration is the use of the test scores, because different usages might require different test blueprints. A final consideration is the time available for testing. For example, a 45-minute testing period would limit a multiple-choice test to approximately 60 items.

Test Administration

Clemans (1971) notes three major sources of error that can occur during the process of administering a test. One, the test author may fail to be specific in writing the directions for test administration. Two, the test administrator may not be thorough in presenting the directions to the students taking the test. Three, the examiner may fail to see that the directions are properly carried out by the students. For the most part, the physical education teacher is the test author, administrator, and examiner. Thus, it is essential that the test directions be carefully thought out ahead of time and specified on the test paper.

The instructions to the student should include several points. The test directions for each section of the test should be clearly stated. For example, true-false items may be designed so that the student must correct all false statements. If the teacher wishes to have only a certain section of the statement corrected, he must underline the portion that may be corrected and instruct the student to correct only the underlined portions of the statements that are marked false. These instructions should be written on the test, and repeated verbally by the teacher.

The verbal directions should also include a statement on guessing. If the student will be penalized for guessing, he should be so informed. If the score will not be corrected for guessing, the student should be told to attempt to answer every question. The concept of correction for guessing will be discussed in detail later in this chapter.

The time limit for the test should be announced at the beginning of the testing period. During the test, the teacher may provide information on the remaining time at suitable intervals. If some portions of the test are weighted more heavily than others, this information should be brought to the student's attention so that he can allocate his time wisely.

The testing environment, including such factors as lighting and noise, should be controlled as much as possible. Special problems can be introduced in a physical education class when a teacher wishes to give a brief written test at the end of a class period. Moving the students from the gymnasium to the classroom would be time-consuming, and the teacher may often elect to give the test in the gymnasium. The student may then be required to use the gymnasium floor or the bleachers to write answers to the test questions. Lap boards can reduce the student's discomfort somewhat. The disadvantage for the student is probably not great if the test is objective and merely requires marking answers on a test sheet. However, if the test requires a considerable amount of writing, the gymnasium environment could handicap some students, especially those who are slow writers under the best conditions.

If the students are prepared for a particular type of test ahead of time, the test directions given at the beginning of the test period should be understood quickly and easily by the students. In addition, advance warning about the test allows the student to study with the knowledge that the test will be of a specified type.

The administration of the test, then, requires the careful consideration of the teacher previous to the actual testing period. If students are allowed to make their own interpretations of the instructions, the reliability of the test is greatly reduced.

Selection Test Items

In a test consisting of selection test items, the student is required to select one of a given number of alternatives. Three types of selection items will be described in this section: alternate-choice, multiple-choice, and matching.

Alternate-Choice Items

Wesman (1971) describes five varieties of the alternate-choice item:

The true-false variety
The right-wrong variety
The yes-no variety
The cluster variety
The correction variety

The first two varieties are essentially equivalent since either true or right, or false or wrong, could be used as an answer for the same statement. The yes-no variety is slightly different in that it is characterized by a direct question. The cluster variety consists of an incomplete stem with several suggested completions. In the correction variety, every false statement is made true by suggesting a substitute for the underlined words. A sample of each variety is given in Table 8–1.

TABLE 8–1 • Samples of Alternate-Choice Items

The true-false variety.
The mean is a measure of central tendency.   *T   F*

The right-wrong variety.
When aiming in field archery, the correct anchor point for the hand is directly under the chin.   *R   W*

The yes-no variety.
Is "dunking" the ball legal in college basketball   *Y   N*

The cluster variety.
A badminton serve that lands in the proper court is legal when the shuttle-cock is hit:

T	*F*	1.	by the frame of the racket
T	*F*	2.	above the racket hand
T	*F*	3.	below the waist
T	*F*	4.	while on one foot.

The correction variety.
The skill with which a tennis serve is executed can be measured by determining the accuracy of the serve.   *(accuracy and force)*

Usefulness of alternate-choice items. The use of alternate-choice items has received a great deal of criticism. While there are some limitations to the use of these items, some of the criticisms seem unwarranted. It is worth noting that the use of this type of item is highly recommended by Ebel (1965, 1971) and Payne (1968), both eminent figures in the study of educational measurement. Nonetheless, an examination of the criticisms is worthwhile in that most of the adverse comments are based on pitfalls that should be avoided in the construction of alternate-choice items.

Alternate-choice items are often criticized because a student is supposed-ly forced to answer the questions by rote. Although questions requiring mere recall can be constructed very easily, their faults lie not with the type of question but rather with the test constructor. It is undoubtedly possible to measure higher levels of cognitive behavior using alternate-choice items. For excellent rebuttals to the criticism that answering this type of item requires only memorization, see Ebel (1956) and Wesman (1971).

Another criticism of alternate-choice tests is that they expose students to error. That is, including false items in a test that the student may not recognize as false reinforces the incorrect concept in the student's mind. However, the student is primed to be critical in a testing situation, and he knows some of the items will be false. The situation might be different if the student were exposed to false statements in a textbook. In this case, some students might accept without question everything they read. However, in a testing situation the expectation certainly would not be one of total acceptance.

A valid objection to alternate-choice items is that they are less reliable than multiple-choice tests of the same length. Although this is true, more alternate-choice items than multiple-choice items can be answered during a given time period. By increasing the number of alternate-choice items, the reliability of the test is increased.

The alternate-choice statement has no standard of comparison and thus must be judged in isolation. In contrast, a multiple-choice item presents several alternatives that can be compared with one another. The correct multiple-choice alternative, then, can be the one that represents the greatest degree of truth. The alternate-choice item, on the other hand, must be clearly true or false. For this reason, the alternate-choice question is difficult to construct. Even so, if the question is ambiguous, the fault still lies with the test constructor. After all, it is the quality of the item that is important. Clarity and meaningfulness are two important attributes of the alternate-choice item. An ambiguous alternate-choice item will not necessarily be improved by increasing the number of alternatives. As Ebel notes, "When a messenger knocks, it is the message he bears that is usually significant, not whether he knocked three times or two" (1971, p. 419). The meaningfulness of the item rather than the number of alternatives is the important consideration.

A frequently expressed objection to the use of alternate-choice items is that students can receive good scores merely by guessing the responses to the items. If a student guesses on every item, he has a fifty-fifty chance of answering any given item correctly. In reality, however, few if any students guess blindly on all questions. A student may not always be certain he is answering correctly, and may answer on the basis of an "educated guess," but when this factor is taken into account, the probability of answering correctly is no longer fifty-fifty. However, certainly some guessing takes place, introducing a degree of chance error that reduces the reliability of the test. A teacher may wish to correct for guessing, but he should only do so under conditions that will be described in a later section. The best solution to the problem of guessing is to prevent it rather than applying a correction factor after the test has been given.

The alternate-choice item has several distinct advantages. It is a simple, direct, and fundamental test of a student's knowledge. This type of test can be used to measure high as well as low levels of cognitive behavior. The scoring of alternate-choice items is fast and efficient. Also, many teachers find it easier to write alternate-choice items than multiple-choice items.

Suggestions for writing alternate-choice items. A number of suggestions for writing a good alternate-choice item will be presented in this section. Other sources are recommended for more detailed discussions of appropriate procedures and for numerous examples of alternate-choice items (Ebel, 1965, 1971; Wesman, 1971; Wood, 1960).

1. Avoid trivial items. Write items that measure meaningful content and behavior.
2. Avoid using sentences from textbooks as questions.
3. Avoid ambiguity.
4. Include an equal number of true and false items. (The tendency in constructing true-false tests is to include more true items than false. At the same time, the student tends to mark an item true if he is uncertain of the correct answer. In addition, the false items discriminate better than the true items.)
5. Order the items on the test in a random pattern. If the order of items is systematic, an extra clue is given to the test-wise student.
6. Express only a single idea in the statement.
7. Avoid negative statements. If an occasional item lends itself to the negative form, underline the negative terms in the statement.
8. Avoid the use of specific determiners like "sometimes," "usually," or "often" in true statements, or "always," "never," or "impossible" in false statements.
9. Make false statements plausible.
10. Make true statements clearly true, so that experts would agree on the answer.

Weighting responses to alternate-choice items. Ebel (1965) suggests a method for controlling the possibility of getting a correct response on alternate-choice items by chance. In Table 8–2, Ebel's table of confidence-weighted responses is presented. Note that a student who is confident that his answer is correct receives more credit for answering correctly than one who is uncertain. The confident student receives double credit for a correct answer, at the risk of an equal penalty for an error. If he has some basis for his response, but is not confident that the response is correct, he is encouraged to answer for less credit. If he has no basis for his response, he is discouraged from blind guessing by being allowed to omit the question for 0.5 credit.

TABLE 8–2 • Confidence-Weighted Response to True-False Test items*

Response Number	Significance of the Response	Score Value		
		Right	Wrong	Omit
1	The statement is probably true.	2	−2	
2	The statement is possibly true.	1	0	
3	I have no idea.			0.5
4	The statement is possibly false.	1	0	
5	The statement is probably false.	2	−2	

*Robert L. Ebel, *Measuring Educational Achievement* (Englewood Cliffs, N. J.: Prentice-Hall, Inc., 1965), p. 131, Table 5.1, by permission of the publisher.

Multiple-Choice Items

The multiple-choice item contains a *stem*, an introductory question or incomplete statement, and a set of *alternatives,* or suggested options. The correct alternative is referred to as the *answer,* and the incorrect alternatives are called *distracters*. Although there are many varieties of multiple-choice tests (Wesman, 1971), the three most common varieties are the correct-answer the best-answer, and the multiple-answer varieties.

In the *correct-answer* variety, only one alternative is correct. More than one alternative is correct in the *best-answer* variety, but one answer is better than the others. In the *multiple-answer* variety, more than one answer may be correct. A sample item for each variety is given in Table 8–3.

TABLE 8–3 • Samples of Multiple-Choice Items

The correct-answer variety.

When a fencer attacks to the high left side of his opponent's target area, the appropriate defensive action is

    a. Parry 2
    b. Parry 4
    c. Parry 6
    d. Parry 8   (b)

The best-answer variety.

To develop skill in shooting a basketball from a given distance, a player must learn to reproduce the correct

    a. vertical angle of projection

    b. horizontal angle of projection
    c. trajectory
    d. velocity   <u>(c)</u>

The multiple-answer variety.
The reliability of a written test can be raised by increasing the
    a. range of ability
    b. length of the test
    c. number being tested
    d. level of ability   <u>(a b)</u>

The stem. The stem is written either as a direct question or as an incomplete sentence. Generally, the incomplete sentence consists of fewer words than the direct question and thus is more economical. However, some measurement specialists (Ebel, 1965; Payne, 1968) note that the less experienced test constructor often utilizes the direct question more effectively. When the stem is an incomplete sentence, each alternative must be written to complete the stem satisfactorily. When the direct question is used, the task is simplified somewhat because the alternatives are written only to conform to each other.

    The stem should present the problem clearly and briefly. Many readers can probably recall taking a multiple-choice test in which the stem was so long that by the time the alternatives were reached, the nature of the problem was lost, forcing the reader to go back to reread the stem. However, one should guard against too much brevity. A stem such as

"Conscious relaxation is . . .."

is too brief. A better approach would be

"The major characteristic of the technique of conscious relaxation is . . .."

As with alternate-choice questions, stereotyped phrases should be avoided. Generally, the stem should be written in positive, not negative, form.

    The alternatives. The recommended number of choices varies between three and five. As Wesman (1971) notes, the effectiveness of the alternatives is more important than the number. Tversky (1964) has shown that the use of three alternatives will maximize the discriminability, power, and information that can be obtained in a given period of time. There is no special reason why one must have the same number of alternatives for each item in a test. Thus, the teacher should not struggle unnecessarily to write a fourth or fifth alternative. If five meaningful alternatives can be written, a teacher should include five. If, after genuine effort on the part of the teacher, five alternatives cannot be written, it is better to settle for fewer alternatives than to write obviously poor ones in order to reach a quota.

As the number of alternatives increases, the reliability of the test increases and the chance level for getting an item correct is reduced. On the other hand, the greater the number of alternatives, the fewer the number of items, as the test must be given within a specified time limit. Actually a test with more items and fewer choices will have approximately the same degree of reliability as one with fewer items and more choices.

Sometimes the correct answer is easy to write, but the distracters are difficult to develop. The distracters should seem to be reasonable answers, both logically and grammatically. A useful approach to writing distracters is to have a group of students similar to those who will be tested answer the items without any alternatives. Some of their answers will be incorrect, and yet will seem plausible. These answers should suggest good distracters.

The distracters should be parallel in grammatical form and approximately of the same length. As with alternate-choice questions, specific determiners such as "never" and "always" should be avoided. "None of the above" and "all of the above" should be used sparingly, and not as a substitute for the fifth alternative that is difficult to write.

The alternatives should be listed in random order so that the correct answer cannot be systematically determined by the test-wise student. A teacher may feel that by ordering the alternatives differently from item to item, he can be sure that no pattern exists for the location of the correct answer. However, although the ordering may seem arbitrary, the pattern may reflect a hidden bias that is not recognized by the teacher. Random order can easily be achieved by drawing numbers out of a container, with the first number representing the alternative that will be listed first, and so forth. This process must be repeated for each item.

Usefulness of multiple-choice items. Multiple-choice, like alternate-choice items, can suffer from ambiguity. For example,

A five-category rating scale is used to assess a gymnastics skill, with five representing the best performance and one, the poorest. What type of measurement scale is represented by the data?
- a. nominal
- b. ordinal
- c. interval
- d. ratio

The use of the word *category* would cause most students to think of *nominal* as the correct answer. For the student with a surface knowledge of measurement scales, the answer given would probably be *nominal*. If he is knowledgeable about scaling, however, he would recognize that there is a meaningful order associated with the categories, although the data are not representative of pure ordinal data. No answer is correct, and the student is faced with the dilemma of marking an incorrect answer or no answer at all. If he chooses to mark an answer, should he mark nominal or ordinal? If he does not answer the question, he will be penalized.

The fact that multiple-choice questions can be ambiguous does not mean such items should not be used. Rather, the test constructor must guard against ambiguity. Wood (1960) notes that, for each item a continuum of degrees of truth exists. The advantage of multiple-choice over alternate-choice items is that the correct answer for the former does not have to be totally true, but must have a greater degree of truth than the distracters. In any case, the students' judgments of an alternate-choice answer must agree with that of the teacher. When teacher-made tests are used within a single classroom, any ambiguity that exists may be dealt with by the teacher after the test has been given. If he listens fairly and openly to student reactions to the test items, ambiguous questions may be identified and omitted. This is not the case when a standardized test is given. Unfortunately, judgments based on the results of a standardized test are often of much greater significance to the student than those based on classroom tests. When a teacher gives an unfair test, he will still have many opportunities to revise his judgments about the student throughout the year, so that a single instance of poor testing will not have long-lasting effects on the student. One would assume that standardized tests are developed with such rigorous controls that ambiguity could not be a factor, although Hoffman (1964) has noted instances in which ambiguity exists in test items developed by national testing organizations.

A disadvantage of multiple-choice questions is that the correct alternative can be chosen for the wrong reason. A test item can be designed to measure a specified level of cognitive behavior. However, the teacher does not know if the student who answered the item correctly used the desired process. In fact a student who did not answer correctly may have used the desired process, but did not clearly understand the content. While this disadvantage should be recognized by educators, the use of multiple-choice questions need not be abandoned for it. Rather, the measurement of process should be systematically explored to clarify these questions. This type of test item is a useful measurement tool for the teacher, and, although difficult to construct, an efficient evaluation instrument.

Matching Items

Matching items consist of two columns of words or phrases, with the column on the right containing the alternatives. The student is instructed to select an alternative from the right column to go with each item in the left column. A sample matching question is given in Table 8–4. The number of alternatives in the second column should be greater than the number of items in column one. If the numbers in both columns are the same, the student may be able to answer the last one or two items through the process of elimination. Between five and fifteen items are recommended. When more than fifteen items are used, the task of reading through all of the items becomes tedious for the student.

TABLE 8–4 • Sample Matching Questions*

Directions: Place the *letter* of the appropriate organization in the space

____1. Organization governing amateur sports in   (a)   AAHPER
America.   (b)   AAU
____2. Organization governing college athletics in   (c)   DGWS
America.   (d)   NCAA
____3. National professional physical education   (e)   USGA
association.   (f)   USLTA
____4. Governs women's collegiate athletics.
____5. Rules governing body for golf.

Directions: Place the *letter* of the appropriate person in the space provided to the
left of each statement.

____1. Grandfather of physical education.   (a)   Aristotle
____2. First president of P. E. professional   (b)   Catherine Beecher
organization.   (c)   Isadora Duncan
____3. Thought aim of education was happiness.   (d)   Martha Graham
____4. Instrumental in growth of measurement   (e)   Luther Gulick
in physical education.   (f)   Guts Muth
____5. Developed athletic achievement tests with   (g)   Margaret H'Doubler
YMCA.   (h)   Edward Hitchcock
____6. Founded interpretive dancing.   (i)   Dio Lewis
____7. Gave first "modern dance" concert.   (j)   Dudley Sargent
____8. Day's order of exercises in public schools   (k)   Jesse F. Williams

*Reprinted from Example 37 of M.J. Haskins, *Evaluation in Physical Education* (Dubuque, Iowa: Wm. C. Brown Company, Publishers, 1971), p. 244, by permission of the author and publisher.

A variation of the matching question uses a small number of alternatives, but each can be used more than once. This is a popular form of testing for knowledge of rules in physical education. Several samples of this variation are given in Table 8–5.

Supply Test Items

When answering supply-type items, the student must provide the words, numbers, or other symbols that constitute the response rather than choosing

TABLE 8–5 • **Sample of Variation of Matching Question***

VOLLEYBALL

Directions: Indicate the official's decision in the following situations, using the key
letters for your answers. There is only one best answer. Assume that no
conditions exist other than those stated.

P —point   L —legal, or play continues
SO —side out   R —re-serve, or serve over

____1. Server steps on the end line as the ball leaves her fist.

____2. On the service, the ball touches the top of the net and lands on the boundary
line of the receiving team's court.

____3. A player on the receiving team spikes the ball before it crosses to her side of the
net. She does not touch the net.

____4. A forward on the serving team in spiking the ball, returns to the floor across the
center line. On the same play, a forward of the receiving team who attempts to
block the ball steps on the center line.

____5. As a player on the serving team attempts to contact the ball, it touches her upper
arm.

SOCCER

Directions: Place the appropriate letter in the space provided.

A —Free kick for opposing team E —Free kick on penalty circle
B —Kick-in for opposing team   F —Penalty kick
C —Roll in   G —No penalty
D —Corner kick   H —Score

____1. On a kick-in player A dribbles the ball rather than kicking it.

____2. A team "B" player, taking a kick-in, sends the ball between the goal posts.

____3. "A" is tackling "B" who has the ball; it goes out of bounds off both players.

____4. During play the ball is lofted into the air, and the left inner bounces it off his knee
through the goal posts.

*Reprinted from Example 38 of M.J. Haskins, *Evaluation in Physical Education* (Dubuque,
Iowa: Wm. C. Brown Company, Publishers, 1971), p. 245, by permission of the author and publisher.

from several designated alternatives. Short-answer tests and essay tests are
two common varieties of the supply-type test. The scoring of supply items is
usually more subjective than the scoring of selection items.

Short-Answer Items

The short-answer test is preferred by many teachers because the items
are easy to construct. However, these tests have drawbacks. More than one
response to a question may be correct. The student may be able to think of
several appropriate words or phrases, and then must try to determine the

answer the teacher has in mind. Also, if the item really requires a short answer, it almost always measures the student's memory for fact.

Wesman (1971) describes three varieties of the short-answer test: the question variety, the completion variety, and the identification or association variety. The *question* variety consists of a direct question, whereas the *completion* variety is written as an incomplete statement. The *identification or association* variety contains a list of words or phrases that the student must identify in the designated way. Samples of these varieties are presented in Table 8–6.

TABLE 8–6   •   Samples of Short-Answer Items

The question variety.
If a bowler gets a strike in the first frame and six pins in the second frame, what is his second frame score?

(22) _____

The completion variety.
The extension of the foil arm in fencing is called the

(thrust) _____

The identification or association variety.
After each name write the sport in which he (or she) achieved fame.

Jerry West	(Basketball) _____ .
Bobby Jones	(Golf) _____
Knute Rockne	(Football) _____
Yvonne Goolagong	(Tennis) _____
Patty Berg	(Golf) _____
Vida Blue	(Baseball) _____

Short-answer questions should be used only when the desired answer is clear to experts, and when the answer can be given in a word or two. The question should be posed simply enough that reading is not a major factor in answering.

Essay Questions

An essay question is defined as

a test item which requires a response composed by the examinee, usually in the form of one or more sentences, of a nature that no single response or pattern of responses can be listed as correct, and the accuracy and quality of which can be judged subjectively only by one skilled or informed in the subject. The most significant features of the essay question are the freedom of response allowed the examinee and the fact that not only can no single answer be listed as complete and correct, and given to clerks to check, but even an expert cannot usually classify a response as categorically right or wrong. Rather, there are different degrees of quality or merit which can be recognized (Stalnaker, 1951, p. 495).

The use of essay questions has been strongly advocated by many educators because this type of question is generally believed to be the best test of the student's ability to express ideas and to analyze and synthesize concepts. However, an essay test is not necessarily superior to an objective test in measuring higher levels of cognitive behavior. On the surface, essay tests might seem superior in this respect, but this form of testing also has limitations.

Limitations of the essay test. One of the major limitations of essay tests is the error associated with the rating of essay questions. Although the following quotation was made with reference to rating term papers, the same lack of objectivity occurs in rating essay tests.

The papers used in this study were 300 essays written by college freshmen on either of two topics, "Who Should Go to College?" and "When Should Teenagers Be Treated As Adults?". In selecting papers for the study, the investigators deliberately included a disproportionately large number of papers written by high-ability and low-ability students. This was done in order to make the discriminations stand out sharply. There were 150 papers on each of the two subjects. . . . 101 of the 300 papers received all nine possible grades and . . . no paper received fewer than five different grades (Miller, 1968, pp. 27–28).

One problem associated with the rating of an essay question is that different raters tend to assign different grades to the same paper. In addition, a single rater tends to assign different grades to the same paper on different occasions. These differences tend to increase as the essay question permits greater freedom of response (Coffman, 1971).

The lack of objectivity on the part of raters exists for several reasons. In the first place, some raters are more severe than others. Some will habitually give lower ratings to all answers than their higher-marking colleagues. Second, the raters may differ in the extent to which they distribute grades over the score scale. One rater may give grades that cluster around the average, while a second may use the full range of possible scores. A bright student might be penalized by the first rater, while an unprepared student would receive an advantage by being scored by the same rater. Finally, raters may differ in the relative values they assign to different papers because each rater uses a different criterion. One rater may judge more on writing form and style, while another rater looks primarily for content.

Another aspect of scorer unreliability is the halo effect. The halo effect will lower objectivity when, for example, a teacher is influenced by the past performance of a student in grading that student's exam. A good essay written by a usually poor student may receive a lower rating than the same quality paper written by generally good student. This effect may be controlled to some extent by concealing the name of the student until after the papers have been rated. The halo effect is also operating when a high rating is given to a paper that has overall good quality, but is in fact poor on specific answers.

Extraneous factors such as handwriting, spelling, and organization can also reduce rater objectivity. A teacher should carefully describe the degree to which these factors will be taken into account in scoring the exam. Otherwise, the student may assume that only content is being graded.

Despite the mass of evidence indicating lack of agreement among raters of essay exams, it is possible to obtain high correlations among raters. Gosling (1966) reports coefficients of 0.98, 0.96, and 0.97 among raters of English composition exams in Australia. The raters were given a list of criteria and a set of 10 reference compositions chosen from a pilot study to represent points on a 15-point rating scale. Essay tests can be as reliable and valid as objective tests, but the cost involved is generally greater.

Another source of error in the use of essay tests is that associated with the sampling of the questions. The greater the number of questions, the higher the reliability of the test. However, since the testing time is limited, the number of essay questions cannot be very large. Therefore, the sample of content and behavior will be limited and the reliability of the test may be low.

Finally, although the student cannot blindly guess on the essay test, a corresponding weakness is bluffing. If a student does not know the answer to a question, he may attempt to write around the answer in such a manner that it will seem as if he answered the question. The technique of bluffing is humorously described in excerpts from the following letter:

> . . . The summation of what is called the liberal arts course is reached with such subjects as political theory, philosophy, etc. Here the air is rarer and clearer and vision easy. There is no trouble at all in circling around the examiner at will. The best device is found in the use of quotations from learned authors of whom he has perhaps —indeed, very likely—never heard, and the use of languages which he either doesn't know or can't read in blurred writing. We take for granted that the examiner is a conceited, pedantic man, as they all are —and is in a hurry to finish his work and get back to a saloon.
>
> Now let me illustrate.
>
> Here is a question from the last Princeton examination in Modern Philosophy. I think I have it correct or nearly so.
>
> "Discuss Descartes' proposition, 'Cogito ergo sum', as a valid basis of epistemology."
>
> Answer:
>
> Something of the apparent originality of Descartes' dictum "cogito ergo sum",

disappears when we recall that long before him Globulus had written, "Testudo ergo crepito", and the great Arab scholar Alhelallover, writing about 200 Fahrenheit, has said, "Indigo ergo gum". But we only have to turn to Descartes' own brilliant contemporary, the Abbé Pate de Foie Gras, to find him writing, "Dimanche, lundi, mardi, mercredi, jeudi, vendredi, samedi" which means as much, or more, than the Descartes assertion. It is quite likely that the Abbe himself was acquainted with the words of Pretzel, Wiener Schnitzel, and Schmierkase; even more likely still he knew the treatise of the low German, Fisch von Gestern, who had already set together a definite system or scheme. He writes: "Wo is mein Bruder? Er ist in dem Haus. Habe ich den Vogel gesehen? Dies ist ein gutes Messer. Holen Sie Karl und Fritz und wir werden alle ins Theater gehen. Danke Bestens".

There, one can see how easy it is. I know it from my own experience. I remember in my fourth year in Toronto (1891) going into the exam room and picking up a paper which I carelessly took for English Philosophy; I wrote on it, passed on it and was pleasantly surprised two weeks later when they gave me a degree in Ethnology. I had answered the wrong paper. This story, oddly enough, is true.*

Stephen Leacock

Construction of essay tests. The essay test seems easy to construct in contrast to the difficult task of developing an objective test. On the other hand, the scoring of the objective test is fast and simple, but that of the essay exam requires a great deal of time and expertise. The essay exam must be rated by a qualified person, usually the teacher, whereas a paraprofessional can efficiently grade an objective test. However, the scoring process of essay exams is greatly facilitated if sound construction techniques are adopted.

In constructing essay exams, the teacher may be tempted to put together a few questions in the shortest possible amount of time. To avoid hasty construction, Wood (1960) suggests taking at least as much time to construct an essay test as the students will take to answer it. The objectives of the test should be carefully defined, and questions should be formulated based on these objectives. General questions, such as

"Discuss the mechanical principles of swimming,"
should be avoided. The student has no reasonable focus and may write the answer in a broad surface manner. The question should be delimited, perhaps in the following way:

"Discuss the principle of buoyancy as it applies to the breast stroke. Include the following points:

1. Definition of principle of buoyancy.

2. Application with regard to coordination of body parts.

3. Application with regard to position of body parts."

The Daily Princetonian (Princeton, New Jersey), from Stephen Leacock letter dated January 26, 1938. Reprinted by permission.

It is preferable to include from 10 to 15 questions that require relatively short answers rather than two or three with longer answers. The greater the number of questions, the better the sampling of content will be.

When the questions have been carefully developed, the teacher should construct a model answer for each question. The model answers should be formed in the amount of time the students will have for the test. If the teacher cannot answer the questions in the desired amount of time, the students cannot be expected to do so.

An essay test may be designed to allow the student to choose a set number of questions to answer out of the total number. At first glance, this procedure seems quite democratic. However, there are drawbacks to the use of this process. It is impossible to know the degree of difficulty for each question, and the difficulty level quite likely varies over a given set of questions (Coffman, 1971; Ebel, 1965). A student who chooses a certain set of questions may have an advantage over a student choosing another set. In effect, the students are being compared on different measures. For purposes of comparability, then, choices of questions should be avoided unless the students taking the test have markedly different backgrounds.

Scoring essay tests. Ebel (1965) has described six deficiencies that commonly occur in the scoring of essay tests.

1. Incorrect statements were included in the answer.
2. Important ideas necessary to an adequate answer were omitted.
3. Correct statements having little or no relation to the question were included.
4. Unsound conclusions were reached, either because of mistakes in reasoning or because of misapplications of principles.
5. Bad writing obscured the development and exposition of the student's ideas.
6. There were . . . errors in spelling and the mechanics of correct writing (Ebel, 1965, p. 103).

There are two well-described methods of scoring essay exams. One is an analytical system in which a detailed guide to rating is developed. In this system, scoring categories are designated and weights are assigned to each category. In the top category, perhaps designated as five, the desired elements of a quality answer are specified. The bottom category, probably zero, reflects the absence of any of the desired elements. When the analytical system is used, the teacher must guard against a reliance on recall. For example, when the desired elements in category five include the number of names, dates, and places a student can recall and exclude such behaviors as analyzing and synthesizing ideas, the inherent benefits of the essay exam are lost.

The second system uses global ratings with many raters. Each rater is asked to read the essay question through rapidly, formulate his reaction, and rate the question on his immediate reaction. This system is based on the premise that no matter how well a scoring system is defined, there will always be a halo effect on the part of the raters. If a large number of raters is used, the halo effect will be taken into account by averaging the scores of all the raters. The global system has been shown to be reliable and more efficient than the analytical system, and yields similar results (Coffman, 1971). Of course, the analytical system is more appropriate for the average teacher due to the lack of availability of other raters.

Whatever system is used for scoring, each question should be rated for all students before moving on to the next question. A poor first answer may influence the rater negatively when scoring subsequent sections if the total test is scored for a given student before the next test is rated. During the process of grading a set of essay tests, it is helpful to occasionally recheck earlier papers to be sure one's standards have not changed.

Weighting Test Components

Although the weighting of items on a test may be handled in complex, mathematical ways, some concepts of weighting are fairly simple and yet basic to the job of constructing a good test. For instance, if more items are included on a particular topic, that topic is automatically weighted more heavily than other topics in the test. Although this statement may seem obvious, sometimes teachers neglect to check on the proportion of items per topic on a test. If several topics vary in importance in the eyes of the teacher, these topics should be weighted proportionally. Assigning weight according to plan has meaning in the test structure, while arbitrary weighting does not.

If an item is included that all students answer correctly, the item is essentially weighted zero. The score for that item simply raises each student's score by the same amount. Thus, the item has no value as a discriminating instrument. The same effect occurs if an item is included that *no* student can answer correctly.

Correction for Guessing

A correction for guessing may be applied to the scores of certain objective tests. When an alternate-choice test is used, the appropriate correction formula is

$$S = R - W \qquad \textbf{(Formula 8-1)}$$

$$\text{where } S = \text{corrected score}$$
$$R = \text{number of right answers}$$
$$W = \text{number of wrong answers}$$

For multiple-choice tests, the correction for guessing formula is

$$S = R - \frac{W}{n-1} \qquad \textbf{(Formula 8-2)}$$

$$\text{where } n = \text{number of alternatives per item}$$

Note that Formula 8-1 is a special case of Formula 8-2 where $n = 2$.

There are several considerations that are pertinent to the use of a correction factor. Correcting for guessing is only effective if some items are omitted by the students taking the test. Otherwise the corrected scores will correlate perfectly with the uncorrected scores (Ebel, 1965; Thorndike, 1971). Therefore, in a *power* test, which characteristically has no time limit, every student has adequate time to attempt to answer every question, and correcting for guessing will be ineffective. In a *speed* test, which is designed so that no student will be able to answer all the items in a given time, an undue advantage is given to the student who answers without reading the items. This student will get some answers right by chance. In this case, the application of a correction factor is useful.

Another consideration is classified by Cureton (1969) as the all-or-none assumption. When scores are corrected for guessing, the assumption is that the student either knows the material and answers correctly or omits it or guesses. This assumption can be questioned since a student might have partial knowledge on a topic and thus be able to answer a question based on an "educated guess."

Ebel (1965) suggests that the results of using a correction for guessing are not momentous in terms of practical consequences. The corrected scores will usually rank students in the same relative position as the uncorrected. In addition, the odds under the formula favor the student who guesses (Cureton, 1969; Ebel 1965; Thorndike, 1971). Thus, most measurement specialists recommend using the correction formula only for speed tests. Otherwise, students should be directed to attempt to answer every question.

Item Analysis

After a set of tests has been scored for a given group of students, an item analysis should be applied to the test to provide the teacher with information on the effectiveness of the test. If the test is designed for single usage, several aspects of the item analysis can be computed by hand. However, if the test will be used year after year, the additional information that can be obtained through computer analysis would be useful.

When a test will be used for more than one class over a period of years, a pilot study is desirable. The trial test should be approximately twice the desired length of the final form so that poor items can be dropped from the test without making the test too short.

The minimum sample size for the pilot study should be one hundred. If test papers from two or three classes are not available, the teacher can collect papers over several years until the desired number is obtained. Ideally, the trial test is given to a group similar to the one being used, but such students may not be available to many teachers. It is of interest to note that Educational Testing Service uses a minimum sample of 420 for pilot studies. The reason fairly large numbers of students are needed is that sampling stability is needed for the *incorrect* answer as well as the correct one. To achieve this stability, at least fifteen people must choose *each* incorrect alternative.

Item Difficulty

The item difficulty is determined by the proportion of students answering an item correctly.

$$p = \frac{\# R}{N}$$ (Formula 8–3)

where p = item difficulty
$\# R$ = number answering correctly
N = total number in group

The item difficulty does not identify the individuals who answer correctly. Therefore, we have no information on the degree to which the item discriminates between good and poor scorers on the test. However, the difficulty level does affect the maximal discrimination that can be achieved.

Maximal discrimination can be achieved at the 50 percent difficulty level. If items are too easy or too hard, we learn nothing about the relative levels of achievement of the students. Ebel (1965) suggests that a middle difficulty level (30 to 70 percent) discriminates almost as well as a level of 50 percent. Note that this standard does not apply to criterion-referenced tests, where a difficulty level of 90 percent may be desirable. The relationship of the difficulty level to the index of discrimination is given in Table 8–7. The column entitled "Bits of Differential Information" shows that more information can be obtained when $p = 50$ percent and the maximum value of D equals one hundred. If two students answered a question right and two answered the same question wrong, four bits of differential information are provided. The fact that Student 1 has more ability than Students 3 and 4 yields two bits of information. By the same reasoning for Student 2, two additional bits of information are obtained.

TABLE 8–7 • Relation of Item Difficulty Level to Maximum Value of D and to Bits of Differential Information Provided*

Percentage of Correct Response	Maximum Value of D**	Bits of Differential Information
100	0.00	0
90	0.20	36
80	0.40	64
70	0.60	84
60	0.80	96
50	1.00	100
40	0.80	96
30	0.60	84
20	0.40	64
10	0.20	36
0	0.00	0

*Robert L. Ebel, *Measuring Educational Achievement* (Englewood Cliffs, N.J.: Prentice-Hall, Inc., 1965), p. 353, Table 11.1, by permission of the publisher.
**Index of Discrimination

Index of Discrimination Computed by Hand

The index of discrimination, D, yields information on the proportion of high and low scorers on a test who answer an item correctly. On an item that discriminates well, more high scorers answer the item correctly than low scorers. If the reverse occurs—more low scorers answer the item correctly—the item is poorly constructed (Johnson, 1951).

When determining the index of discrimination, the following steps are appropriate:

Step 1:   Separate two subgroups of test papers, an upper group, consisting of approximately 27 percent of the total group, who received highest scores on the test, and a lower group, consisting of an equal number of papers from those who received lowest scores.

Step 2.   Count the number of times each possible response to each item was chosen on the papers of the upper group. Do the same separately for the papers of the lower group.

Step 3.   Record these response counts opposite the responses they refer to on a copy of the test.

Step 4.   Subtract the lower group count of correct responses from the upper group count of correct responses. Divide this difference by the maximum possible difference, that is, the number of papers in the upper (or lower) group.

This quotient, expressed as a decimal fraction, is the index of discrimination (Ebel, 1965, p. 347).

$$D = \frac{R_u - R_l}{N_u} \qquad \textbf{(Formula 8–4)}$$

where D = index of discrimination
R_u = number of correct responses in upper group
R_l = number of correct responses in lower group
N_u = total number in upper group

Twenty-seven percent of the upper and lower extremes is usually recommended so that the differences between the extremes will be maximal (Kelley, 1939). However, Ebel (1965) suggests that 27 percent, although optimal, is not that much better than 25 or 33 percent. Thus a teacher may select extremes using whatever percentage he prefers as long as he stays within the 25 to 33 percent range. If the total sample size is small, the top 9 percent and the bottom 9 percent may be counted twice.

The index of discrimination can be as high as 1.00, although in reality an index that high is never obtained. How high should the index be to reflect adequate discrimination? The generally accepted standards are given in Table 8–8.

TABLE 8–8   •   Evaluation of the Size of the Index of Discrimination*

Index of Discrimination	Item Evaluation
0.40 and up	Very good items
0.30 to 0.39	Reasonably good but possibly subject to improvement
0.20 to 0.29	Marginal items, usually needing and being subject to improvement.
Below 0.19	Poor items, to be rejected or improved by revision

*Robert L. Ebel, *Measuring Educational Achievement* (Englewood Cliffs, N. J.: Prentice-Hall, Inc., 1965), p. 364, by permission of the publisher.

The index of discrimination is also related to the reliability coefficient. The greater the mean item discrimination, the higher the reliability of the test, as shown in Table 8–9.

**TABLE 8-9 •   Relation of Item Discrimination to Test Reliability for a
One-Hundred Item Test***

Mean Index of Discrimination	Standard Deviation of Scores	Reliability of Scores
0.1225	5.00	0.000
0.16	6.53	0.420
0.20	8.16	0.630
0.30	12.25	0.840
0.40	16.32	0.915
0.50	20.40	0.949

*Robert L. Ebel, *Measuring Educational Achievement* (Englewood Cliffs, N. J.: Prentice-Hall, Inc., 1965), p. 366, Table 11.4, by permission of the publisher.

Index of Discrimination Obtained by Computer

When a computer program is available for a complete item analysis, more precise information can be obtained about the discriminating power of each item. The correlation between each alternative of an item with the total test score is computed using biserial or, sometimes, tetrachoric correlation methods. The correlation between the *correct* alternative and the total score will be high and positive if those who answer the item correctly also have a high score on the total test. If this correlation is high and negative, the low scorers answered this item correctly. Thus, a high positive correlation (0.30 or greater) between the correct answer and the total score is desired. A coefficient of 0.70 is considered very good (Harris, 1968).

For each *incorrect* alternative, or distracter, moderate negative correlations are desired, since those who mark this alternative as correct should be the low scorers on the test, *if* the item discriminates well. The correlation between the incorrect alternative and the total score should be in the –0.20 to –0.30 range or greater (Harris, 1968).

Note that the correlation between the alternative and the total score will be spuriously high, because the item is a part of the test and the item score enters into both variables. The smaller the number of items, the greater the spuriousness; that is, the shorter the test, the higher the correlation between alternatives and total test score. A correction factor can be used to adjust for this (Henrysson, 1971). If the correction factor is not applied in shorter tests, the index of discrimination should be greater than 0.30 for the correct answers.

Other measures of discrimination obtained through computer analysis are X_{50} and β, as depicted in Figure 8-1. The symbol X_{50} represents the "point of the criterion scale where item choice has maximum discrimination. . . . Subjects with a criterion score equal to X_{50} have a 50–50 chance of choosing that response" (Harris, 1968, p.11). Notice in Figure 8-1 that

X_{50} is expressed in standard deviation units. An X_{50} value of $+1.65$ standard deviation units discriminates well between good scorers but not between poor scorers, while $X_{50} = -1.65$ discriminates well between poor scorers and not between good ones.

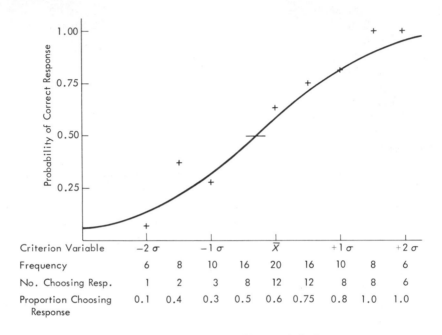

Criterion Variable		$-2\,\sigma$		$-1\,\sigma$		$\bar{X}$		$+1\,\sigma$		$+2\,\sigma$
Frequency		6	8	10	16	20	16	10	8	6
No. Choosing Resp.		1	2	3	8	12	12	8	8	6
Proportion Choosing Response		0.1	0.4	0.3	0.5	0.6	0.75	0.8	1.0	1.0

FIG. 8–1   A Typical Item Characteristic Curve

The symbol β, beta, represents the slope of the item characteristic curve at the X_{50} point. Beta represents the discriminating power of the item, and is interpreted in the same manner as the biserial or tetrachoric r. If $\beta = 0$, the item has no discriminating power. Figure 8–2 gives examples of items having various item characteristics.

Summary

The physical education teacher often uses written tests to measure the understanding of movement. By developing a test blueprint, the teacher can approach the construction of a written test in a systematic way. The blueprint is determined by the purposes of the test and the group for which the test is designed. When the blueprint has been completed, the appropriate

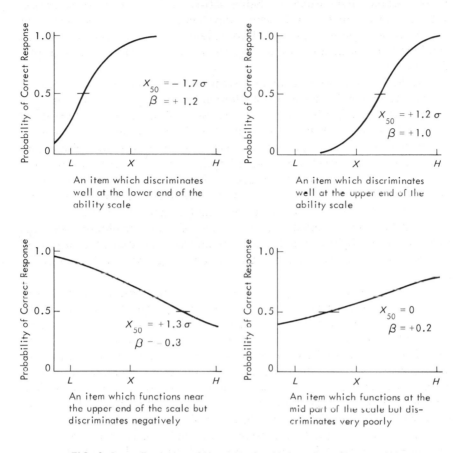

An item which discriminates
well at the lower end of the
ability scale

An item which discriminates
well at the upper end of the
ability scale

An item which functions near
the upper end of the scale but
discriminates negatively

An item which functions at the
mid part of the scale but discriminates very poorly

FIG. 8-2   Examples of Items Having Various Item Characteristics

content and behaviors may be recorded in a table of specifications. The teacher may then proceed with the actual construction of the test.

When developing a written test, the directions for test administration
should be clearly stated. Otherwise, measurement error can occur owing to
faulty administration procedures. The teacher should carefully consider the
administration of the test previous to the actual testing period.

One broad category of test items is that of *selection* items, in which
the student is required to select as the answer one of a given number of alternatives. Within this category, three types of items—alternate-choice,
multiple-choice, and matching—are commonly used.

An alternate-choice item is usually either right or wrong. This type of
item has frequently received much criticism. However, a well-constructed

alternate-choice item would probably satisfy all but the harshest critics. Still, the teacher must guard against developing items that measure only low levels of cognitive behavior. Two advantages of this type of item are objectivity of scoring and ease of construction (as compared with multiple-choice items).

Multiple-choice items contain a stem (an introductory question or an incomplete sentence) and a set of alternatives or suggested options. The correct alternative is referred to as the *answer,* and the incorrect alternatives are called *distracters.* Between three and five alternatives are recommended. The distracters should appear to be reasonable answers, both logically and grammatically. The teacher must guard against ambiguity when constructing multiple-choice items. The advantage of multiple-choice over alternate-choice items is that the correct answer for the former does not have to be totally true, but must have a greater degree of truth than the distracters.

Matching items consist of two columns of words or phrases, with the columns on the right containing the alternatives. The student is instructed to select an alternative from the right column to go with each item in the left one.

A second broad category of test items is *supply* items, in which the student must provide the words, numbers, or other symbols that constitute the response rather than choosing from several designated alternatives. Two commonly-used varieties of the supply test items are short-answer items and essay items. Many teachers prefer to develop *short-answer* tests because the items are relatively easy to construct. However, these tests have several inherent disadvantages. One of these is that more than one response to a question may be correct. Another is that an item requiring a short answer very often measures only the student's memory for fact.

The use of essay questions is often advocated by many educators because such questions are believed to be the best test of the student's ability to express ideas and to analyze and synthesize knowledge. Nonetheless, the essay test has several notable limitations, such as the lack of objectivity associated with the rating of essay questions and the error associated with the sampling of the questions. Since the number of essay questions in a given test cannot be very large, the reliability of the test may be low. A final limitation is that some students are encouraged to bluff on essay-type tests.

Although the construction of an essay test seems easy, the scoring requires a great deal of time and expertise and must be scored by a qualified person. However, the process of scoring is greatly facilitated if sound construction techniques are followed. A model answer may be constructed for each question. One of two scoring methods may be used. One is an analytical system in which a detailed guide to rating is developed. In this system, scoring categories are designated and weights are assigned to each category. The second system uses global ratings by many raters. Each rater is asked to read the essay question through rapidly, formulate his reaction, and rate the question on his immediate reaction.

A correction for guessing may be applied to the scores of certain objective tests. However, correcting for guessing is only effective if some items are omitted by the students taking the test. Thus, the application of a correction factor is useful for *speed* tests but not for *power* tests. In a power test, students should be directed to attempt to answer every question.

Whenever a test is utilized for the first time, an item analysis should be applied to it in order to provide the teacher with information on the test's effectiveness. The determination of item difficulty and the index of discrimination are useful aspects of the item analysis. The *item difficulty* is determined by the proportion of subjects answering an item incorrectly. The *index of discrimination* yields information on the proportion of high and low scorers on a test who answer an item correctly. If an item discriminates well, more high scorers answer the item correctly than low scorers. Maximal discrimination can be achieved at the 50 percent difficulty level.

More precise information can be obtained about the discriminating power of each item. However, a simple item analysis conducted in the classroom (have students in upper and lower groups raise hands for correct answers) may provide the teacher with all of the information he needs for improving his test.

Bibliography

BAKER, F. B. "Origins of the Item Parameters X_{50} and β as a Modern Item Analysis Technique," *Journal of Educational Measurement,* II (1965), pp. 167–80.

BAKER, F. B. "Automation of Test Scoring, Reporting, and Analysis," in *Educational Measurement,* ed. R. L. Thorndike. Washington, D. C.: American Council on Education, 1971.

BROWN, D. J. *Appraisal Procedures in the Secondary Schools.* Englewood Cliffs, N. J.: Prentice-Hall, Inc., 1970.

CLEMANS, W. V. "Test Administration," in *Educational Measurement,* ed. R. L. Thorndike. Washington, D. C.: American Council on Education, 1971.

COFFMAN, W. E. "Essay Examinations," in *Educational Measurement,* ed. R. L. Thorndike. Washington, D. C.: American Council on Education, 1971.

CURETON, E. E. "Measurement Theory," in *Encyclopedia of Educational Research,* ed. R. L. Ebel. New York: The Macmillan Company, 1969.

EBEL, R. L. *Measuring Educational Achievement.* Englewood Cliffs, N. J.: Prentice-Hall, Inc., 1965.

EBEL, R. L. "How to Write True-False Items," *Educational and Psychological Measurement,* XXXI (1971), pp. 417–26.

GOSLING, G. W. W. *Marking English Compositions*. Victoria: Australian Council for Educational Research, 1966.

HARRIS, M. L. "Some Methodological Suggestions for Construction of an Objective Measurement Instrument." Technical Memo from the Wisconsin Research and Development Center for Cognitive Learning. The University of Wisconsin, Madison, December 1968.

HASKINS, M. J. *Evaluation in Physical Education*. Dubuque, Iowa: Wm. C. Brown Company Publishers, 1971.

HENRYSSON, S. "Gathering, Analyzing, and Using Data on Test Items," in *Educational Measurement*, ed. R. L. Thorndike. Washington, D. C.: American Council on Education, 1971.

HOFFMAN, B. *The Tyranny of Testing*. New York: Collier Books, 1964.

JOHNSON, A. P. "Notes on a Suggested Index of Item Validity: The U-L Index," *Journal of Educational Psychology*, LXII (1951), pp. 499–504.

KELLEY, T. L. "The Selection of Upper and Lower Groups for the Validation of Test Items," *Journal of Educational Psychology*, XXX (1939), pp. 17–24.

LEACOCK, S. *The Daily Princetonian*. Princeton, N. J., January 26, 1938.

MILLER, A. P. *In Cold Red Ink*. New York: Adams Press, 1968.

PAGE, E. B. "Grading Essays by Computer: Progress Report," in *Proceedings of the 1966 Invitational Conference on Testing Problems*. Princeton, N. J.: Educational Testing Service, 1967, pp. 417–26.

PAYNE, D. A. *The Specification and Measurement of Learning Outcomes*. Waltham, Mass.: Blaisdell Publishing Company, 1968.

STALNAKER, J. M. "The Essay Type of Examination," in *Educational Measurement* ed. E. F. Lindquist. Washington, D. C.: American Council on Education, 1951.

THORNDIKE, R. L. "The Problem of Guessing," editor's note in *Educational Measurement*, ed. R. L. Thorndike. Washington, D. C.: American Council on Education, 1971.

TINKELMAN, S. N. "Planning the Objective Test," in *Educational Measurement*, ed. R. L. Thorndike. Washington, D. C.: American Council on Education, 1971.

TVERSKY, A. "On the Optimal Number of Alternatives at a Choice Point," *Journal of Mathematical Psychology*, I (1964), pp 386–91.

WESMAN, A. G. "Writing the Test Item," in *Educational Measurement*, ed. R. L. Thorndike. Washington, D. C.: American Council on Education, 1971.

WOOD, D. A. *Test Construction*. Columbus, Ohio: Charles E. Merrill Books, Inc., 1960.

9

the assessment
of physical fitness

Physical fitness is recognized by the general public as well as by professional physical educators as one of the goals of a physical education program. The literature on physical fitness ranges from material in popular magazines to technical articles on research in medical and physiological journals. Clearly, a sizable proportion of the American population is concerned about physical fitness. If an individual recognizes the importance of physical fitness and knows how to improve his level of physical fitness, he will quite likely want to know how fit he is. How can he assess his level of physical fitness? If physical fitness is considered one of the goals of a physical education program, how can the physical educator determine the degree to which this goal is being met? In this chapter, instead of a wide variety of available fitness tests, selected tests that are widely used will be presented and analyzed.

Definition of Physical Fitness

Although physical fitness has been defined in many ways, two definitions seem to be most commonly used. From a medical point of view, physical fitness is defined as the capacity to adapt to and recover from strenuous exercise. A more general definition considers physical fitness as "the ability to carry out daily tasks with vigor and alertness, without undue fatigue, and with ample energy to enjoy leisure time pursuits and to meet unforeseen emergencies" (Clarke, 1971, p.1). In several physical education texts, physical fitness is differentiated from motor fitness in that motor fitness includes abilities that are not components of physical fitness (Johnson and Nelson, 1969; Mathews, 1969). According to these authors, physical fitness reflects cardiorespiratory fitness. In this chapter, the distinction between motor fitness and physical fitness will not be made. Physical fitness, however, is differentiated from motor ability, which is sometimes referred to as general athletic ability. Even though some of the tests designed to measure motor ability represent commendable efforts, little is known about motor ability as a construct. Since there is no new material on motor ability that is not already available in other books (Barrow and McGee, 1972; Haskins, 1971; Johnson and Nelson, 1969; Mathews, 1969), motor ability tests are not included in this text.

Components of Physical Fitness

In the first issue of the *Physical Fitness Research Digest,* July 1971 (Clarke, 1971), three components of physical fitness were described as commonly accepted elements of fitness. They are muscular strength, muscular endurance, and cardiorespiratory endurance. Other components that are often identified as elements of physical fitness are muscular power, agility, speed, flexibility, and balance. These components may be generally defined as follows:

> *Muscular strength:* contraction force of muscles.
>
> *Muscular endurance:* continuous muscular contraction until muscle is fatigued.
>
> *Circulatory-respiratory endurance:* moderate contractions of large muscle groups until predetermined circulatory-respiratory state is reached.
>
> *Muscular power:* ability to release maximum muscular force in the shortest time.
>
> *Agility:* speed in changing body positions or in changing directions.
>
> *Speed:* rapidity with which successive movements of the same kind can be performed.
>
> *Flexibility:* range of movement in a joint or a sequence of joints.
>
> *Balance:* ability to maintain body equilibrium.

These definitions, although general, serve as an orientation to the study of fitness. Most scholarly discussions of physical fitness break down each component of fitness into subcomponents.

Strength

Strength has been divided into at least three subcomponents: static strength, dynamic strength, and explosive strength. *Static strength* is "the maximum effective force that can be applied once to a fixed object by an individual from a defined, immobile position" (Van Huss and Huesner, 1970, p.4). A common measure of this type of strength is the hand dynamometer. Other measurement techniques are described in Johnson and Nelson, 1969; Mathews, 1969; Van Huss and Huesner, 1970.

Dynamic strength can be defined as "the maximum load which can be moved once, through a specified range of motion of a joint, with the body in some defined position" (Van Huss and Huesner, 1970, p.5). The military press in weight lifting is an example of dynamic strength.

Explosive strength is defined as "the ability to exert maximum energy in one explosive act" (Fleishman, 1964, p. 29). Strength defined in this way is also referred to as power. The shot put and the high jump are examples of explosive strength.

Endurance (Muscular)

Two types of muscular endurance have been identified: static and dynamic. *Static muscular endurance* is "the length of time a given intensity of a defined contraction can be maintained" (Van Huss and Huesner, 1970, p.5). Holding a heavy object is an example of this type of muscular endurance.

Dynamic muscular endurance "ranges from [the ability] to perform a minimum of two repetitions of a task involving a high intensity of work to that required to repeat a task involving a low intensity of work many times" (Van Huss and Huesner, 1970, p.6). Van Huss and Huesner (1970) subdivide this category into three subclassifications. These classifications, with accompanying examples, are:

> *Dynamic muscular endurance—short (short duration, high intensity)*
>   Chins (college men)
>   20–yard dash (college men)
>   50–yard sprint in swimming (college men)
>   25–yard sprint in swimming (children)
> *Dynamic muscular endurance—medium (medium duration, moderate intensity)*
>   440–yard dash
>   880–yard dash
> *Dynamic muscular endurance—long (long duration, low intensity)*
>   Distance cycling
>   Distance running
>   Distance swimming

For the most part, school testing should be limited to the first subclassification, Dynamic muscular endurance—short (Van Huss and Huesner, 1970). The following measures are recommended: 100–yard dash, and number of repetitions in 20 seconds of pullups, push-ups, and bent-knee sit-up tests.

For high school boys, increasing the length of the dash to 220 yards is re-commended. The pullup and push-up tests are not recommended for girls. Time limits are suggested for pullups, push-ups and sit-ups since timed and untimed measures are highly correlated. Other advantages of a time limit are that test administration time is saved, the effects of motivation are mini-mized, and extreme muscle soreness from prolonged testing is avoided.

When interpreting the results of strength and muscular endurance tests, not only age and sex, but also body weight, should be taken into account because weight is correlated with both strength and endurance. For example, heavier individuals tend to perform better than light individuals on static strength measures, while the reverse is true for static muscular endurance measures.

A brief discussion of *isometric* and *isotonic* exercise is appropriate. The main advantage of *isometric* exercise is that it can be done anywhere within a short period of time. Studies have shown that a strength gain of one to two percent per week can be obtained with a single daily six-second contraction against resistance equal to two-thirds of the muscle's strength. However, isometrics must be applied throughout the range of motion of the joint. Otherwise, strength is developed only at one point (Clarke, 1971).

There are several advantages of *isotonic* exercise. Generally, motivation is better. As compared with isometrics, both recovery from muscular fatigue and development of muscular endurance are faster with isotonics. (Clarke, 1971). When isometric exercises are performed, the circulation to the con-tracting muscle is occluded, which interferes with the oxygen supply. This phenomenon does not occur with isotonic exercise. In heart disease patients, "isometric exercise as contrasted with [isotonic] is more prone to produce irregular heart beats, premature ventricular contractions, and abnormally fast heart beats" (Clarke, 1971, p.11). Although these results can not be generalized to the healthy individual, it does seem that isometric exercise and testing are of little value in the school if the same benefits can be obtained from isotonics, for which there is greater motivation.

In a discussion of *endurance,* Welch (1970) distinguishes between endurance tests and cardiovascular tests. The former are performance tests that are affected by motivation, while the latter are tests of physiological capacity. He recommends using the 12-Minute Run Test (which is described later in this chapter) in the public schools, but cautions against applying adult standards to an adolescent population. For students in junior high school, a shorter test of eight minutes or one mile may be desirable. In any case the teacher should develop his own norms. For elementary school children, Welch (1970) suggests that the best measure of endurance is the 600-yard run-walk, although he questions the use of any endurance test for this age group because of motivational problems.

Cardiorespiratory Fitness

Circulatory-respiratory fitness is defined as "the capacity of circulatory-respiratory system to function during sports or other physical activities which require sustained effort" (Montoye, 1970, p. 41). This type of fitness can be estimated by measuring maximal oxygen uptake while performing to exhaustion on the treadmill, the bicycle ergometer, or in a bench test.

Because these methods are not practical for use in the schools, a submaximal test may be used as a satisfactory substitute. In submaximal testing, heart rate and work load are used to obtain a rough estimate of maximal oxygen uptake. The postexercise heart rate is measured, as in the Harvard Step Test (Brouha, 1943). Montoye (1970) recommends using the Harvard Step Test or a modification of it for normal children from 8 to 22 years of age. Modifications of the test for different age groups are suggested. A shortcut can be used whereby the pulse beats from 30 seconds to one minute after exercise are counted instead of calculating the Harvard Step Test score by the recommended formula. Using this modification in scoring, teachers would have to develop their own performance standards.

Flexibility

Flexibility is defined as the range of movement about a joint. Fleishman (1964) refers to two types of flexibility: extent flexibility and dynamic flexibility. Extent flexibility refers to the ability to extend or stretch some part of the body as far as possible in various directions. Dynamic flexibility involves the ability to make repeated flexing or stretching movements. This type of flexibility consists of three subdivisions: speed of limb movement, speed of change of directions, and running speed.

A commonly used test of flexibility is touching the floor with finger tips, keeping the knees straight. A variation of this test is performed standing on a bench, from which the subject reaches down as far as possible on an attached scale. This type of measure is criticized for several reasons. The foremost reason is that flexibility is highly specific, and thus the measurement of the flexibility of a few joints provides no indication of an indivdual's overall flexibility (Harris, 1969; Sigerseth, 1970). In addition, the ability to touch the floor is dependent upon the lengths of body segments. The process of scoring requires subjective judgment, and no scoring ranges are provided since a pass-fail or deviation score is used. Finally, this type of measure is not restricted to the measurement of individual joints.

Sigerseth (1970) recommends determining flexibility by measuring the movements of body segments in degrees. The flexometer is an instrument that can be used in a school situation. Reliability coefficients for the instrument range from 0.901 to 0.983 (Sigerseth, 1970). Since flexibility is highly task specific, it is doubtful that the measurement of this component is useful within the typical school setting. Although the flexometer is not an expensive device, the cost in terms of the amount of time required for administering the tests would be prohibitive. For detailed information on measurement techniques and norms for males and females at selected ages, see Sigerseth (1970).

More sophisticated devices are available for measuring flexibility. One is the electrogoniometer (elgon), that records in degrees the changes in the angles of joints during movement. The manual goniometer records the angles of joints in stationary positions. These devices are not practical for use in most teaching situations, and therefore will not be described in detail in this chapter.

Balance

There are indications that balance has the same degree of specificity as flexibility. For example, Sanborn and Wyrick (1969) found no relationship between the ability to perform the same balance task at different heights. Fleishman (1964) however, isolated three types of balance in his schema: static balance, dynamic balance, and balancing objects. *Static balance* is the ability to maintain body equilibrium in some fixed position. *Dynamic balance* is the ability of an individual to maintain balance while performing some task. *Balancing objects* involves balancing an object for a given period of time.

Summary

Due to the large number of subcomponents of physical fitness, the measurement of total fitness is extremely difficult. Evaluation of measures of fitness should be made with these subcomponents in mind.

Administration of Physical Fitness Tests

Tests of motor performance may involve even more administrative problems than written tests. Not only must the student understand the directions to the test, but he must also be able to follow the directions while taking the test. For example, in the shuttle run, a student may make numerous errors because he does not understand the directions or cannot follow them. He may throw the block across the line instead of placing it on the ground or forget the number of times he must change directions. In either case the trial should be thrown out—an easy statement to make, but an unpleasant suggestion for the teacher with large numbers of students who must be tested within a short period of time. The solution lies primarily in adequate preparation for testing.

Preparation for Testing

When fitness tests are administered, we want to know what the *best* performance level of each student is. Thus, a student should be thoroughly familiar with the test. To expose a student to the shuttle run on the day of the test is asking the student to perform a novel task. In that case, it would be his ability to perform a new task that is measured. Part of his energy and attention are devoted to *how* to perform the test. If we are interested in his ability to learn a new task, this procedure might be a satisfactory one. However, this is probably not our major concern in physical fitness testing. Very likely we are interested in his *level of fitness*. If so, the nature of the test must not interfere with his ability to perform.

On the other hand, the idea of preparation can be carried to extremes. Such a procedure as requiring a student to practice the shuttle run day after day as a part of his regular physical education program can hardly be justified. If practicing the shuttle run increases the student's agility, then *some* practice is legitimate. However, we also assume that other means of improving agility exist that will contribute to the student's overall agility level. This is an assumption and not a known fact because there is no satisfactory measure of overall agility. Agility, in fact, may be highly task specific. Yet we must recognize that the selection of a single test, such as the shuttle run, as a measure of a component of fitness (agility), indicates that we think this test measures agility in an overall sense. If the test is not an overall measure of agility, and practice on the shuttle run increases test performance while practicing agility in other ways does not, the fault does not lie with the test but with our interpretation of it.

Test preparation also includes practical issues, such as the clothing a student wears for testing. In junior and senior high school where students wear special uniforms for physical education classes, this is not a problem. In the elementary schools where special uniforms are not required, the problem created by inadequate attire can be acute. Whether the testing takes place indoors or outdoors, tennis shoes should be worn. Without them, the student will have trouble approaching his best performance level. If he performs the shuttle run indoors with bare feet, the quick shift of directions can create enough friction between the floor and the bottoms of the feet to be painful. With street shoes, the problem in one of sliding because he is unable to stop. If the testing takes place outdoors, the situation is somewhat better for the student without tennis shoes, but it is far from ideal. As long as the student can move freely, a wide variety of clothing would be satisfactory, but proper shoes are essential. The teacher must stress this point with the students ahead of time.

Because fitness testing is so extensive in nature, assistants are usually needed. Whether the assistants are teachers or students, they should be thoroughly familiarized with the tests which they will administer. Score sheets, clipboards, and pencils should be provided for all assistants.

Data Processing of Physical Fitness Results

The process of administering fitness tests within a school is in itself an enormous task. Once the scores of the tests have been recorded, the teacher is then faced with the job of analyzing them. There is no justification for the administration of tests of any kind if the results are not utilized. If the school district has access to a computer, the scores can be handled for the teachers in a way that requires minimal time and effort. A small proportion of school districts throughout the country already use computers for analyzing fitness data. Several school districts in New York State use data processing equipment to process fitness results. The procedures used by these schools have been described in Straub and Hungerford (1969).

Number of Trials

In administering a given fitness test, the number of trials needed is determined by the reliability of the test. The practice of selecting the best trial out of the total number administered may be appropriate in competition, but is inappropriate in a physical education class where we are concerned with a reliable estimate of a student's performance. One trial, in most cases, will not be reliable.

If we want to have a stable representation of performance, we must eliminate the effects of practice, learning, and fatigue. In other words, we want to eliminate any trend effect. (The trend effect was discussed in the chapter on reliability, in which methods of removing the effect of trend when computing the reliability coefficient were presented.) In a group of trials in which trend occurs, does the average of the trials represent stable performance? If, for example, six trials formed the pattern depicted in Figure 9–1, which trials should be selected to represent stable performance? (The number of trials selected must *still* have a satisfactory reliability coefficient.)

The effect of trend appears to be evident in the first three trials, while performance seems to level off in Trial 4 and remain stable. Should we use the mean of *all* trials for the student's score, or the mean of the last three trials? This decision cannot be made arbitrarily. However, we can compute the reliabilities for different combinations of trials and then make our decision.

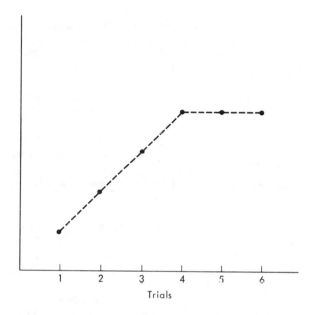

FIG. 9–1   Group of Six Trials with First Three Affected by Trend

Baumgartner and Jackson (1970) computed reliabilities for measures in which a trend exists across trials, and then computed a second reliability coefficient for each measure with the trials causing the trend removed. The results of their study are presented in Table 9–1. Note the reliability of the standing broad jump performed by junior high school boys compared with the reliability of the jump performed by senior high boys. All took six trials of the broad jump on one day. The high school boys displayed a practice effect on the first three trials, and leveled off on the last three, similar to the pattern shown in Figure 9–1. The highest reliability estimate for the senior high boys was obtained using the last three trials, where $R = 0.97$. Thus, a senior high school teacher would have to administer six trials, but use only the average of the last three for the student's score.

On the other hand, the junior high boys performed in a stable manner on the *first* three trials, and performance dropped off systematically over the last three trials, as shown in Figure 9–2. Presumably, the junior high boys fatigued after the third trial. At any rate, the best estimate of reliability is based on the first three trials ($R = 0.97$), indicating that only three

TABLE 9–1 • Results of Two Measurement Schedules for All Groups*

Group	Test	No. of Trials	$\overline{X}$	F^a	Trials selected	$\overline{X}$	F^a	R
		All trials			**Best trial grouping**			
Junior high	Standing broad jump	6	68.94	2.05	1–3	69.31	1.21	0.96
	40-yd. shuttle run	4	10.61	3.45ᵇ	2–3	10.52	1.41	0.76
Senior high	Standing broad jump	6	81.87	11.03ᵇ	3–6	82.68	0.37	0.97
	40-yd. shuttle run	4	9.86	12.78ᵇ	3–4	9.73	0.62	0.82
College men I	Standing broad jump	6	89.41	5.57ᵇ	3–6	89.90	0.24	0.95
	50-yd. shuttle run	4	11.23	17.90ᵇ	3–4	11.14	1.10	0.85
College men II	Agility side step	5	28.59	71.37ᵇ	3–5	29.87	8.96ᵇ	0.95
Physical education majors	Grip	4	55.21	3.30ᵇ	1–3	55.41	1.13	0.97
	Elbow flexion	3	24.80	0.76	1–3	24.80	0.76	0.99
	Knee extension	5	49.53	3.02ᵇ	2–5	49.70	0.89	0.99
	Knee flexion	5	23.47	3.20ᵇ	2–5	23.56	1.82	0.97
	Ankle plantar flexion	5	51.04	9.06ᵇ	2–5	51.43	0.47	0.97
	Jump and reach	6	22.98	21.43ᵇ	2–6	23.15	1.16	0.98
	Running jump and reach	5	24.86	2.87ᵇ	2–5	24.91	2.32	0.98
	Standing broad jump	5	91.86	7.53ᵇ	2–5	92.22	1.07	0.97
	Timed softball throw	5	0.21	0.29	1–5	0.21	0.29	0.90
	Timed volleyball throw	4	0.20	9.70ᵇ	2–4	0.19	0.95	0.74
	Timed basketball pass	4	0.461	7.02ᵇ	2–4	0.458	0.97	0.92
	Timed soccer ball pass	4	0.23	2.54	1–4	0.23	2.54	0.60
	20-yd. sprint	2	2.84	2.98	1–2	2.84	2.98	0.79
	50-yd. sprint	2	6.22	5.61ᵇ	1–2	6.22	5.61ᵇ	0.95
	Left boomerang	5	7.15	25.95ᵇ	3–5	7.10	1.33	0.93
	Dodging run	5	6.88	46.97ᵇ	3–5	6.80	2.34	0.96
	Shuttle run	5	5.15	32.67ᵇ	4–5	5.07	5.82ᵇ	0.88

a This is the F for testing trial-to-trial variation
b Significant at 0.05 level

*Reprinted from Table 1 of T. Baumgartner and A. Jackson, "Measurement Schedules for Tests of Motor Performance," *Research Quarterly,* XLI (1970), 10–14, and by permission of the authors and publisher.

trials need to be given to this age group, but that the average of the three must be used for the student's score.

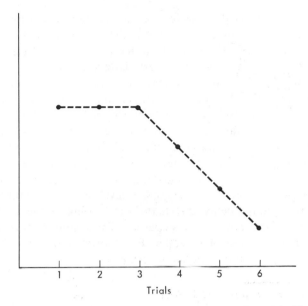

FIG. 9 2   Group of Six Trials with Last Three Affected by Trend

The high school teacher may wish to settle for a lower reliability estimate and use fewer trials, because of the time element involved, but he should recognize that he is not measuring the most stable performance of his boys. The practice of using fewer trials than actually administered in order to obtain maximum reliability (*not* to select the best performance score) needs further study for a wide range of tests over all age groups and for both sexes.

Baumgartner (1969) has investigated the stability over time of the standing broad jump and the side step performed by college men. Three trials of the broad jump were given on each of three days, and five trials of the side step test were administered over the same time period. The standing broad jump scores were stable over the first two days, but increased significantly on the third day. The side step test scores increased significantly from trial to trial as well as from day to day. In another study, elementary school children took twelve trials of the standing broad jump on each of two days, and 60 percent of the children performed their best jump on the second day (Kane and Meredith, 1952). The children had had no previous experience with the standing broad jump. These studies indicate that we cannot assume stability of performance over a given number of days, and that the conditions under which stability occurs need extensive exploration.

Kraus-Weber Test of Physical Fitness

Historically, physical fitness receives great emphasis during times of war. The first widespread interest in physical fitness for the nation as a whole came about as a result of the use of the Kraus-Weber Test (1953). This test was designed as a medical-clinical test battery to examine adult patients with functional low-back pain. Patients who were free from organic disease were treated with the therapeutic exercise, and as back pain decreased the test results improved. When the patient stopped exercising, the low back pain returned and test failures increased. The test was then used as a measure of the minimal level of muscular physical fitness of United States' and European children. European children proved to be markedly superior to United States children on the test items. The use of the test battery was justified on the assumption that there is a level of strength and flexibility of certain muscle groups below which the functioning of the whole body as a healthy organism seems to be impaired. The results of this testing were brought to the attention of President Eisenhower and were of widespread concern to many lay and professional people.

Description of the Kraus-Weber Test

The Kraus-Weber Test consists of six items. The original battery was scored on a scale of from one to ten. However, the tests were subsequently scored on a pass-fail basis by many physical educators.

> **Test 1. Strength of the abdominal plus psoas muscles.** The subject is in a supine position, hands behind the neck. The examiner holds his feet down. The test is to perform one sit-up.
>
> **Test 2. Strength of the abdominal muscles without psoas.** The subject is in the same position as in Test 1, except the knees are bent with the heels close to the buttocks. The test is to perform one sit-up.
>
> **Test 3. Strength of the psoas and lower abdominal muscles.** The subject is supine with hands behind the neck. The legs are fully extended with the heels ten inches off the table. The test is to hold this position for ten seconds.
>
> **Test 4. Strength of the upper back muscles.** The subject lies prone with a pillow under hips and lower abdomen, hands behind the neck. The examiner holds his feet down. The subject must raise his chest, head, and shoulders and hold them without touching the table for ten seconds.
>
> **Test 5. Strength of the lower back.** The subject is in the same position as in Test 4, except that the examiner holds his chest down. The subject must raise his legs off the table, with knees straight, and hold this position for ten seconds.
>
> **Test 6. Length of back and hamstring muscles.** The subject stands erect in stocking or bare feet, hands at his side, feet together. The subject leans down slowly and touches the floor with the finger tips. This position is held for three

seconds. Bouncing is not permitted. The examiner should hold the knees of the person being tested in order to prevent any bend and to detect a slight bend in case it occurs.

Critique of the Kraus-Weber Test

The most comprehensive critique of the Kraus-Weber Test was written by Kendall in 1965. Tests 1 and 2, both sit-up tests, can be evaluated within the same framework. Four types of sit-ups can be described. One type is the sit-up with the back flexed and knees extended. In this case, the abdominal muscles are flexed, and then the hip flexor muscles flex. A second type is the sit-up with the back flexed and the knees flexed. Here, the same two muscle groups act, but the hip flexors work through a different arc of motion in this exercise than in the first one. A common misconception is that the psoas muscles do not contribute when executing sit-ups with the knees flexed (Kendall, 1965; Soderberg, 1966). However no sit-up would occur if the hip flexors were not acting. The third type of sit-up is the one with the back arched and knees extended. Here the pelvis is tilted and the upper trunk is brought to a sitting position by the hip flexors. The fourth type of sit-up is done with the back arched, and the knees flexed. Again, the hip flexors are not eliminated. In each of these types of sit-ups, the feet may be held. If the feet are held, weakness of the abdominal muscles may be obscured. If an individual is not able to curl the trunk while attaining the sitting position, quite likely the hip flexors are doing all the work. Kendall recommends that the feet not be held in the initial phase of the movement. She cites a study which was conducted in an elementary school in which sixty-nine students were tested on sit-ups. All could perform the sit-ups with feet held. Eleven could not perform any sit-ups when the feet were not held. Two had only 50 percent of their potential upper abdominal strength and still did sit-ups with the feet held. Kendall suggests that the feet be held only in the final phase of sit-ups if the body build requires it, in other words, if the torso is heavy in relation to the legs. Many men need this support but most women and adolescent boys and girls do not.

Kendall states that Test 3 is useful for determining the strength of the lower abdominals, but not as used here. Lifting the legs is the action of the hip flexor muscles. "The test is whether the abdominal muscles can maintain the posterior pelvic tilt to keep the low back flat on the table, while the legs are raised or lowered" (Kendall, 1965, pp. 190–91). She suggests that the legs be raised to a 90 degree angle. The subject should hold the lower back down on the table, and slowly lower the legs. The moment the lower back begins to arch and pelvis starts to tilt forward, note the angle of the legs with the table. A 60 degree angle would equal 60 percent abdominal strength. A 40 degree angle would indicate 80 percent abdominal strength. A 20 degree angle (roughly ten inches off the table) would equal 90 percent abdominal strength. Most school children would fall between 60 percent and 80 percent abdominal strength. As it is, Test 3 measures endurance of the hip flexor muscles, and length of time the abdominal muscles can tolerate strain.

Test 4 is a good test of back extensors but not of the upper back. The action occurs in lower back muscles. Very few weaknesses occur in this area so this test is basically unnecessary.

Test 5, which is purported to measure strength of the lower back, is in fact not localized to the low-back area. The gluteal muscles are used also. Again, because of the low failure rate, this is not a discriminating test.

Test 6, measuring the back and hamstring muscles, can be useful but children between the ages of ten and fourteen might be harmed. At these ages there is a discrepancy between leg length and trunk length. The test is satisfactory for young children and for adults. One other point should be considered here. One of the two muscle groups may be short, the other having compensated by elongation. This can easily be checked by placing the individual in a sitting position. In fact, Kendall recommends testing the hamstrings in a sitting position. This is a better test because it is easier to keep the knees straight, and also tilting or rotating of the pelvis will be prevented.

Some additional comments on the Kraus-Weber Test are appropriate here. Only one standard is applied for all age levels and for both sexes. Because of the differences between boys and girls and the differences among the various age levels, the application of only one standard to any age or either sex is questionable. The abdominal minus psoas test is failed most often by girls. The flexibility test is failed most often by boys. The low failure rate on back tests makes these test items indiscriminate. Because strength failures on the Kraus-Weber Test decrease with age and flexibility failures increase with age, these two items when scored on the pass-fail system counteract each other to the extent that it appears no changes occur as age increases. The test emphasizes strength, and then only at a minimal level. Items such as endurance, balance, and agility are not measured at all.

AAHPER Youth Fitness Battery

In 1958, the AAHPER Youth Fitness Battery was published as the first nationwide attempt to formulate a battery of fitness tests (Hunsicker, 1958). Both the age and classification norms were revised (Hunsicker and Reiff, 1966) and presented in the 1965 test manual. The battery included seven items:

Pullups (boys) and flexed-arm hang (girl): measures arm and shoulder strength.
Sit-ups: measures efficiency of abdominal and hip flexor muscles.
Shuttle run: measures speed and change of direction.
Standing broad jump: measures explosive muscle power of leg extensors.
50-yard dash: measures speed.
Softball throw: measures skill and coordination.
600-yard run-walk: measures cardiovascular efficiency.

The organization of a battery of tests and the development of national norms represent commendable efforts. However, no validation procedures were described for the test items aside from a general statement of expert opinion regarding the important components of fitness. In addition, reliabilities for the various age groups on the battery items were not reported in the test manual. Therefore, in the following section an attempt will be made to consolidate some of the evidence that has been reported on the reliability and validity of the test.

Test Descriptions*

1 • Flexed-Arm Hang (girls)

EQUIPMENT. A horizontal bar approximately $1\frac{1}{2}$ inches in diameter is preferred. A doorway gym bar can be used; if no regular equipment is available, a piece of pipe can serve the purpose. A stop watch is needed.

DESCRIPTION. The height of the bar should be adjusted so it is approximately equal to the pupil's standing height. The pupil should use an overhand grasp (Fig. 9–3). With the assistance of two spotters, one in front and one in back of pupil, the pupil raises her body off the floor to a position where the chin is above the bar, the elbows are flexed, and the chest is close to the bar (Fig. 9–4). The pupil holds this position as long as possible.

RULES. 1. The stop watch is started as soon as the subject takes the hanging position.
2. The watch is stopped when (a) pupil's chin touches the bar, (b) pupil's head tilts backward to keep chin above bar, (c) pupil's chin falls below the level of the bar.

*AAHPER Youth Fitness Manual (Washington, D.C.: AAHPER, 1965), 8–15, by permission of the publisher.

SCORING. Record in seconds to the nearest second the length of time the subject holds the hanging position.

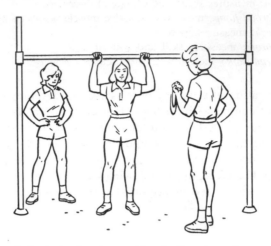

FIG. 9–3   Starting position for flexed-arm hang

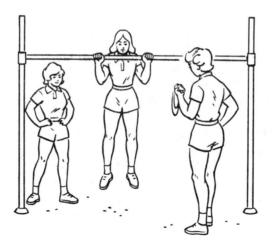

FIG. 9–4   Flexed-arm hang

1 • Pullups (boys)

EQUIPMENT. A metal or wooden bar approximately $1\frac{1}{2}$ inches in diameter is preferred. A doorway gym bar can be used, and, if no regular equipment is available, a piece of pipe or even the rungs of a ladder can also serve the purpose (Fig. 9–5).

DESCRIPTION. The bar should be high enough so that the pupil can hang with his arms and legs fully extended and his feet free of the floor.

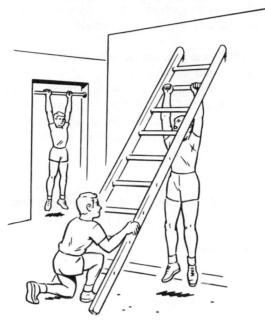

FIG. 9–5 Improvised equipment for pullup—doorway gym bar in background, ladder in foreground.

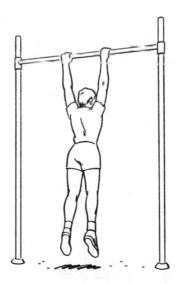

FIG. 9–6 Starting position for pullups

He should use the overhand grasp (Fig. 9–6). After assuming the hanging position, the pupil raises his body by his arms until his chin can be placed over the bar and then lowers his body to a full hang as in the starting position. The exercise is repeated as many times as possible.

RULES. 1. Allow one trial unless it is obvious that the pupil has not had a fair chance.
2. The body must not swing during the execution of the movement. The pull must in no way be a snap movement. If the pupil starts swinging, check this by holding your extended arm across the front of the thighs.
3. The knees must not be raised and kicking of the legs is not permitted.

SCORING. Record the number of completed pullups to the nearest whole number.

2 • *Sit-up (boys and girls)*

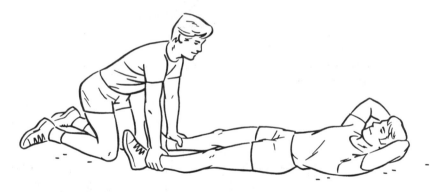

FIG. 9–7   Starting position for sit-up.

EQUIPMENT. Mat or floor.

DESCRIPTION. The pupil lies on his back, either on the floor or on a mat, with legs extended and feet about two feet apart. His hands are placed on the back of the neck with the fingers interlaced. Elbows are retracted. A partner holds the ankles down, the heels being in contact with the mat or floor at all times (Fig. 9–7). The pupil sits up, turning the trunk to the left and touching the right elbow to the left knee, returns to starting position, then sits up turning the trunk to the right and touching the left elbow to the right knee. The exercise is repeated, alternating sides (Fig. 9–8).

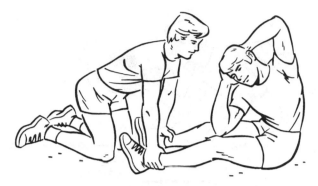

FIG. 9–8   Sit-up.

RULES. 1. The fingers must remain in contact behind the neck throughout the exercise.
2. The knees must be on the floor during the sit-up but may be slightly bent when touching elbow to knee.
3. The back should be rounded and the head and elbows brought forward when sitting up as a "curl" up.
4. When returning to starting position, elbows must be flat on the mat before sitting up again.

SCORING. One point is given for each complete movement of touching elbow to knee. No score should be counted if the fingertips do not maintain contact behind the head, if knees are bent when the pupil lies on his back or when he begins to sit up, or if the pupil pushes up off the floor from an elbow. The maximum limit in terms of number of sit-ups shall be: 50 sit-ups for girls, 100 sit-ups for boys.

3 • Shuttle Run (boys and girls)

EQUIPMENT. Two blocks of wood, 2 inches x 2 inches x 4 inches, and stopwatch. Pupils should wear sneakers or run barefooted.

DESCRIPTION. Two parallel lines are marked on the floor 30 feet apart. The width of a regulation volleyball court serves as a suitable area. Place the blocks of wood behind one of the lines as indicated in Fig. 9–9. The pupil starts from behind the other line. On the signal "Ready? Go" the pupil runs to the blocks, picks one up, runs back to the starting line, and *places* the block behind the line; he then runs back and picks up the second block, which he carries back across the starting line. If the scorer has two

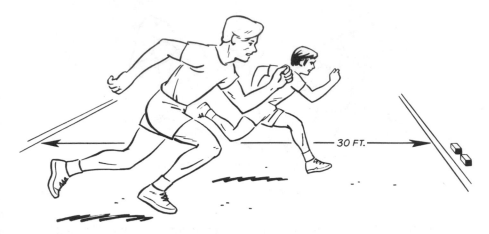

FIG. 9–9   Starting the shuttle run.

stopwatches or one with a split-second timer, it is preferable to have two pupils running at the same time. To eliminate the necessity of returning the blocks after each race, start the races alternately, first from behind one line and then from behind the other.

RULES. Allow two trials with some rest between.

SCORING. Record the time of the better of the two trials to the nearest tenth of a second.

4 • Standing Broad Jump (boys and girls)

EQUIPMENT. Mat, floor, or outdoor jumping pit, and tape measure.

DESCRIPTION. Pupil stands as indicated in Fig. 9–10, with the feet several inches apart and the toes just behind the take-off line. Preparatory to jumping, the pupil swings the arms backward and bends the knees. The jump is accomplished by simultaneously extending the knees and swinging forward the arms.

RULES. 1. Allow three trials.
2. Measure from the take-off line to the heel or other part of the body that touches the floor nearest the take-off line (Fig. 9–10).
3. When the test is given indoors, it is convenient to tape the tape measure to the floor at right angles to the take-off line and have the pupils jump along the tape. The scorer

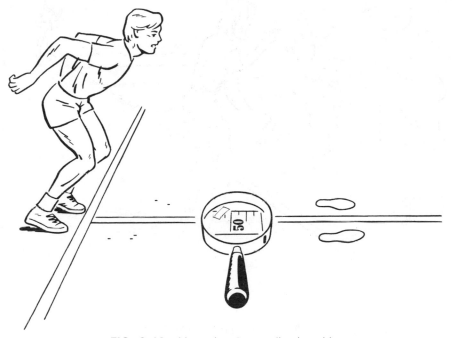

FIG. 9-10   Measuring the standing broad jump.

stands to the side and observes the mark to the nearest inch.

SCORING. Record the best of the three trials in feet and inches to the nearest inch.

5 • 50 yard Dash (boys and girls)

EQUIPMENT. Two stopwatches or one with a split-second timer.

DESCRIPTION. It is preferable to administer this test to two pupils at a time. Have both take positions behind the starting line. The starter will use the commands "Are you ready?" and "Go!" The latter will be accompanied by a downward sweep of the starter's arm to give a visual signal to the timer, who stands at the finish line.

RULES. The score is the amount of time between the starter's signal and the instant the pupil crosses the finish line.

SCORING. Record in seconds to the nearest tenth of a second.

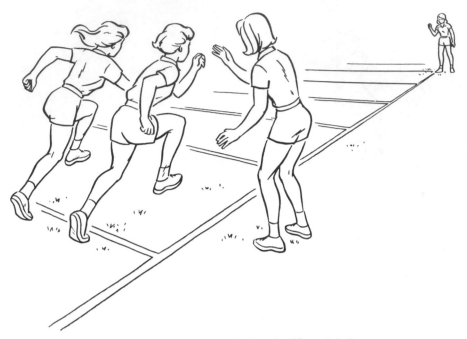

FIG. 9–11   Starting the 50-yard dash.

6 • *Softball Throw for Distance (boys and girls)*

EQUIPMENT. Softball (12-inch), small metal or wooden stakes, and tape measure.

DESCRIPTION. A football field marked in conventional fashion (five-yard intervals) makes an ideal area for this test. If this is not available, it is suggested that lines be drawn parallel to the restraining line, five yards apart. The pupil throws the ball while remaining within two parallel lines, six feet apart (Fig. 9–12). Mark the point of landing with one of the small stakes. If his second or third throw is farther, move the stake accordingly so that, after three throws, the stake is at the point of the pupil's best throw. It was found expedient to have the pupil jog out to his stake and stand there; and then, after five pupils have completed their throws, the measurements were taken. By having the pupil at his particular stake, there is little danger of recording the wrong score.

RULES. 1. Only an overhand throw may be used.
2. Three throws are allowed.
3. The distance recorded is the distance measured at right angles from the point of landing to the restraining line (Fig. 9–12).

SCORING. Record the best of the three trials to the nearest foot.

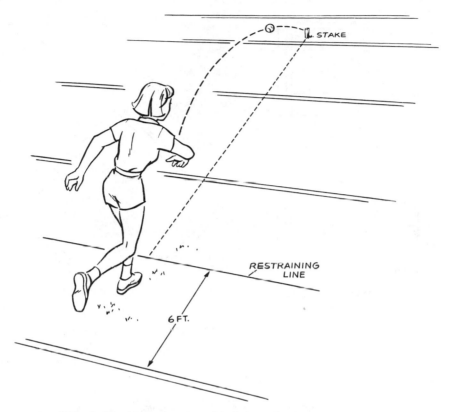

FIG. 9–12   Measuring the softball throw for distance.
Wherever ball lands, measure distance perpendicular to starting line.

7 • *600-yard Run-Walk (boys and girls)*

EQUIPMENT. Track or area marked according to Fig. 9–13, 9–14, 9–15 and stopwatch.

DESCRIPTION. Pupil uses a standing start. At the signal "Ready? Go!" the pupil starts running the 600-yard distance. The running may be interspersed with walking. It is possible to have a dozen pupils run at one time by having the pupils pair off before the start of the event. Then each pupil listens for and remembers his partner's time as the latter crosses the finish. The timer merely calls out the times as the pupils cross the finish.

RULES. Walking is permitted, but the object is to cover the distance in the shortest possible time.

SCORING. Record in minutes and seconds.

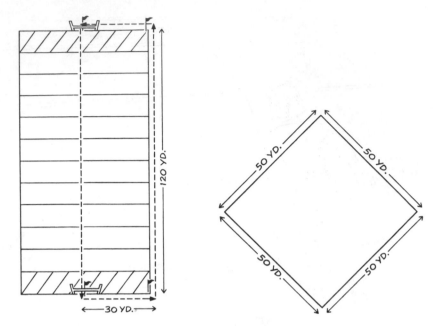

FIG. 9–13 Using football field for 600-yard run-walk.

FIG. 9–14 Using any open area for 600-yard run-walk.

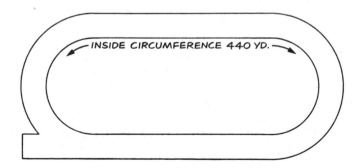

FIG. 9–15 Using inside track for 600-yard run-walk.

Reliability

Only one study has reported reliabilities for all ages and both sexes on the multitrial items of the Youth Fitness Test, which consist of the standing broad jump, the shuttle run, the 50-yard dash, and the softball throw (Marmis et al., 1969). The correlation coefficients for between-trial comparisons, along with differences in trial means, were studied to determine the number of trials needed for a reliable performance. A summary of the results indicates that the following number of trials are needed:

Standing Broad Jump: Instead of three trials, two would be sufficient.
Shuttle Run: Instead of two trials, at least three are necessary.
50-yard Dash: Two, as prescribed, are necessary.
Softball Throw: Instead of three trials, two would be sufficient.

Other reliability coefficients that have been reported in the literature are presented in Table 9–2. More research has been done on the 600-yard run-

TABLE 9–2 • Reliabilities for AAHPER Youth Fitness Test Items

Item	Source	Sample	Trials (t) and Days (d)		Reliability Coefficient	
Pullups	Klesius	150 10th grade males	1t,	2d	0.89,	0.82
Flexed-arm hang	Cotten and Marwitz	14 female P. E. majors	2t,	1d	0.74	
Standing Broad Jump	Klesius	150 10th grade males	2t,	1d	0.94,	0.93
	Fleishman	Adult males	2t		0.90	
	Kane and Meredith	100 males, age 7	12t*,	1d	0.97	
		100 females, age 7	12t*,	1d	0.98	
		100 males, age 8	12t*,	1d	0.98	
		100 females, age 8	12t*,	1d	0.98	
		100 males, age 9	12t*,	1d	0.99	
		100 females, age 9	12t*,	1d	0.98	
		75 males, age 7	12t,	2d**	0.83	
		75 females, age 7	12t,	2d**	0.86	
50-yard dash	Baumgartner and Jackson	76 male P. E. majors	2t,	1d	0.949***	
	Klesius	150 10th-grade males	2t,	1d	0.86,	0.83
Softball Throw	Klesius	150 10th-grade males	2t,	1d	0.93	0.90
	Fleishman	adult males	2t		0.93	
600-yard run-walk	Klesius	150 10th-grade males	1t,	2d	0.80,	0.80
	Wilgoose, et al.	70 junior high males	1t,	2d	0.92	
		70 junior high females	1t,	2d	0.92	
	Askew	71 senior high males	1t,	2d	0.762	
		46 senior high females	1t,	2d	0.653	
	Doolittle and Bigbee	9 9th-grade males			0.92	
Sit-ups	Klesius	150 10th-grade males	1t,	2d	0.57	0.68
Shuttle run	Klesius	150 10th-grade males	1t,	2d	0.68,	0.75

*Best of 12 correlated with second-best.
**Best of 12 on one day correlated with best of 12 on second day.
***Intraclass correlation coefficient.

walk test than on the other items, although reliabilities for some of the remaining items can be found in studies of motor ability, growth and development, and strength.

Validity

The validity of each item in the AAHPER Youth Fitness Battery will be considered separately. In some cases, suggested modifications of selected items will be described, although the modified item should be used as a part of the battery only after norms have been developed for the students.

Pullups. Esslinger (1960) suggested that pullups might not be an adequate measure of arm strength. More recently, Berger and Medlin (1969) noted that using chin-ups as a test of absolute strength is not valid because body weight is inversely related to the number of chins performed. Thus, body weight must be taken into account. These investigators developed a formula by which the number of chins can be used to predict maximum chinning strength. Validity has been established for college men and for seventh, eighth, and ninth graders.

Kendall (1965) questioned the adequacy of pullups because this measure yields too many zero scores. When too many students make scores of zero, the measure does not discriminate.

Flexed-arm hang. Cotten and Marwitz (1969) studied the validity of the flexed-arm hang for girls by comparing performance on the AAHPER test with a pullups test and a modified flexed-arm hang test. Pullups were measured using the overhand grip and partial scores were given up to one (0.25, 0.50, 0.75). The reliability of the pullups test was 0.89. The correlation between this test and the AAHPER Flexed-arm Hang was 0.72. In the modified flexed-arm hang test which was developed by Cotten and Marwitz, the hanging position was identical to that of the AAHPER test, but the stopwatch ran until the angle at the elbow became greater than 90 degrees. The reliability for the modified test was 0.83. The correlation between the modified hang and pullups was 0.93. The results of this study indicate that the modified test may be a better measure of the kind of arm strength measured by pullups than the standard flexed-arm hang test. However, this conclusion must be regarded with caution due to the small sample size ($N =$ fourteen college women) used in this study.

Standing broad jump. The standing broad jump is generally accepted as an adequate measure of explosive power, although there is an element of timing involved in executing this jump that does not exist to the same extent for other measures of explosive power such as the vertical jump. The validity of the broad jump might be improved by standardizing the directions for executing the jump. At present, the jump can be measured indoors or outdoors, with or without a jumping pit or mat.

Softball throw. Cotten and Chambers (1968) experimented with variations in the softball throw test. The variations were in the positions from which the ball was thrown. The first variation was called a "feet-in-place throw," where the feet remained flat on the ground during the throw. The second variation was a "knees-in-place throw," where the ball is thrown from the kneeling position with the knees remaining on the ground during the throw. These variations were compared with the standard AAHPER test, the stride throw, in which a step may be taken. The results, based on performance by male college students, suggest that any method of administration is appropriate, but the investigators suggest that the "knees-in-place throw" is easier to administer. There are fewer illegal throws, and less space is required. Also, the coordination and skill factors are reduced, and the explosive strength and arm-shoulder involvement are emphasized. However, either variation probably measures something different from the original softball throw.

The use of a distance measure to assess the throw reduces the validity of this test. Two balls might be thrown with quite different trajectories, yet the distances thrown could be the same, and thus both throws would receive the same score. If the softball throw is included in the battery as a measure of skill and coordination, probably the ball with the lower trajectory would be considered the better throw, but the score would not reflect this difference.

50-yard dash. The 50-yard dash is a very reliable measure, but the greatest source of error occurs during the first 20 yards of the dash. Jackson and Baumgartner (1969) computed intraclass reliability coefficients for the dash from 0 to 50 yards ($R = 0.949$) and from 20 to 50 yards ($R = 0.975$). For the most reliable measure of running speed, the teacher might wish to time only the last 30 yards of the 50-yard dash. Here again, appropriate norms must be developed if the modified test is used.

Sit-ups. See under Kraus-Weber Test above.

Shuttle run. No studies have been conducted on the validity of the shuttle run test. The test directions are more complex than most of the other tests in the battery, and the reliability estimates may tend to be somewhat lower. In addition, this test may be more unfamiliar to students than many of the other items in the battery.

600-yard run-walk. Before administering the 600-yard run-walk, a certain amount of warm-up and preparatory training is desirable. Several investigators have examined the relationship between maximal oxygen uptake and the 600-yard run-walk. These correlations are given in Table 9–3. The correlations indicate that the 600-yard run-walk test is a fair predictor of cardiorespiratory endurance.

Several investigators have examined the relationship between maximal oxygen uptake and the entire battery of the Youth Fitness Tests. For 12-and 13-year old boys, the AAHPER test was found to provide an adequate means of predicting oxygen uptake (Metz and Alexander, 1970). Using the entire battery, the maximal multiple correlation ($R = 0.777$) was obtained. Using the two items from the total battery, pullups and 50-yard dash, a multiple correlation coefficient of 0.739 was obtained. No combination of the tests was considered an adequate predictor for 14-and 15-year old boys; however, the investigators did not consider any coefficient below 0.70 as adequate. Olree et al. (1965) obtained a maximal multiple correlation coefficient of 0.62 for a combination of the shuttle run, 50-yard dash, and the 600-yard run-walk. Corroll (1969) investigated the relationship of the Youth Fitness items to maximal oxygen uptake. He found that the Youth Fitness items plus height plus weight equals 0.648 of the variance of maximal oxygen uptake. The highest contributions were made by the 600-yard run-walk, pullups and body weight.

TABLE 9–3 • Validity of the 600-yard Run-walk Test

Source	Sample	Correlation between 600-yard Run-walk and VO₂ max.
Falls, et al.	Adult	—0.64
Olree	Males, ages 16–17	—0.53
Metz and	30 males, ages 12–13	—0.66
Alexander	30 males, ages 14–15	—0.27
Safrit	Males, age 11	—0.71
	Females, age 11	—0.68
Doolittle and Bigbee	9 9th-grade boys	—0.62

A two-count one-minute step test has been suggested as a practical alternative to the 600-yard run-walk (Manahan and Gutin, 1971). This test is scored by counting the number of steps in a prescribed period of time. The step test correlated –0.824 with the 600-yard run-walk test, as performed by forty 9th-grade girls. However, using a modified step test as a substitute for the 600-yard run-walk test is of value only if the test is a valid measure of cardiorespiratory endurance. Comparing the two–count one–minute step test with another step test of established validity would determine whether this was so. When in fact the modified test was compared with the Skubic-Hodgkins Step Test, which is scored by counting three postexercise pulses, the maximum correlation between the two tests was 0.399. Thus, a step test that is scored by counting the number of steps may not be a good predictor of cardiorespiratory endurance.

Analysis of Total Youth Fitness Battery

Seven tests of physical fitness were selected for the AAHPER battery because each test was considered a valid measure of an important component of fitness. In a study by Ponthieux and Barker (1963), factor analytic techniques were applied to the Youth Fitness Tests. The factor analysis yielded three factors which the authors labeled as circulo-respiratory endurance, gross body coordination, and muscular explosiveness. The factor named *circulo-respiratory endurance* included three items: pullups, sit-ups, and 600-yard run-walk. The factor labeled *muscular explosiveness* also included three items: shuttle run, standing broad jump, and 50-yard dash. The softball throw appeared alone, and the factor was named *gross body coordination*. Although other factor analysis models should be applied to Youth Fitness Test data as a check on this factor solution, the results indicate that the AAHPER test is measuring fewer than seven factors.

Kendall suggests that there are several omissions in the available fitness tests. One is tightness of shoulder abductor muscles. The second is tightness of hip flexor muscles. The third is tightness of hamstring muscles, separate from forward bending. The fourth is strength of lower abdominal muscles.

The primary difficulty in constructing a test of physical fitness is that many components of fitness cannot be adequately measured by any single test. This point has already been made in an earlier discussion of flexibility. Harris (1969) obtained fourteen common factors in a factor analytic study of flexibility. Her results clearly indicated that flexibility is not a single general characteristic of the entire human body, but rather is specific to single body segments. Other investigators have concluded that there is no one type of balance, and that balance is also specific to various body parts. In addition, there appear to be differences in performing these same balance items at different heights, and that the learning curves differ for the different heights (Sanborn and Wyrick, 1969). The nature of agility has also been studied. Several investigators (Hilsendager, et al, 1969) tried to improve agility by working on speed and strength; however, practice on specific agility items resulted in a greater increase in agility than practice on either speed or strength items. Seven agility measures were used in this study. The results indicated that there is a factor unique to agility, and that all agility tests do not measure the same factor.

Twelve-Minute Run Test

Balke (1963) demonstrated that the distance covered during run-walk tests of specific duration was a valid indicator of maximal oxygen uptake and thus of cardiorespiratory fitness. He developed a 15-minute field test, which Cooper modified to a 12-minute run test. The Twelve-Minute Run Test is a sound and practical measure of cardiorespiratory endurance. The test consists simply of running as far as possible in 12 minutes. The distance run is recorded in miles, and the corresponding level of fitness is determined by referring to a table. Very little equipment is required. Other than an accurately measured track, only a stop watch and a whistle are needed.

A summary of validity studies of the Twelve-Minute Run Test is given in Table 9–4. The validity coefficients are determined by correlating Twelve-Minute Run scores (miles covered) with maximal oxygen uptake as determined by a laboratory test. The initial study by Cooper reported a validity coefficient of 0.897, indicating that the Twelve-Minute Run Test is a good substitute for the lab test for adult males. One other study reported an equally high validity coefficient (Doolittle and Bigbee, 1968), but the sample contained only nine 9th-grade boys. In another report (Maksud and Coutts, 1971), the validity coefficients were lower, suggesting that until further research is conducted, caution should be used in predicting maximum aerobic capacity from Twelve-Minute Run performance.

TABLE 9–4 • Validity of the Twelve-Minute Run Test

Source	Sample	Correlation between 12-minute run and VO_2 max.
Cooper	Adult males	0.897
Doolittle and Bigbee	9 9th-grade males	0.90
Maksud and Coutts	17 males, ages 11–14	0.65

The reliabilities reported for the Twelve-Minute Run Test are presented in Table 9–5. Generally they are high. Even though the evidence is again somewhat sketchy, indications are that the test will be reliable for adolescent males and females as well as adults.

TABLE 9–5 • Reliability of the Twelve-Minute Run Test

Source	Sample	Reliability Coefficient	
Doolittle and Bigbee	9 9th-grade males	0.94	
Doolittle, Dominic, and Doolittle	100 9th-and 10th-grade females	0.89	
	45 9th-grade females	0.89	
Wanamaker	48 college males (volunteers)	0.82,	0.88
	48 college physical education majors (selected)	0.91,	0.95
Maksud and Coutts	14 males, ages 11–14	0.92	

The standards for the Twelve-Minute Run Test have been developed by Cooper for adult males and females. There is little evidence that these standards are appropriate for adolescents. Two studies have reported data on the average distances covered by individuals in the adolescent age range (Doolittle and Bigbee, 1968; Maksud and Coutts, 1971). These distances are given in Table 9–6. The mean scores are more useful when examined in conjunction with the standard deviations, as reported by Maksud and Coutts.

TABLB 9–6 • Mean Distances on the Twelve-Minute Run

Source	Sample		Standard Deviation
Doolittle, et al.	100 9th-and-10th grade females	2022 yd (1.16 mi)	*
	45 9th-grade females	2296 yd (1.31 mi)	*
Maksud and Coutts	44 males, ages 11–12	2308 yd (1.31 mi)	357 yd (.203 mi)
	36 males, ages 13–14	2507 yd (1.42 mi)	371 yd (0.211 mi)

*Not reported.

However, in both cases the reader is provided with an indication of the average performance for selected adolescent samples, although generalizations cannot be drawn from these results. Nonetheless, the data indicate that the average scores of these samples are close to, if not within, the average range reported by Cooper for adult males.

Harvard Step Test

Measures of cardiovascular endurance are considered by many to be the best measures of physical fitness. One of the most valid and reliable tests of this nature is the Balke Treadmill Test. The test consists of having a subject walk at a constant speed on a treadmill, increasing the slope each minute, and measuring his heart rate each minute. However, the test requires a treadmill and an electrocardiograph, plus a trained administrator. Thus, it is not practical for most school physical education programs unless the school has an exercise physiology laboratory.

A popular test in many school settings is the Harvard Step Test developed by Brouha during World War II (1943). The subject exercises on a 20-inch bench for as long a period as possible up to five minutes. The cadence is 30 steps per minute. The pulse is counted during three recovery periods from 1 to $1\frac{1}{2}$ minutes, from 2 to $2\frac{1}{2}$ minutes and from 3 to $3\frac{1}{2}$ minutes after cessation of the exercise. Then, the duration of exercise measured in seconds and the sum of pulse counts in the three recovery periods are applied to a formula from which the index of physical efficiency is computed. The major criticism of the Harvard Step Test is that it is very strenuous and that fatigue and cramps often occur in the large leg muscles. Therefore, a team of researchers from Ohio State University (Kurucz, Fox and Mathews, 1969) have attempted to develop a modified Step Test which would estimate the ability to tolerate maximal work, but which would also be practical and less strenuous than the Harvard Step Test.

This test utilizes a split-level bench (the heights of the two levels are fifteen and twenty inches) with an adjustable hand bar, a metronome, and a stop watch. The test consists of 18 innings of 50-second duration, a total of 15 minutes. Each inning consists of a 30-second work period and a 20-second rest period. The pulse is taken for 10 seconds beginning with the second five and ending at the second fifteen. The 18 innings are divided into three work loads: phase one—6 innings at 24 steps per minute on the 15-inch bench, phase two—6 innings at 30 steps per minute on the 15-inch bench, phase three—6 innings at 30 steps per minute on the 20-inch bench. These phases are taken continuously. The subject stops when the pulse rate reaches 25 beats in the 10-second period or 150 beats per minute. If the subject completes 18 innings before this pulse rate is reached, the test is ended. The score is the inning in which the subject's pulse reaches 150 beats per minute. The correlation between this test and the Balke Treadmill Test is 0.94, indicating high validity. The test-retest reliability coefficient is 0.94. The advantage of the OSU Test is that exercise progresses gradually, so that those in poor condition can be evaluated, but is also strenuous enough in the end so that the highly fit can be measured. A modification of the OSU Test has been developed in which a 17-inch bleacher step is used (Cotten, 1971). The validity of the modified test is slightly lower than that of the OSU Test ($r = 0.84$). However, the modification requires a minimum of special equipment. The reliabilities of the Harvard Step Test and the modifications of this test are given in Table 9–7.

TABLE 9–7 • Reliability of Harvard Step Test and Modifications

Source	Sample	Reliability Coefficient
Kurucz, Mathews, and Fox	75 males, ages 19–56	0.94*
Meyers	31 male college freshmen	0.77**
	119 8th-grade males	0.65**
Cotten	34 male p.e. majors	0.95*
	46 9th-to 12th-grade boys	0.75*

*Modification of Harvard Step Test.
**Combination of rater and subject reliability.

The coefficients reported by Meyers (1969) are essentially representative of the reliability of the subjects along with the objectivity of the raters on the Harvard Step Test. In the first testing situation, college men were tested on two days, yielding a reliability coefficient of 0.65. However, the variability in performance from one testing period to another might be a result of change in a subject's condition or inconsistency in counting a subject's pulse. (In one case, the pulse was counted by the subject's partner.) In the second testing situation, the reliability of the 30-second pulse count taken in a sitting position after five minutes of rest was 0.77. All counts were made by the same tester. However, two sources of error again exist—the inconsistency of the subjects and the lack of objectivity of the rater. In the third setting, the counts were made by 8th-grade boys, yielding a coefficient of 0.65. If the objectivity of the raters had been determined previous to the reliability, perhaps the reliability coefficient would be a more accurate reflection of the stability of the subjects.

Fleishman's Physical Fitness Battery

To date, the most thorough battery of physical fitness tests in terms of sound test construction has been developed by Fleishman (1964). Using factor analytic techniques he developed a battery of nine physical fitness tests. These tests, as well as their reliability coefficients, are given below.

Test 1. Extent Flexibility Factor. Ability to flex or stretch the trunk and back muscles as far as possible in either a forward, lateral or backward direction. The subject stands with left side toward, and at arms length from, the wall. With feet together and in place, he twists back around as far as he can, touching wall with his right hand at shoulder height

$$r = 0.90$$

Test 2. Measures dynamic flexibility factor. The ability to make repeated, rapid, flexing movements in which the resiliency of the muscles in recovery from strain or distortion is critical. With his back to the wall and hands together, the subject bends forward, touches an X between his feet, straightens, twists to the left and touches a X behind him on the wall. He repeats the cycle, alternately twisting to the right and to the left, doing as many as possible in the time allowed.

$$r = 0.92$$

Tests 3 and 4. Measures explosive strength factor. The ability to expend a maximum of energy in one or a series of explosive acts. This factor is distinguished from other strength factors in requiring mobilization of energy for a burst of effort, rather than continuous strain, stress, or repeated exertion of muscles. Although the two tests of this factor are significantly correlated with each other, . each emphasizes different specific muscle groups or activities. Thus, shuttle run involves legs, speed, and gross body movement, while softball throws represent a more specific arm-shoulder involvement. In the shuttle run test, a 20-yard distance is covered five times for a 100-yard total. In the softball throw test, the subject throws the 12-inch softball as far as possible without moving his feet.

$$r = 0.85 \text{ for shuttle run}$$
$$r = 0.93 \text{ for softball throw}$$

Test 5. *Static Strength Factor.* Measures the maximum force which the subject can exert, even for a brief period, where the force is exerted continuously up to this maximum. In contrast to other strength factors, this is the force that can be exerted against external objects (for example, lifting heavy weights, pulling against a dynamometer) rather than in supporting or propelling the body's own weight. In the hand-grip test, the subject squeezes a grip dynamometer as hard as possible.

$$r = 0.91$$

Test 6. *Dynamic Strength Factor.* Measures the ability to exert muscular force repeatedly or continuously over a period of time. It represents muscular endurance and emphasizes the resistance of the muscle to fatigue. The common emphasis of tests measuring this factor is on the power of the muscles to propel, support, or move the body repeatedly or to support it for prolonged periods. In the pullups test the subject hangs from a bar with palms facing his body, and does as many pullups as possible.

$$r = 0.93$$

Test 7. *Trunk Strength Factor.* This is a second, more limited, dynamic strength factor specific to the trunk muscles, particularly the abdominal muscles. In the leg-lift test, while flat on his back, the subject raises his legs to a vertical position, and lowers them to the floor as many times as possible within the time limit.

$$r = 0.89$$

Test 8. *Gross Body Coordination Body Factor.* Measures the ability to coordinate the simultaneous actions of different parts of the body while making gross body movements. In the cable-jump test, the subject holds in front of him a short rope held in each hand. He attempts to jump through this rope without tripping, falling, or releasing the rope.

$$r = 0.70$$

Test 9. *Gross Body Equilibrium Factor.* Measures the ability of an individual to maintain his equilibrium, despite forces pulling him off balance, where he has to depend mainly on nonvisual (for instance, vestibular and kinesthetic) cues. Although also measured by balance tests where the eyes are kept open, it is best measured by those conducted with the eyes closed. In balance A test, the subject balances for as long as possible on a $\frac{3}{4}$ inch wide rail with his hands on his hips, using his preferred foot.

$$r = 0.82$$

Test 10. *Stamina (cardiovascular endurance) Factor.* Measures the capacity to continue maximum effort, requiring prolonged exertion. In the 600-yard run-walk test, the student attempts to cover a 600-yard distance in as short a time as possible.

$$r = 0.80$$

Jackson (1971) reanalyzed Fleishman's three-factor strength model (dynamic, static, and explosive strength) and hypothesized nine strength factors instead of three. His solutions yielded five robust (occurring across all solutions) factors and two tentative factors. Liba (1967) hypothesized eleven strength factors but only included selected measures for eight hypothesized factors. Nine factors were obtained from one solution and eleven from another. In neither study did the factor patterns resemble the one obtained in the Fleishman model. However, in terms of procedure, the development of the Fleishman model can still serve as a model for constructing test batteries that measure attributes such as physical fitness.

Summary

Although many other tests of physical fitness have been developed, only selected measures of muscular and cardiovascular fitness have been reviewed in this chapter. The AAHPER test has received the greatest publicity, but although it has made a valuable contribution to the testing of physical fitness, some revisions would seem appropriate. It is possible that the Twelve-Minute Run Test is the best measure of overall fitness, although whether this is true for all ages and both sexes must be determined by future studies.

Bibliography

ASKEW, N. R. "Reliability of the 600-yard Run-Walk Test at the Secondary School Level," *Research Quarterly,* XXXVII, No. 4 (1966), pp. 451–54.

BALKE, B. "A Simple Field Test for the Assessment of Physical Fitness," *CARI Report.* Oklahoma City, Okla.: Civil Aeromedical Research Institute, Federal Aviation Agency, 1963.

BARROW, H. M. and R. McGEE. *A Practical Approach to Measurement in Physical Education.* Philadelphia: Lea and Febiger, 1972.

BAUMGARTNER, T. A. "Stability of Physical Performance Test Scores," *Research Quarterly,* XL, No. 2 (1969), pp. 257–61.

BAUMGARTNER, T. A. and A. S. JACKSON. "Measurement Schedules for Tests of Motor Performance," *Research Quarterly,* XLI, No. 1 (1970), pp. 10–14.

BERGER, R. A. and R. L. MEDLIN. "Evaluation of Berger's 1-RM Chin Test for Junior High School Males," *Research Quarterly,* XL (1969), pp. 460–63.

BROUHA, L. "The Step Test: A Simple Method of Measuring Physical Fitness for Muscular Work in Young Men," *Research Quarterly,* XIV (1943), pp. 31–36.

CLARKE, H. H. ed. *Physical Fitness Research Digest.* Washington, D. C.: President's Council on Physical Fitness and Sports, July 1971.

COOPER, K.H. *The New Aerobics.* New York: Bantam Press, 1970.

CORROLL, V. "Relationship of the AAHPER Youth Fitness Test Items and Maximal Oxygen Intake." Doctoral Dissertation, University of Illinois, Urbana, 1969 (Microcard PE 1004, University of Oregon, Eugene).

COTTEN, D. J. "A Modified Step Test for Group Cardiovascular Testing," *Research Quarterly,* XLII, No. 1 (1971), pp. 91–95.

COTTEN, D.J. and E. CHAMBERS. "A Comparison of Three Methods of Administering the Softball Throw," *Research Quarterly,* XXXIX, No. 3 (1968), pp. 788–89.

COTTEN, D.J. and B. MARWITZ. "Relationship between Two Flexed-Arm Hangs and Pull-Ups for College Women," *Research Quarterly,* XL, No. 2 (1969), pp. 415–16.

COUTTS, K. and M. G. MAKSUD. "Physiological Responses of the 'Inner-City' Child to Standardized Exercise." Unpublished report, University of Wisconsin, Milwaukee, 1969.

DOOLITTLE, T. L. and R. BIGBEE. "The Twelve-Minute Run-Walk: A Test of Cardiorespiratory Fitness of Adolescent Boys," *Research Quarterly,* XXXIX, No. 3 (1968), pp. 491–95.

DOOLITTLE. T. L., J. C. DOMINIC and J. DOOLITTLE. "The Reliability of Selected

Cardio-Respiratory Endurance Field Tests with Adolescent Female Population," *American Corrective Therapy Journal*, XXIII, No. 5 (1969), pp. 135–38.

ESSLINGER, A. A. "Perspectives on Testing," *Journal of Health, Physical Education and Recreation*, XXXI (1960), pp. 36–37.

FALLS, H. B., A. H. ISMAIL and D. F. MacLEOD. "Estimation of Maximum Oxygen Uptake in Adults from AAHPER Youth Fitness Test Items," *Research Quarterly*, XXXVII (1966), pp. 192–201.

FLEISHMAN, E. A. *The Structure and Measurement of Physical Fitness*. Englewood Cliffs, N. J.: Prentice-Hall Inc., 1964.

HARRIS, M. L. "A Factor Analytic Study of Flexibility," *Research Quarterly*, XL, No. 1 (1969), pp. 62–70.

HASKINS, M. J. *Evaluation in Physical Education*. Dubuque, Iowa: Wm. C. Brown Company Publishers, 1971.

HILSENDAGER, D. R., M. H. STRAW and K. J. ACKERMAN. "Comparison of Speed, Strength, and Agility Exercises in the Development of Agility," *Research Quarterly*, XL (1969), pp. 71–75.

HUNSICKER, P. "AAHPER Physical Fitness Test Battery," *Journal of Health, Physical Education and Recreation*, XXIX (1958), pp. 24–25.

HUNSICKER, P. and G. REIFF. "A Survey and Comparison of Youth Fitness 1958–1965," *Journal of Health, Physical Education and Recreation*, XXXVII (1966), pp. 23–25.

JACKSON, A. S. "Factor Analysis of Selected Muscular Strength and Motor Performance Tests," *Research Quarterly*, XLII, No. 2 (1971), pp. 164–71.

JACKSON, A. S. and T. A. BAUMGARTNER. "Measurement Schedules of Sprint Running," *Research Quarterly*, XL, No. 4 (1969), pp. 708–11.

JOHNSON, B. L. and J. K. NELSON. *Practical Measurements for Evaluation in Physical Education*. Minneapolis: Burgess Publishing Company, 1969.

KANE R. J. and H. V. MEREDITH. "Ability in the Standing Broad Jump of Elementary School Children, 7, 9, and 11 Years of Age," *Research Quarterly*, XXIII, No. 1 (1952), pp. 198–208.

KENDALL, F. P. "A Criticism of Current Tests and Exercises for Physical Fitness," *Journal of the American Physical Therapy Association*, XLV, No. 3 (1965), pp. 187–97.

KLESIUS, S. E. "Reliability of the AAHPER Youth Fitness Test Items and Relative Efficiency of the Performance Measures," *Research Quarterly*, XXXIX, No. 3 (1968), pp. 809–11.

KRAUS, H. and R. HIRSCHLAND. "Muscular Fitness and Health," *Journal of Health, Physical Education and Recreation*, XXIV (1953), pp. 17–19.

KURUCZ, R. L., E. L. FOX, and D. K. MATHEWS. "Construction of a Submaximal Cardiovascular Step Test," *Research Quarterly*, XL, No. 1 (1969), pp. 115–22.

LIBA, M. R. "Factor Analysis of Strength Variables," *Research Quarterly*, XXXVIII, No. 4 (1967), pp. 649–62.

MAKSUD, M. G. and K. D. COUTTS. "Application of the Cooper Twelve-Minute

Run-Walk Test to Young Males," *Research Quarterly*, XLII (1971), pp. 54–59.

MANAHAN, J. E. and B. GUTIN. The One-Minute Step Test as a Measure of 600-yard Run Performance," *Research Quarterly*, XLII, No. 2 (1971), pp. 173–77.

MARMIS, C. et al. "Reliability of the Multi-Trial Items of the AAHPER Youth Fitness Test," *Research Quarterly*, XL, No. 1 (1969), pp. 240–45.

MARTENS, R. and B. J. SHARKEY. "Relationship of Phasic and Static Strength and Endurance," *Research Quarterly*, XXXVII (1966), pp. 435–37.

MATHEWS, D.K. *Measurement in Physical Education*. Philadelphia: W. B. Saunders Company, 1969.

METZ, K. F. and J. F. ALEXANDER. "An Investigation of the Relationship between Maximum Aerobic Work Capacity and Physical Fitness in Twelve- to Fifteen-Year-Old Boys," *Research Quarterly*, XLI, No. 1 (1970), pp. 75–81.

MEYERS, C. R. "A Study of the Reliability of the Harvard Step Test," *Research Quarterly*, XL, No. 2 (1969), p. 423.

MONTOYE, H. J. "Circulatory-Respiratory Fitness," in *Physical Fitness, An Introduction to Measurement in Physical Education* (Vol. 4), ed. H. J. Montoye. Indianapolis: Phi Epsilon Kappa Fraternity, 1970.

OLREE, H. et al. "Evaluation of the AAHPER Youth Fitness Test," *Journal of Sports Medicine and Physical Fitness*, V (1965), pp. 67–71.

PONTHIEUX, N. A. and D. G. BARKER. "An Analysis of the AAHPER Youth Fitness Test," *Research Quarterly*, XXXIV (1963), pp. 525–26.

SAFRIT, M. J. "The Physical Performance of Inner City Children in Milwaukee, Wisconsin." Unpublished report, University of Wisconsin, Milwaukee, 1969.

SANBORN, C. and W. WYRICK. "Prediction of Olympic Balance Beam Performance from Standardized and Modified Tests of Balance," *Research Quarterly*, XL, No. 1 (1969), pp. 174–84.

SIGERSETH, P. O. "Flexibility," in *Physical Fitness, An Introduction to Measurement in Physical Education* (Vol. 4), ed. H. J. Montoye. Indianapolis: Phi Epsilon Kappa Fraternity, 1970.

SODERBERG, G. L. "Exercises for the Abdominal Muscles," *Journal of Health, Physical Education and Recreation*, XXXVII (1966), pp. 67–70.

STRAUB, W. F. and B. W. HUNGERFORD. "Guidelines for the Data Processing of Physical Education Test Results," *New York State Journal of Health, Physical Education and Recreation*, XXI, No. 3 (1969), pp. 15–18.

VAN HUSS, W. D. and W. W. HUESNER. "Strength, Power, and Muscular Endurance," in *Physical Fitness, An Introduction to Measurement in Physical Education* (Vol. 4), ed. H. J. Montoye. Indianapolis: Phi Epsilon Kappa Fraternity, 1970.

WELCH, H. G. "Endurance," in *Physical Fitness, An Introduction to Measurement in Physical Education* (Vol. 4), ed. H. J. Montoye. Indianapolis: Phi Epsilon Kappa Fraternity, 1970.

WILLGOOSE, C. E., N. R. ASKEW and M. P. ASKEW. "Reliability of the 600-yard Run-Walk at the Junior High School Level," *Research Quarterly*, XXXII, No. 2 (1961), pp. 264–66.

10

norms and scales

When Mary, who is fifteen years old, is tested on the standing broad jump in her physical education class, she jumps five feet. A score of five feet undoubtedly has some meaning for Mary. She knows that her score is average, above-average, or below-average compared with her typical performance on the jump. She may be able to estimate roughly how well she jumps in comparison with others in her class. However, both Mary and her teacher may wish to know more precisely how her score compares with other girls in her age group outside of Mary's class. By referring to the *AAHPER Youth Fitness Test Manual* (1965), Mary and her teacher can utilize the table of national norms for girls on the standing broad jump (See Table 10–1). Mary's raw score is located in the column for 15-year old girls. Her standing broad jump score of five feet has a percentile rank of 55. This means that 55 percent of the national sample have scores equal to or lower than Mary's. Mary's score falls in the middle of the distribution of standing broad jump scores. Although her score may be low when compared with other girls in her class, it is an average score compared with the national sample of girls her age. Norms, therefore, can be useful in interpreting raw scores.

The percentile rank is one type of normative score. This type, along with several others, will be described in this chapter. For a more complete discussion of norms and scales, see Angoff (1971) and Lyman (1970) listed in the bibliography.

Raw Scores and Derived Scores

A *raw score* is the actual score an individual obtains on a test. When the raw scores of a test are transformed to another scale, the scores are referred to as *derived scores*. Transforming the raw scores can also be described as "rescaling" the scores; thus, a set of derived scores may be referred to as a *scale*.

If a student's raw score is the only information we are given about his test performance, interpretation of the score is difficult. If we wish to compare the student's score on one test with his score on another test, the direct comparison of raw scores will be meaningless. For instance, if Mary's score on the 50-yard dash is 7.8 seconds, does this score represent a higher or lower level of ability than her broad jump score? The raw scores should be transformed into derived scores before direct comparisons are made.

A common method of transforming raw scores is to convert them to percentage-correct scores. Percentage-correct scores are determined by dividing the highest possible test score by the score actually obtained on the test. This type of score is used for mastery tests. Percentage-correct scores are probably more useful for tests of motor skill than for written tests. When a test is scored using the percentage-correct method, the teacher usually decides upon a certain percentage score that reflects an adequate mastery of the material. For example, an 80 percent mastery level may be set. Using this procedure, the teacher is required to make an absolute judgment about the difficulty level of the items on a written test. The difficulty levels of two written tests may vary considerably, and the teacher has no real basis for determining the appropriate difficulty level for each test. Teachers have been found to be notably unreliable in determining difficulty levels (Angoff, 1971; Ebel, 1965). Thus, percentage-correct scores are considered useful for written tests only if certain defined limits of knowledge are to be tested. Even in this case, different standards for different groups will probably be necessary. For example, if a knowledge test on softball rules were administered, a desired percentage-correct score might be 80 percent for students in a physical education class, but 95 percent for the student aides who will be officiating in softball games.

The use of percentage-correct scores for tests of motor skill can be viewed somewhat more positively than the use of such scores for written tests. When a skill test is given, we are not dealing with a test that consists of different items that may represent different difficulty levels. Rather, the skill test consists of a given number of trials on the *same* item. Thus, the difficulty level remains the same over all trials. While no one mastery level is appropriate for all tests of motor skill, the proper levels of mastery can be determined through experience. A percentage-correct score cannot be used for direct comparisons of several tests. For example, the maximum number of sit-ups for boys is set at 100 in the AAHPER Youth Fitness Test. If a boy performs 60 sit-ups, his percentage-correct score is 60 percent. The maximum number of sit-ups designated for girls is 50. A girl who performed 30 sit-ups would also receive a percentage-correct score of 60 percent. In reality, however, their scores are not comparable. Whether motor or mental tests are given, the percentage-correct score does not allow for the direct comparison of a student's scores for several tests, or of two different groups on the same test. Derived scores must be used when direct comparison is desired.

Norms

Norms are derived scores that are determined from the raw scores obtained by a specific group on a specific test. A norm should not be viewed as a standard against which a student is to be judged. Whenever norms are determined for a given group of people, half of the people will fall above the middle of the distribution and half will fall below. There is no inherent value attached to any given norm score. The norm identifies a person in relation to a given sample whose norms have been determined. Any judgment made about the norm is made by the person using the norm score.

Grade Norms

Grade norms are computed by determining the average of the raw scores for each grade, and using the grade equivalent in place of that average. If, for example, the average distance a class of fifth grade boys could throw the softball was 96 feet, 96 feet would be given a grade norm of 5. However measures of physical performance are rarely transformed to grade norms. One reason is that a given grade will include different ages, and the older children, being more advanced in physical growth and development, will have a natural advantage over the younger ones in many motor skills.

There are several limitations to the use of grade norms for tests of both mental and physical abilities. The units from one grade norm to another are not equal over different parts of the scale. Thus achievement from grade two to grade three may be greater than or less than achievement from grade eight to grade nine. Reading skills, for instance, may increase in great amounts from grade to grade in the elementary school. However, this skill may level off previous to entrance into high school, and thus the significance of a grade norm of 11 for a ninth grade student is not nearly as great as that of a grade norm of four for a second grade student.

In addition, grade units may be unequal from test to test. A sixth grade student with grade norms of 10 on reading and eight on mathematics would appear to be better in reading than in mathematics. However, there may be a greater range of reading scores than mathematics scores for a given grade, and the student may actually have very high percentile ranks on both tests.

Grade norms are useful for reporting growth in the basic academic skills at the elementary school level. However, because of the ease with which this type of norm can be misinterpreted, other types are usually preferred.

Age Norms

Age norms are determined by computing the average score for a given age. The raw score is interpreted in terms of an age equivalent. If the average standing broad jump for 17-year old boys is 7ft 3in., then 7ft 3in. is given an age norm of 17. Age norms have the same characteristics and limitations as grade norms. This type of norm is also rarely used for physical education tests, since skeletal maturation is a more significant factor in physical performance than age. In growth and development scales, a type of age norm is often used to describe sequences of motor behavior. This is one of the few places where a form of age norms is used that would be of interest to physical educators.

Percentile Norms

Percentile ranks are used in the norm tables for the AAHPER Youth Fitness Test (1965), the AAHPER Cooperative Physical Education Tests (1970), and the AAHPER Sports Skill Tests (1967). All of the tables of norms are multiple-group tables. In the Youth Fitness Test Manual, the norms are presented according to age and classification groups determined on the basis of age, height, and weight. Classification groups are used in an attempt to take the level of physical maturation into account. The Knowledge Test norms are presented according to grade groups, while tables of norms for the Skill Test series use age groups. Grouping by age or grade should not be confused with age norms and grade norms. In the latter case, age and grade are the *norms;* in the former case the percentile rank is the norm.

A *percentile rank* is based on the position an individual occupies in a group. No matter what the range of raw scores is, the percentiles will range from zero to one hundred. If 30 is the highest score made on a given test, then 30 is the hundredth percentile. If 50 is the highest score made, 50 is the hundredth percentile.

> The insensitivity of percentile ranks to general level of group performance might seem to be a disadvantage, and would be if the apparent level of group performance were not so largely determined by unintentional, and to a considerable

degree uncontrollable, variations in the difficulty of the test. It is unfortunately true that dependable standards of measurement are seldom provided by the examiner's a priori judgments of how difficult a question is likely to be, and, if it requires the exercise of subjective judgments in scoring, his judgments of how well the student has answered it. The typical unreliability of measures obtained by these means has been demonstrated quite convincingly (Ebel, 1965, p. 255).

Percentiles divide a frequency distribution into one hundred groups of equal size. Whereas raw scores may form a bell-like distribution, percentiles form a rectangular one as shown in Figure 10–1. It is evident that percentiles are not equally spaced throughout the distribution because more people are clustered in the middle of a distribution than at the extremes. Only if the same number of persons obtains each raw score are the percentiles equally spaced. However, such a distribution is not likely to occur. Therefore, although percentiles seem easy to interpret, we are likely to overemphasize differences near the median and underemphasize differences near the extremes. An individual must improve more to move from the eighty-fifth to the ninety-fifth percentile than he would have to improve to move from the fiftieth to the sixtieth percentile. Figure 10–2 shows the relationship of percentiles to other types of derived scores.

Percentile ranks may be averaged by first converting the percentiles to z scores. These conversions can be made using tables that are available in most statistics textbooks. The z scores are then averaged, and the average z score is converted back to a percentile rank using the same table. When percentiles are averaged, the raw score distribution is assumed to be normal. Also, all percentiles must have been obtained from the same

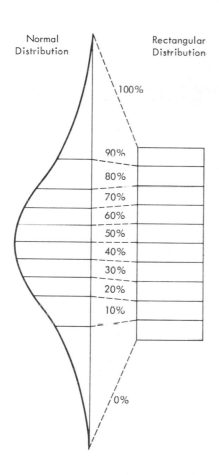

FIG. 10–1   Relation between Normal and Rectangular Distributions

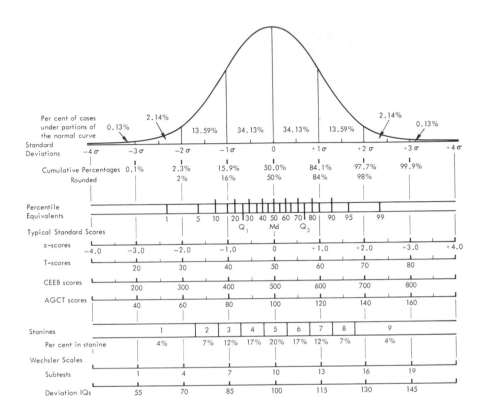

FIG. 10–2   The Normal Curve: Percentiles and Standard Scores

norm group. A table of norms using percentiles is given in Table 10–1.

Percentile bands are useful aids in interpreting percentiles. When a percentile band is presented in a table of norms, a band is given for each percentile. Each band includes the range of percentile ranks surrounding an individual percentile rank. The upper limit of the percentile band is determined by computing the percentile rank for a score that is one standard error of measurement above an individual's raw score. The lower limit of the band is the percentile rank for one standard error of measurement below the actual test score. Since we know that measurement error exists in any measurement process, the percentile band provides a more reasonable interpretation of an individual's score than the percentile rank taken alone because the existence of measurement error is taken into account. The assumption is that a person's

Table 10–1 • **Standing Broad Jump for Girls.**
Percentile Scores Based on Age*

Percen-tile	Age								Percen-tile
	10	11	12	13	14	15	16	17	
100th	6′ 2″	7′ 1″	6′ 11″	6′ 8″	6′ 11″	7′ 0″	7′ 2″	7′ 0″	100th
95th	5′ 4″	5′ 7″	5′ 8″	5′ 9″	6′ 0″	6′ 2″	6′ 5″	6′ 6″	95th
90th	5′ 1″	5′ 4″	5′ 6″	5′ 7″	5′ 9″	6′ 0″	6′ 0″	6′ 2″	90th
85th	4′ 11″	5′ 2″	5′ 3″	5′ 5″	5′ 7″	5′ 9″	5′ 11″	6′ 0″	85th
80th	4′ 10″	5′ 0″	5′ 2″	5′ 4″	5′ 6″	5′ 6″	5′ 8″	5′ 10″	80th
75th	4′ 8″	4′ 11″	5′ 0″	5′ 2″	5′ 4″	5′ 4″	5′ 6″	5′ 8″	75th
70th	4′ 7″	4′ 10″	4′ 11″	5′ 1″	5′ 2″	5′ 3″	5′ 5″	5′ 7″	70th
65th	4′ 6″	4′ 8″	4′ 10″	5′ 0″	5′ 1″	5′ 2″	5′ 3″	5′ 5″	65th
60th	4′ 5″	4′ 8″	4′ 9″	4′ 11″	5′ 0″	5′ 0″	5′ 2″	5′ 3″	60th
55th	4′ 4″	4′ 6″	4′ 7″	4′ 9″	4′ 10″	5′ 0″	5′ 1″	5′ 2″	55th
50th	4′ 3″	4′ 6″	4′ 6″	4′ 8″	4′ 9″	4′ 10″	5′ 0″	5′ 0″	50th
45th	4′ 2″	4′ 4″	4′ 6″	4′ 7″	4′ 8″	4′ 9″	4′ 11′	5′ 0″	45th
40th	4′ 1″	4′ 3″	4′ 5″	4′ 6″	4′ 7″	4′ 8″	4′ 10″	4′ 10″	40th
35th	4′ 0″	4′ 2″	4′ 3″	4′ 5″	4′ 6″	4′ 7″	4′ 9″	4′ 8″	35th
30th	3′ 10″	4′ 0″	4′ 2″	4′ 4″	4′ 5″	4′ 5″	4′ 8″	4′ 7″	30th
25th	3′ 9″	3′ 11″	4′ 1″	4′ 3″	4′ 4″	4′ 4″	4′ 6″	4′ 6″	25th
20th	3′ 8″	3′ 10″	4′ 0″	4′ 2″	4′ 2″	4′ 3″	4′ 4″	4′ 4″	20th
15th	3′ 6″	3′ 8″	3′ 10″	3′ 11″	4′ 0″	4′ 1″	4′ 3″	4′ 2″	15th
10th	3′ 4″	3′ 6″	3′ 9″	3′ 9″	3′ 10″	4′ 0″	4′ 0″	4′ 0″	10th
5th	3′ 2″	3′ 3″	3′ 5″	3′ 6″	3′ 6″	3′ 8″	3′ 10″	3′ 7″	5th
0	2′ 5″	2′ 5″	2′ 9″	2′ 7″	2′ 3″	3′ 0″	2′ 6″	3′ 1″	0

*Reprinted from Table 4 of *AAHPER Youth Fitness Manual* (Washington, D.C.: AAH-PER, 1965), p. 21, by permission of the publisher.

score will never be free of measurement error, and thus a person's true score will never be known. The percentile band identifies an area that will be likely to encompass the true score. Percentile bands were developed in conjunction with percentiles for the AAHPER Cooperative Physical Education Tests as shown in Table 10–2.

Standard Score Norms

Standard score norms, like percentile norms, are widely used for measures of physical performance, although they are generally not used to determine national norms. *T* scores are used in the Scott Motor Ability Test (1959), the Barrow Motor Ability Test (1972), the Wear Physical Education Attitude Inventory (1951), the French-Stalter Badminton Tests (1959), the

TABLE 10–2 • AAHPER Cooperative Physical Education Norms: Grades 10, 11, and 12*

CONVERTED SCORE	GRADE 10 Percentile Band	GRADE 10 Percentile Rank	GRADE 10 Stanine	GRADE 11 Percentile Band	GRADE 11 Percentile Rank	GRADE 11 Stanine	GRADE 12 Percentile Band	GRADE 12 Percentile Rank	GRADE 12 Stanine
295–297									
292–294									
289–291									
286–288				99.8—99.9	99.9	9			
283–285				99.5—99.9	99.9	9	99.5—99.9	99.9	9
280–282	99.8—99.9	99.9	9	99.1—99.9	99.9	9	99.2—99.9	99.8	9
277–279	99.5—99.9	99.9	9	99.0—99.9	99.8	9	98.0—99.9	99.8	9
274–276	99.1—99.9	99.9	9	98.0—99.9	99.6	9	97.0—99.9	99.6	9
271–273	98.0—99.9	99.8	9	97.0—99.9	99.3	9	96.0—99.9	99.4	9
268–270	98.0—99.9	99.5	9	95.0—99.9	99	9	94.0—99.9	98	9
265–267	96.0—99.9	99.2	9	93.0—99.7	98	9	92.0—99.6	97	9
262–264	95.0—99.9	99	9	91.0—99.4	97	9	89.0—99.4	96	8
259–261	93.0—99.6	98	9	89.0—99	95	8	86.0—99	94	8
256–258	91.0—99.3	96	9	85.0—98	93	8	83.0—97	92	8
253–255	88.0—99	95	8	82.0—97	92	8	79.0—96	90	8
250–252	85.0—98	94	8	78.0—96	89	7	75.0—95	87	7
247–249	82.0—97	91	8	73.0—94	86	7	70.0—93	84	7
244–246	78.0—96	89	8	68.0—93	83	7	66.0—91	80	7
241–243	73.0—95	86	7	64.0—90	79	6	60.0—89	76	7
238–240	68.0—92	83	7	59.0—88	74	6	55.0—85	72	6
235–237	64.0—90	79	7	53.0—85	70	6	50.0—82	67	6
232–234	59.0—88	75	6	49.0—81	65	6	45.0—78	62	6
229–231	54.0—84	69	6	44.0—77	60	6	41.0—74	56	5
226–228	48.0—81	66	6	39.0—72	56	5	36.0—69	52	5
223–225	43.0—77	61	6	34.0—67	51	5	32.0—64	48	5
220–222	39.0—72	56	5	29.0—62	47	5	28.0—59	43	5
217–219	33.0—68	51	5	25.0—59	42	5	24.0—55	38	5
214–216	29.0—64	46	5	22.0—53	36	4	21.0—50	34	4
211–213	25.0—59	41	5	19.0—49	32	4	18.0—45	30	4
208–210	21.0—54	36	4	16.0—44	27	4	15.0—41	26	4
205–207	18.0—48	31	4	13.0—39	24	4	13.0—36	23	4
202–204	17.0—43	27	4	12.0—34	21	3	11.0—32	19	3
199–201	14.0—39	23	4	10.0—29	18	3	10.0—28	16	3

Score									
196—198	2.0—33	20	3	9.0—25	15	3	8.0—24	14	3
193—195	0.0—29	13	3	7.0—22	13	3	7.0—21	12	3
190—192	8.0—25	15	3	6.0—19	11	3	6.0—18	11	2
187—189	6.0—21	13	3	5.0—16	9	2	5.0—15	9	2
184—186	5.0—18	11	3	4.0—13	8	2	4.0—13	8	2
181—183	4.0—16	9	2	3.0—11	6	2	3.0—11	6	2
178—180	3.0—13	7	2	3.0—10	6	2	3.0—9	5	2
175—177	3.0—1	6	2	2.0—8	5	2	2.0—8	4	2
172—174	2.0—9	5	1	2.0—7	3	1	2.0—6	4	1
169—171	2.0—8	4	1	1.0—6	3	1	1.0—6	3	1
166—168	1.0—6	3	1	1.0—5	2	1	0.9—5	3	1
163—165	1.0—5	2	1	0.8—4	2	1	0.8—4	2	1
160—162	0.9—4	2	1	0.6—3	2	1	0.6—3	1	1
157—159	0.8—3	2	1	0.4—2	1	1	0.4—3	1	1
154—156	0.6—2	1	1	0.3—2	0.9	1	0.4—2	0.8	1
151—153	0.5—2	0.9	1	0.2—2	0.6	1	0.4—1	0.6	1
148—150	0.4—2	0.8	1	0.1—1	0.4	1	0.3—1	0.5	1
145—147	0.4—1	0.6	1	0.1—0.9	0.3	1	0.3—0.8	0.4	1
142—144	0.3—1	0.5	1	0.1—0.7	0.2	1	0.3—0.7	0.4	1
139—141	0.2—0.8	0.5	1	0.1—0.5	0.1	1	0.2—0.5	0.3	1
136—138	0.2—0.7	0.4	1	0.1—0.3	0.1	1	0.2—0.4	0.3	1
133—135	0.1—0.5	0.3	1	0.1—0.3	0.1	1	0.1—0.4	0.3	1
130—132	0.1—0.5	0.3	1	0.1—0.1	0.1	1	0.1—0.3	0.3	1
127—129	0.1—0.4	0.2	1	0.1—0.1	0.1	1	0.1—0.3	0.2	1
124—126	0.1—0.3	0.1	1	0.1—0.1	0.1	1	0.1—0.3	0.1	1
121—123	0.1—0.3	0.1	1	0.1—0.1	0.1	1	0.1—0.2	0.1	1
118—120	0.1—0.2	0.1	1	0.1—0.1	0.1	1	0.1—0.2	0.1	1
115—117				0.1—0.1					
112—114				0.1—0.1					
109—111				0.1—0.1					
106—108				0.1—0.1					
Number of Students	3106			2534			2504		
Mean	216			221			223		
Standard Deviation	24			24			25		
Upper Quartile	233			239			242		
Median	218			224			227		
Lower Quartile	203			206			209		

Wilson Intermediate Swimming Tests (1962), and others. T scales are also used in the Brown Revised Golf Skill Test (1969) and the Dyer Backboard Test of Tennis Ability (1938). Stanines (see p. 208) are used in the AAHPER Cooperative Physical Education Tests (1970).

All standard scores are based on the z score, which is the most basic of standard scores. The z score is described in Chapter 4. Many test users do not find z scores convenient to use because the scores are expressed in decimal places. In addition, all scores below the z score mean are negative numbers.

Because of the difficulty associated with interpreting the z score, the T score is more commonly used and is determined by the equation

$$T = 10\,z + 50$$

Multiplying the z score by 10 removes the decimal, and adding 50 makes all of the numbers positive. The T score distribution, then, has a mean of 50 and a standard deviation of 10. Regardless of what the mean and standard deviation of a distribution of raw scores are, the mean is set at 50 and the standard deviation is set at 10 when converting raw scores to T scores. When T score transformations are used, several test scores can be compared for a given individual.

The T score distribution generally ranges from 20 to 80. Since performances of four standard deviations above or below the mean are rare, T scores of 10 or 90 are equally rare. Thus, we should be somewhat suspicious of a T score that is higher than 80 or lower than 20. Although it is possible to obtain scores outside of the typical T score range, such occurrences would be care.

Many other transformations can be made using the z score distribution. Some commonly used transformations are:

College Entrance Examination Board Score $= 100z + 500$
Wechsler IQ Score $= 15z + 100$
Stanford-Binet IQ Score $= 16z + 100$

Actually, the z score may be rescaled in any way one wishes, but the underlying meaning of the scale does not change. The mean of the College Entrance Examination Board scores is simply transformed to 500. The standard deviation is rescaled to 100. This distribution will approximate the distribution of raw scores, as would the T score, the z score, the Wechsler IQ score, and the Stanford-Binet IQ score distributions, if all these transformations were applied to the same set of raw scores.

T scores are sometimes confused with T scales and percentiles because all three scales utilize numbers of the same sizes. However, the T score reflects the raw score distribution, while both percentiles and T scales alter (normalize) the raw score distribution unless this distribution is normal to begin with. If the raw score distribution is normal, T scores and T-scaled scores will be identical.

Normalized standard scores such as the T-scaled score appear similar to the standard scores described above, but are computed like a percentile rank. Normalized standard scores are obtained by computing percentiles, and then substituting normalized standard score values for the normal probability distribution. In essence, the *median* of a percentile distribution is set at a z score of zero (or a T-scaled score of 50), and standard score values are then set for other points on the distribution. When the raw score distribution is not normal, the normalized standard score distribution tends to more closely approximate the normal probability distribution, as shown in Figure 10–3. Thus, normalized standard scores are more appropriate for a skewed distribution. (In a skewed distribution, the mean is pulled further toward the skewed end of the distribution than the median, and the median is considered to be a better measure of central tendency.)

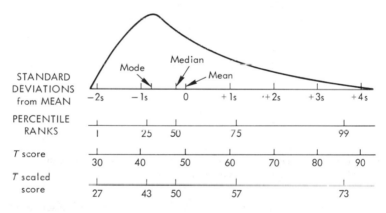

FIG. 10–3   Relationships of Selected Scores in a Normal Distribution and a Positively Skewed Distribution

The *T-scaled* score is the same as the T score only if the distribution is normal. We must keep in mind that the mean of T score distribution is determined by setting the *mean* of the raw score distribution at 50, while the mean of the T-scaled score is determined by setting the *median* of the raw score distribution at 50. Thus, the differences between the T score and the T-scaled score increase as the distribution of raw scores becomes increasingly skewed. The T-scaled distribution has a mean of 50 and a standard deviation of 10. An example of a table of norms using the T-scaled score for the Dyer Tennis Test is given in Table 10–3.

TABLE 10–3 • T Scale For New Method Scoring*

T Scale	Test Score	T Scale	Test Score	T Scale	Test Score	T Scale	Test Score
100	67	75	50	50	33	25	16
99	66	74	49	49	32	24	15
98		73		48		23	
97	65	72	48	47	31	22	14
96	64	71	47	46	30	21	13
95		70		45		20	
94	63	69	46	44	29	19	12
93	62	68	45	43	28	18	11
92		67	44	42	27	17	10
91	61	66		41		16	
90	60	65	43	40	26	15	9
89	59	64	42	39	25	14	8
88		63		38		13	
87	58	62	41	37	24	12	7
86	57	61	40	36	23	11	6
85		60		35		10	
84	56	59	39	34	22	9	5
83	55	58	38	33	21	8	4
82		57		32		7	
81	54	56	37	31	20	6	3
80	53	55	36	30	19	5	2
79		54		29		4	
78	52	53	35	28	18	3	1
77	51	52	34	27	17	2	
76		51		26		1	

*Reprinted from J. Dyer, "Revision of Backboard Test of Tennis Ability," *Research Quarterly*, XI, (1938), p. 25, by permission of the author and publisher.

Another type of normalized standard score is the stanine score. Stanine scores were developed during World War II to provide the maximum information that could be punched in a single column of an IBM card. Stanine refers to a *stan*dard score of *nine* units. Each stanine, except for the extremes of 1 and 9, is one–half standard deviation in width. The mean of the stanine scale is 5, the midpoint of the middle stanine, and the standard deviation is 2. The stanine of five is determined by the middle 20 percent of the raw scores. The remaining stanines account for increasingly smaller percentages of the raw score distribution.

Stanine Scale

1	2	3	4	5	6	7	8	9
4%	7%	12%	17%	20%	17%	12%	7%	4%

A stanine of four, then, represents the next 17 percent of the raw score distribution that falls below the stanine of five.

Stanines are rather coarse representations of the raw score distribution. If a test is surrounded by a great deal of measurement error, the stanine scale is probably adequate, because precisely pinpointing the individual's position is impossible. However, for a highly reliable test, stanines are probably unnecessarily coarse. A further limitation is the difficulty in interpreting stanines because the percentages of scores vary across stanines. Table 10–2 gives an example of the use of stanines in physical education.

Choice of Type of Scale

The choice of the type of derived score that should be used depends in part upon the needs of the test constructor. Probably no one type of scale can be considered best. Lyman (1970), however, expresses a preference for percentiles and percentile bands because of their ease of interpretation and consideration of measurement error. The *APA Standards* (1966) recommends the use of standard scores since such scores may be utilized statistically in more ways than percentiles, so that more information can be obtained from test results. Whenever standard scores are used, the test constructor should specify whether linear transformations of raw scores (as in T scores) or normalized scores (as in T-scaled scores) are used. For the physical education teacher who develops local norms, percentiles and percentile bands are probably more convenient if the scales are to be used to interpret individual student's raw scores. For other purposes, such as group comparisons, the mean and standard deviation will probably be computed making the use of standard scores more convenient.

Criteria for Selecting Norms

Before a teacher uses a test that is accompanied by a table of norms, the table should be carefully examined. Five questions are appropriate for the examination of a norms table (Gronlund, 1965).

1. Are the norms relevant for the students?
2. Are the norms based on a representative sample?
3. Are the norms up-to-date?
4. Are the norms comparable from test to test?
5. Are the norms adequately described?

The question of relevance can be answered by examining the nature of the sample on which the norms are based. The norm group should be similar in type to the students who will be taking the test. If, for instance, a physical education teacher who deals with high school boys is interested in using the table of norms for a battery of skill tests, and the norms were developed for college men, should the teacher use these norms? Probably not. Preferably, the norms should be developed using a sample of high school boys. However, if the high school students are seniors in a school area where most of the students go on to college, the norms might be useful for general comparisons. In most high school situations, however, the use of norms developed for college students would be questionable.

If the norms are developed for high school students, is the sample of high school students a *representative* one? For example, norms developed using high school students in California would not be representative of the typical high school population. Because the climate is conducive to regular physical activity throughout the year, many physical performance norms based on the California sample would not be representative of high schools in other parts of the country. Thus, comparisons with students from depressed economic areas where the climate is harsh would not be proper. If the norms are national norms, all areas of the country should be sampled, as well as all sizes of schools, in order to have a representative sample. If the norms are developed using students from only one school, the area from which the norm sample was drawn and the size of the school should be similar to the area and school size of the students whose scores are to be compared.

Norms developed ten years ago may no longer reflect the ability of the population they concern. Thus, norms should be reexamined periodically and revised if necessary. The AAHPER Youth Fitness Test norms were first published in 1958. When the items were reexamined at a later date (1966), the raw scores for a given norm were higher in almost every case than in the 1958 tables of norms. Based on this information, the norms were revised in the 1965 *Test Manual*. The teacher using norms should be satisfied that the norms are reasonably up-to-date.

When norms are given for several tests in a battery, the norms for all tests should be based on the same sample so that comparisons from test to test are meaningful. If the norms for the flexed-arm hang are determined using a sample of girls from twenty-five schools, and the norms for the standing broad jump were determined using a sample of girls from twenty-five *different* schools, the two samples are not necessarily comparable and, thus, neither are the two sets of norms.

Whenever a norms table is published, the following information should be included for the teacher:

1. Method of sampling.
2. Number and distribution of cases included in the norm sample.
3. Characteristics of the norm group with regard to such factors as age, sex, race, scholastic aptitude, educational level, socioeconomic status, types of schools represented, and geographic location.
4. Extent to which standard conditions of administration and motivation were maintained during the testing.
5. Date of the testing, whether it was done in the fall or spring (Gronlund, 1965, p. 298).

Local Norms and National Norms

A table of norms presented by a test publisher is usually based on a large sample of students who are representative of the specified population. The norms for both the AAHPER Youth Fitness Test and the AAHPER Cooperative Physical Education Knowledge Tests are based on large national samples. However, little information is given by the publishers on the details of drawing the sample. Assuming national norms meet selection criteria adequately, they can be useful for certain purposes. A teacher may wish to compare his students' levels of ability with the national sample as partial evidence when justifying a physical education program. If the norms are high, the program is operating satisfactorily with respect to whatever ability is being tested. If the norms are low, perhaps certain aspects of the program need to be expanded. National norms are also useful for comparisons among distinct subpopulations within an area. For example, in a large metropolitan area, comparisons of performance levels of "inner city" students, "fringe" area students, and suburban students with national norms may be useful.

On the other hand, national norms are limited in the type of information they can provide. In a school with a good physical education program, *all* of the students may score above the middle of the distribution on the tables of national norms. While this information may be useful in justifying a physical education program, the individual student receives little information on his performance relative to the other students in his school. *Local norms* would provide more useful information in this case. A student who is above-average on national norms may be average or even below-average compared with local norms. Local norms must be developed by the teachers within a school district. It may be necessary to collect scores over a period of several years in order to obtain adequate data to develop norms. Local norms should be revised periodically so that they are up-to-date.

Summary

Norms are developed by transforming the raw scores of a given norm group into some type of derived scores so that they may be interpreted more easily. Raw scores can be converted to percentage-correct scores, in which the score actually obtained on the test is divided by the highest possible test score. This type of conversion is useful for tests of motor skills and abilities, but cannot be used for comparisons among tests.

Four types of norms have been most commonly used: grade, age percentile, and standard score norms. *Grade norms* are determined by computing the average of the raw scores for each grade, and using the grade equivalent in place of the average. *Age norms* are determined by computing the average of the raw scores for each age, and using the age equivalent in place of the average. *Percentile norms* are determined by the percentage of individuals in the norm group who fall below an individual's score. *Standard score norms* are represented by the distance of a given raw score above or below the mean of the norm group as expressed in standard deviation units. Although all types of norms have advantages and disadvantages, the use of percentiles (and percentile bands) or standard scores is generally recommended.

The decision to use a table of norms should be based on five criteria: relevance, representativeness, recency, comparability, and descriptive detail. If the norm group is similar to the individuals who will be compared, the norms are *relevant*. If the norm group consists of an adequate sample of the type of individuals described, the norms are *representative*. Norms should be reasonably *up-to-date* so that the present level of ability of students is reflected. Norms for subtests within a battery of tests should be based on the same norm group so that the subtest norms are *comparable*. A table of norms should be accompanied by a *detailed description* of the norm group and the testing circumstances.

Local norms can easily be developed by physical education teachers. Although national norms are useful for general comparison and for the justification of physical education programs, these norms do not provide information on the local group of students within a school or school district. Both national and local norms are useful under certain circumstances. The choice of appropriate norms can best be made using a combination of common sense and knowledge about scales.

Bibliography

American Association for Health, Physical Education and Recreation. *Youth Fitness Test Manual*. Washington, D. C.: American Association for Health, Physical Education and Recreation, 1965.

American Association for Health, Physical Education and Recreation. *AAHPER Sports Skills Tests*, Washington, D.C.: American Association for Health, Physical Education and Recreation, 1967.

American Psychological Association. *Standards for Educational and Psychological Tests and Manuals*. Washington, D. C.: American Psychological Association, Inc., 1966.

ANGOFF, W. H. "Scales, Norms, and Equivalent Scores," in *Educational Measurement*, ed. R. L. Thorndike. Washington. D. C.: American Council on Education, 1971, pp. 508–600.

BARROW, H. M. and R. McGEE. *A Practical Approach to Measurement in Physical Education*. Philadelphia: Lea and Febiger, 1972.

BROWN, H. S. "A Test Battery for Evaluating Golf Skills," *Texas Association for Health, Physical Education and Recreation Journal* (1969), pp. 4–5, 28–29.

Cooperative Tests and Services. *AAHPER Cooperative Physical Education Tests*. Princeton, N.J.: Educational Testing Service, 1970.

DYER, J. T. "Revision of Backboard Test of Tennis Ability," *Research Quarterly*, IX, No. 1 (1938), p. 25.

EBEL, R. L. *Measuring Educational Achievement*. Englewood Cliffs, N. J.: Prentice-Hall, Inc., 1965.

GRONLUND, N. E. *Measurement and Evaluation in Teaching*. New York: The Macmillan Company, 1965.

HUNSICKER, P. and G. G. REIFF. "A Survey and Comparison of Youth Fitness 1958–1965." *Journal of Health, Physical Education and Recreation*, XXXVII (1966), pp. 23–25.

LYMAN, H. B. *Test Scores and What They Mean*, Englewood Cliffs, N. J.: Prentice-Hall, Inc., 1970.

SCOTT, M. G. and E. FRENCH. *Measurement and Evaluation in Physical Education*. Dubuque, Iowa: Wm. C. Brown Company Publishers, 1959.

WEAR, C. L. "The Evaluation of Attitude toward Physical Education as an Activity Course," *Research Quarterly*, XXII (1951), pp. 114–126.

WILSON, M. R. "A Relationship between General Motor Ability and Objective Measures of Achievement in Swimming at the Intermediate Level for College Women." Unpublished Master's thesis, University of North Carolina, Greensboro, 1962.

11

grading in physical education

Because educators make a number of final decisions based on grades, the issue of grading is a controversial one. The controversy is by no means of recent orgin. Throughout the twentieth century, the shortcomings of various systems of grading have been discussed in the educational literature. The same shortcomings exist today. In this chapter, several systems of grading will be examined along with bases for grading. No specific grading system will be recommended. Each system has advantages and disadvantages that should be taken into account by the teacher using it. The bases for determining a grade will also be discussed, although again no specific ones will be suggested, since the teacher's decisions will be at least partially determined by his own philosophy and the philosophy operating within his school system.

Much of the controversy associated with the determination of grades is due to the fact that grades are often misused. The process of grading is in itself complex, being filled with unsolved problems. In addition, as the teacher determines grades, he is required to make judgments that are often irreversible and have definite ramifications for his students. This process is, for many teachers, against human nature. If a teacher likes a student a great deal, he may feel reluctant to give that student a low grade, even if the student deserves the grade. Students are not likely to complain about grades that are higher than they deserve; however, some students raise objections about poor grades that they in fact merit.

Two major shortcomings can be associated with grading. First, the meaning of the grade is not clearly defined. Grades can vary from class to class and from teacher to teacher. Thus, an "A" in one course may be equivalent to a "C" in another course of the same type. Second, grades are often not based on objective evidence. Too often the halo effect operates in the determination of grades. Some teachers have been known to give good grades as a reward and poor grades as punishment. Others simply feel that they can competently grade their students using subjective judgment. Occasionally, a teacher will say that he graded his students subjectively, then determined their grades based on objective evidence, and found that the two sets of grades were the same. Such a conclusion suggests one of two possibilities. Either the teacher, by virtue of collecting the objective evidence, is using information that is much more than purely subjective to judge each student, or the so-called objective evidence is based more on subjective tests than objective ones. At any rate, the use of subjective judgment alone is totally unfair to the student, who has the right to know the bases upon which he is being judged.

In recent years, some teachers have rejected grades because they view grades as poor motivational devices. This may be an indictment of the teacher rather than an indictment of grades because it is far easier for the teacher not to have to make judgments. Then, however, the students cannot know what, if any, standards they have met. If a teacher who objects to grading does little in the way of evaluating students, that teacher's practices can be called into question. Even if no grades are given, the teacher should attempt to provide maximal feedback to the students. If grades must be given, the teacher should use as much evidence as possible in determining them.

Use of Grades

The most common uses of grades are to report the student's status to himself, to his present and future teachers, to his parents, and to the administrators. Also, grades often act as motivational devices for students.

Reporting the Student's Status to Himself

In a physical education class where the teaching-learning process is operating efficiently, the student will continually receive feedback on his performance. However, at the end of any given unit, the student would probably profit from some type of summary of his achievement. A unit grade can provide this sort of information.

Grades are based on the summative evaluation of student learning. Thus, grades reflect the end product of educational units. It is true that the means to that end are more important than the end itself, but as long as grades are used in school settings, they will be important to students. No matter how much the teacher de-emphasizes grades, the students will be concerned about them.

Reporting the Student's Status to Parents.

Although a student may receive feedback from day to day in a physical education class, the student's grade is the major method of communication between the school and the parents and as much information as possible should be given along with it. For example, the major objectives might be listed along with an indication of the student's progress toward meeting them. Whatever grading system is used, the parents should be informed of its bases.

Reporting the Student's Status to Teachers

The student's teacher can make use of his grade in several ways. Class grades can be used to aid in the evaluation of both teaching and the curriculum. Perhaps the most valuable effect of grading is to help the teacher gain a better overall understanding of the student's achievement. Information on grades should also be helpful in providing guidance for the student.

When a teacher begins a new year with a new group of students, grades from the previous year can be used to classify the students into groups. Even if classification is not desired, the information on grades can be used in planning future units. However, the teacher should guard against placing total reliance on previous grades since they might not have been determined objectively.

Reporting the Student's Status to Administrators

The student's grades are used in many ways within a school system. They can be used as evidence that students are meeting stated objectives. Grades are also used for purposes of promotion and graduation, honors, althletic eligibility, and college entrance.

Motivation of Students

Grades are motivational devices for most students. Whether or not teachers like it, the motivation is often to do whatever is needed in order to receive a satisfactory grade.

> If the marks earned in a course of study are made to represent progress toward getting an education, working for marks is *ipso facto* a furtherance of education. If the marks are so bad that the student who works tor and attains them misses an education, then working for marks is a practice to be eschewed. When marks are given, we are not likely to dissuade pupils from working for them; and there is no sensible reason why we should. It simply does not make sense to grade pupils, to maintain institutional machinery for assembling and recording the gradings,

while at the same time telling pupils marks do not amount to much. As a matter of fact they do amount to something and the pupil knows this. If we are dissatisfied with the results of working for marks we might try to improve the marks (Stroud, 1946, p. 632).

Bases for Determining Grades

Measurement authorities in physical education agree that one important basis for determining a grade is improvement in the motor or psychomotor domain. This area includes achievement in skills, playing ability and physical fitness. There is also general agreement that the cognitive domain should provide part of the basis for grading, although perhaps to a lesser extent. The cognitive area includes knowledges and understanding of the principles and mechanics of movement, rules, safety, conditioning, history, and so on. The predominant area of disagreement regarding appropriate bases for grading lies within the affective domain. This area includes social behaviors such as effort, attitude, sportsmanship, and citizenship. The degree to which each of the three domains affects a given grade is largely a matter of philosophy.

Achievement in Motor Skills as a Basis for Grading

The importance of achievement in motor skills as a basis for grading depends upon the objectives of the unit. Probably this area will receive the greatest emphasis in grading in many physical education classes. In a beginning class, much emphasis will probably be placed on skill development, where as in an intermediate class the emphasis on skill development and playing ability may be equal.

One of the overall objectives of a physical education program may be the development of physical fitness. If so, assessment of the student's level of fitness should be incorporated into the final grade. Hanson (1967) suggests using several sets of criteria rather than a single standard of fitness, because of individual differences in body build. These differences may be partially taken into account by using tables of norms based on age, height, and weight.

Improvement in Motor Skills as a Basis for Grading

When a student's performance improves over a given period of time, we assume that learning has taken place, although performance and learning are not necessarily synonymous. We can examine the student's final achievement level, or we can focus on the amount of improvement that has been attained. Although improvement is desired by both the student and the teacher, perhaps more problems develop from attempting to use improvement as a basis for grading than from any other source.

First of all, improvement scores are notably unreliable. To obtain improvement scores, a post-test score must be compared with a pretest score. The difference between them is the improvement score. There will be a degree of unreliability associated with both the pretest and post-test scores. The measurement error associated with each test is compounded in the improvement score. In addition, as the correlation between the pretest and the post-test increases, the reliability of the improvement score decreases, no matter how reliable the tests may be.

At the same time, the potential amount of improvement a given individual can attain depends upon his level of skill. The highly skilled person cannot be expected to improve as much as the poorly skilled, because the highly skilled one has less room for improvement.

Another problem associated with grading on improvement is the necessity for obtaining the student's pretest score. Proper motivation by the teacher is essential to prevent the test-wise student from giving less than his best performance on the pretest in hopes of appearing to make greater gains on the post-test.

Hanson (1967) notes that in order to improve, we must allow adequate time for improvement. Some students need to practice over long periods of time in order to improve. Thus, being limited to a five- or six-week unit may handicap some students. This is also a problem when grading on achievement.

Finally, although an attempt to grade on improvement may motivate the poorly skilled student who feels locked in a certain grade tract, emphasizing the student's improvement score will not conceal his true achievement level. If the student's performance is poor in relation to others in class, he knows it. Grading on improvement, although desirable, should probably be minimized until more appropriate ways are developed to handle improvement scores.

Development of Cognitive Skills as a Basis for Grading

There is general agreement that knowledge and understanding of certain aspects of physical education should be part of the grade. Understanding of the principles and mechanics of movement, along with the application of these principles to specific activities, are among the more important cognitive skills. Lower level cognitive skills such as knowledge of the rules and strategies of a sport can be used in determining grades when appropriate. Other cognitive skills that might be measured are safety factors, the history of a given sport, and principles of conditioning.

Development of Affective Skills as a Basis for Grading

Grades that are based on affective skills, sometimes referred to as the impressionistic method of grading (Weber and Paul, 1971), are determined by such factors as attitude, attendance, sportsmanship, effort, dress, and showers. Unfortunately, these factors constitute the major part of the grade in some physical education classes even though their assessment is generally unreliable and frequently punitive in nature. For this type of grading, certain factors are usually considered as a reflection of attitude, that is, if a student's attitude is good, he will attend class, be a good sport, try hard, wear the proper uniform and shower after class. However, these factors are extremely difficult to measure and the halo effect can play a large part in assessing affective skills. Furthermore, the cognitive and psychomotor skills can be neglected when affective skills are overemphasized. The presence of desired affective skills in no way guarantees achievement in motor skills or understanding of movement. A discussion of some of the affective skills which are often used as a basis for grading follows.

Attendance. According to a report by Mathews (1968), in 80 percent of the schools to which fifty practice teachers were assigned, grades were based solely on being present and in uniform daily. The determination of factors on which the grade is to be based should depend upon the course objectives. Is regular attendance a course objective, or is it a matter of school policy? Attendance should be a matter of school policy, and deviant behavior related to attendance should be dealt with by the principal or other designated authorities. A grade that is based on attendance is punitive.

The practice of grading on attendance has sometimes been supported by observing that a student cannot learn if he is not in class. If, however, the student is able to meet the course objectives satisfactorily, his grade should not be reduced because of attendance. Although disciplinary action should be taken against a student who is in school but does not attend class, whether this action comes from the principal or the teacher, the punishment should not take the form of reducing his achievement grade.

Effort. Effort is extremely difficult to evaluate. Does a student who performs well with seemingly little effort work less than the student with less skill who obviously works hard? Can a teacher judge the amount of effort displayed by an individual based on his facial expression? On how tired he looks? If part of the grade is based on effort, then effort must be evaluated with a reasonable degree of objectivity. A teacher may genuinely feel that he is able to judge effort adequately by using his (subjective) judgment, but his personal values will probably interfere.

We can assume that effort is reflected in achievement. However, if no achievement occurs, is the effort meaningful?

T. L. Kelley (1927) reported that, "In the year 413 B. C. some seven thousand survivors of the ill-fated Athenian army were thrown into the quarries near Syracuse, and it is recorded that in many cases their very lives and their release from the agonies of their imprisonment depended upon their ability to repeat verses of Euripides. There is no record that anyone received A for effort" (Cureton, 1971, p. 1).

Even if effort is one of the affective skills of concern in the course objectives, it should not be graded unless systematic means with which to do so are devised.

Dress and showers. The need for clothing appropriate for physical education classes is obvious. However, the practice of grading on uniforms is questionable. Whether or not a student is in uniform is a matter of departmental (or teacher) policy. If the student has a dirty uniform or no uniform at all, he should be penalized (if the policy requires uniforms), but not by lowering his achievement grade. If grading on dress is essential for disciplinary purposes, this type of grade should be recorded separately from the achievement grade.

The practice of taking showers should also be controlled by departmental policy. Theoretically, showers are easy to check, but for purposes of expediency the shower check often consists of checking to see that the student is wet on some part of his body. If showering is thought to reflect attitude objectives or health objectives, what is an indication of a satisfactory shower? The need for showers can be explained, and the students can be encouraged to take showers, but grading the student on showers is no assurance that the value will become ingrained. At any rate, whether or not showers are mandatory, grades should not be based on them unless a separate grade is reported.

Sportsmanship. Every physical education teacher hopes to implant values associated with good sportsmanship in his students. The development and encouragement of habits that reflect good sportsmanship constitute some objectives of many physical education programs. However, the process of grading this attribute is often haphazard and unreliable. If sportsmanship is to be graded, the teacher must record incidents for each student that reflect varying degrees of sportsmanship in the class situation. Although this may seem like a totally unrealistic task to the teacher, he should keep in mind the degree to which his personal values can affect such judgments. If a systematic approach cannot be taken to the assessment of affective skills, these skills should not be graded. If disciplinary matters are of concern to the teacher, such matters can be recorded and reported separately.

Absolute and Relative Grades

Absolute grades are determined by the achievement of predetermined levels of mastery. This method of grading is associated with the concept of mastery learning (as described in Chapter 3) and the use of percentage-correct scores (see Chapter 10). Relative grades are based on a student's performance in relation to others in class. This system is based on the normal probability curve. Relative grades are related to the idea of norm-referenced measures (Chapter 3) and the standard score distribution (Chapter 10).

Grading on an Absolute Standard

If the traditional five-letter or five-number grading system is used, five categories of percentages must be determined for the absolute grading system. If the mastery level has been identified as 90 percent, then 90 percent–100 percent could be designated as the A category, as shown in Table 11–1. In this table, the percentage-correct score categories are determined using the percentage-correct scores that correspond to the letter grade. The percentages do *not* represent percentages of individuals taking the test. The categories in Table 11–1 are arbitrary in that the mastery level itself may vary from one test to another, or the minimal passing level (D) may vary.

TABLE 11–1 • Example of Grading on an Absolute Standard

Grade	Percentage-correct Score
A	90%—100%
B	80% –89%
C	70%—79%
D	60%—69%
F	Below 60%

The difficulties in using the absolute grading system become evident when several sets of percentage-correct scores must be used to determine final grades. The scores cannot be directly compared across tests, since the level of difficulty for each test will vary. If membership in a category is determined by a given range of points, then a point system can be used to determine the final grade. For example, if a test is designed to measure speed and accuracy, the maximum accuracy and the optimal speed score will yield the highest number of points. Instead of transforming the points to a percentage-correct score, the score ranges can be used to determine the grade categories. (This method is used extensively in the section on "Formative Evaluation in Golf" at the end of Chapter 3.) When the percentage-correct score is used, as shown in Table 11–1, the letter grades for the appropriate categories must be converted to numbers in order to determine the final grade. A conversion table is given in Table 11–2.

TABLE 11–2 • Table for Converting Letter Grades to Numbers

Grade	Number	Grade	Number
A +	12	C	5
A	11	C −	4
A −	10	D +	3
B +	9	D	2
B	8	D −	1
B −	7	F	0
C +	6		

Since some measures will be of greater importance than others in a given unit, the teacher must consider a system of weighting the tests. If the scores of each test are averaged using some transformation, and the tests are similar in difficulty level, each test automatically receives the same weight. When working with percentage-correct scores, the first must be converted into letter grades, and then the letter grades must be converted into numerical values. The tests of greater importance are then given higher weights by the teacher. This system is described in Table 11–3 in which the motor skills are weighted more heavily than any other abilities, since skill development received the greatest emphasis in this situation. This example is somewhat simplified, and is not meant to reflect the complete set of objectives for the course.

TABLE 11–3 • Use of Weights in Determining Grades

Badminton Unit for Beginners

Test	Weight	Grade	Total
Skill Development	3	B−	3 × 7 = 21
Short serve			
Long serve			
Overhead clear			
Development of knowledges	2	C	2 × 5 = 10
Knowledge of rules			
Knowledge of principles			
Playing Ability	1	B+	1 × 9 = 9
	6		40

GRADE = 40/6 = 6.67 = B–

Using Table 11–2, the numerical values for the grades in Table 11–3 are determined. The numerical value for the skills grade of B− is 7. The weight for skill development (3) is multiplied by the numerical value for a B− (7). When this procedure is carried out for all components of the final grade, the total (40) is divided by the sum of the weights (6). In this case, the result is 6.67, which should be rounded off to 7. Referring again to Table 11–2, the appropriate grade for a numerical value of 7 is B—.

The procedure for determining a final grade from percentage-correct scores has some inherent weaknesses. In the process of converting the scores to grades, and the grades to numbers, information is lost about the original scores. For this reason, the system of working with total points rather than percentage-correct scores may be preferred. Other disadvantages of the absolute method of grading are primarily the same as those of using percentage-correct scores. This method requires a level of precision that is difficult to attain, since measurement errors surround every score. The teacher must know how much *can* be learned, and then must determine how much *was* learned.

This system, however, has the advantage of providing a fixed, standard measure of achievement. Achievement, then, is related to predetermined levels of mastery, providing students with clearly defined goals. Another advantage lies in the relative ease of computation. In addition, the use of absolute grades can complement program evaluation and is useful in evaluating motor skills and abilities.

Grading on a Relative Standard

A relative standard of grading can be utilized according to either the percentage method or the standard deviation method. In both cases, any given number of grade categories can be determined. However, since the majority of schools use a five-category grading system, five categories will be used in the examples for each of the two methods.

Percentage method. The percentage method should be differentiated from the percentage-correct method. In the *percentage method,* categories are assigned by designating the percentages of the group taking the test. In Table 11–4, membership in the top category is determined by taking the top 7 percent of the individuals taking the test. Whether the scores are considered good or bad, the top 7 percent of the students will receive A's and the bottom 7 percent will receive F's. The *percentage-correct method* determines the categories in advance. The student is not judged relative to his peers but rather according to the predetermined category into which he falls. Several varieties of the percentage method are given in Table 11–4. Many other varieties are also possible. Note that example 1 in Table 11–4 approximates the normal distribution.

The percentage method has the same disadvantage as percentiles: grades on various tests cannot be directly compared because of the differences that exist among tests.

Standard deviation method. The standard deviation method is based on

TABLE 11–4 • **Examples of the Percentage Method of Grading**

Grade	Example 1	Example 2	Example 3
A	7	10	15
B	24	20	20
C	38	40	30
D	24	20	20
F	7	10	15

the standard deviation of the distribution of scores. This method is good to use because scores on all tests can be transformed into a common scale. The grades can then be averaged to determine a final grade, and scores can be directly compared from test to test. The use of this method for a five-category grading scale is described in Table 11–5.

TABLE 11–5 • **Example of the Standard Deviation Method of Grading**

Grade	Standard deviation range	Percent
A	$1.5s$ or more above mean	7
B	Between $+ 0.5s$ and $+ 1.5s$	24
C	Between $+ 0.5s$ and $- 0.5s$	38
D	Between $- 0.5s$ and $- 1.5s$	24
F	$1.5s$ or more below the mean	7

One disadvantage of this system is that the students set the standard. Not all classes are typical, yet some students in each class will receive A's and some will receive F's. However, this system has been found to be the most reliable of any grading system. In addition, the students are not penalized for differences in instruction. The standard deviation method is useful in physical education classes for evaluating cognitive skills (Weber and Paul, 1971), although some physical educators recommend using this method for psychomotor skills as well (Barrow and McGee, 1964; Broer, 1959).

A point of view on relative standards of grading which is held by many measurement specialists is described in this analogy:

> In most areas of human activity awards go to the individuals who are outstanding in relative, not absolute, terms. There are no absolute standards for speed in running the mile or for distance in throwing the javelin. The winner in any race is determined on a relative basis. Runners on a starting line seldom agree to loaf along simply because there is no absolute standard of speed they have to meet. From the point of view of the individual runner in the 100-yard dash, as well as that of the individual student majoring in history or chemistry, the best way to achieve outstanding success is to put forth outstanding effort (Ebel, 1965, p. 414).

One response to this viewpoint might be that the competitive situation involves a level of motivation that is not present in the average learning situation.

When using the standard deviation method of grading, the test with the greater variability will automatically be weighted the most. For example, a test that is twice as variable as another is weighted twice as much. The variability of each test, then, must be taken into account when developing a system of weights.

Since standard scores can be averaged, less information is lost in the process of determining the final grade. This process is preferable to that of converting the raw scores into letter grades, and the letter grades into numbers in order to determine the final grade.

Other Systems of Grading

Many other systems of grading have been used by educators. Two of these systems—pass-fail grading and a checklist of objectives—will be briefly described in this section.

Pass-Fail Method

The use of a two-grade category, such as pass-fail or satisfactory-unsatisfactory, is sometimes recommended by physical educators so that attempts by students to achieve only for the sake of a grade will be reduced. In addition, this method is thought to reduce the error that occurs when attempting to use a larger number of grade categories. However, this is not really the case. There is considerable evidence that, although the number of incorrect placements is reduced, this method is more unreliable than those using more categories because every incorrect placement is now of much greater significance (Ebel, 1965). In other words, giving an individual a grade of C when the individual's grade should have been a B is a serious matter, but not nearly so severe as giving the individual a grade of Fail when he should have received a Pass. The use of fewer grade categories is *never* more reliable than the use of many categories.

Generally, pass-fail grades are not recommended for physical education classes except as a voluntary system in an elective program, such as that described by Shea (1971). Use of this system, however, does not remove the inequities that exist in other grading systems.

The notion that marking problems can be simplified and marking errors reduced by using fewer marking categories is an attractive one. Its weakness is exposed by carrying it to the limit. If only one category is used, if everyone is given the same mark, all marking problems vanish, but so does the value of marking. A major shortcoming of two-category marking, and to some degree of five-category marking as well, is this same kind of loss of information. To trade more precisely meaningful marks for marks easier to assign may be a bad bargain for education (Ebel, 1965. p. 422).

Checklist of Objectives

A grading system that is commonly used at the elementary school level is a set of symbols that can be used with a list of the major objectives of the program. The following symbols might be used with the list of objectives:

O   (outstanding)
S   (satisfactory)
N   (needs improvement)

The appropriate symbol is placed next to each objective on the list. Table 11–6 gives an example of this system as it might be used in elementary school physical education.

TABLE 11–6 • Sample Checklist of Objectives for Elementary School Physical Education

Symbol	Objective
S	Ability to move at different speeds, using different levels.
S	Ability to handle various sizes of balls in a variety of ways.
N	Ability to use a variety of locomotor patterns.

The student's report card will probably not have adequate space to list the major objectives of each class. Therefore, the physical education teacher may wish to send a letter containing more detailed information to the parents of each child.

Use of Institutional Grading Systems

The use of a common grading system throughout a school is a unanimous recommendation of measurement specialists. When a common grading system is used, the grades will form similar distributions throughout the school. In addition the reliability of the grading system is somewhat increased. The same kind of information is provided for students in all areas of the curriculum. Special areas, such as physical education, should use grades to discriminate to the same degree as other parts of the curriculum so that excellence in performance is recognized in all areas.

Reporting Multiple Grades

The procedure of including more than one grade for each curriculum area is often recommended so that one of the grades can be based purely on achievement. Frequently, a second grade is classified as a "citizenship" grade. In physical education, separating motor skill grades from the grades for cognitive and affective skills would provide useful information for all concerned. Although such a separation is somewhat artificial, the grades will have more meaning than a single grade to their interpreters.

Summary

Much of the controversy associated with grading is the result of their misuse. Even though some individuals may disagree with the practice of giving grades, most school systems require teachers to report grades for students in their classes. Since a student's grade becomes a part of his permanent record and is used in many ways, the teacher should strive for maximal objectivity in reporting grades.

Grades are typically used to provide information on the student's status to his parents, his teachers, the administrators in his school, and the student himself. Because of the ways in which grades are used, they become strong motivational devices for the students.

Grades should be determined according to the degree to which the course objectives are met. A physical education curriculum may include objectives for the development of psychomotor, cognitive, and affective skills. There is general agreement that physical educators should base grades on the development of psychomotor and cognitive skills, although a teacher may wish to report separate grades for the two types of skills. Although objectives based on the development of affective attributes, such as sportsmanship are important, the difficulty in measuring such skills objectively complicates the determination of reliable grades for them.

Two systems of grading, neither of which is appropriate for the same situation, are the absolute system and the relative system. Grades based on an absolute standard are determined by the achievement of predetermined levels of mastery. Grades based on a relative standard are determined by a student's performance in relation to others in class. The former method is appropriate for mastery-type learning, while the latter is useful when maximum discrimination among students is desired. Other systems of grading, such as the pass-fail system and the checklist of objectives, are useful in more limited situations.

> In the last forty years reams of material have been written about marking systems, but most of it has been a discussion of whether we should have marks at all. In actual practice it seems likely that we will have marks for some time to come. We need them for selection for honors, for promotion and for admission to courses of study, as well as for graduation; employers want them; graduate departments use them both for selection of students and for appointment of graduate assistants; students want them for their own guidance. And Jacques Barzun, in 1954 in his *Teacher in America,* wrote about ". . . the student's need to learn how to jump hurdles . . . Examinations are not just things that happen in school. They are a recurring feature of life, whether in the form of decisive interviews to pass, or important letters to write, or life and death diagnoses to make, or meetings to address, or girls to propose to. In most of these crises, you cannot bring your notes with you, and you must not leave your wits behind. The habit of passing examinations is therefore one to acquire early and to keep exercising even when there is a possibility of getting around it" (Cureton, 1971, p. 6).

Bibliography

BARROW, H. M. and R. McGEE. *A Practical Approach to Measurement in Physical Education.* Philadelphia: Lea and Febiger, 1972.

BROER, M. R. "Are Physical Education Grades Fair?" *Journal of Health, Physical Education and Recreation,* XXX (1959), pp. 27, 83.

CURETON, L. W. "The History of Grading Practices," *Measurement in Education,* II, No. 4 (1971).

EBEL, R. L. *Measuring Educational Achievement.* Englewood Cliffs, N.J.: Prentice-Hall, Inc., 1965.

GRONLUND, N.E. *Measurement and Evaluation on Teaching.* New York: The Macmillan Company, 1965.

HANSON, D.L. "Grading in Physical Education," *Journal of Health, Physical Education and Recreation,* XXXVIII (1967), pp. 34–39.

MATHEWS, D. K. *Measurement in Physical Education.* Philadelphia: W.B. Saunders Company, 1968.

SHEA, J. B. "The Pass-Fail Option in Physical Education," *Journal of Health, Physical Education and Recreation,* XLII (1971), pp. 19–20.

STROUD, J. B. *Psychology in Education.* New York: David McKay Co., Inc., 1946.

WEBER, L. J. and T. L. PAUL. "Approaches to Grading in Physical Education," *The Physical Educator,* XXVIII, No. 2 (1971), pp. 59–62.

A

sources for selected sports skill tests

This section is designed to provide the reader with references for a wide variety of sports skills tests that may be of interest to physical educators. Due to changes that have occurred in many sports over the years, some of the older tests may no longer be wholly appropriate for class usage. Nonetheless, numbers of these tests are included in this appendix because of their usefulness to the teacher in developing formative evaluation measures.

Archery

American Association for Health, Physical Education and Recreation. *Archery Skills Test Manual*. Washington, D.C.: American Association for Health, Physical Education and Recreation, 1967.

BOHN, R. W. "An Achievement Test in Archery." Unpublished Master's thesis, University of Wisconsin, Madison, 1962.

HYDE, EDITH I. "An Achievement Scale in Archery," *Research Quarterly*, VIII (1937), pp. 109–16.

ZABICK, R. M. and A. S. JACKSON. "Reliability of Archery Achievement," *Research Quarterly*, XL (1969), pp. 254–55.

Badminton

Department of Physical Education for Women, Badminton Report. An unpublished report prepared by the badminton committee, University of Wisconsin, 1963.

273

FRENCH, E. and E. STALTER. "Study of Skill Tests in Badminton for College Women," *Research Quarterly,* XX (1949), pp. 257–72.

GREINER, M. R. "Construction of a Short Serve Test for Beginning Badminton Players." Master's thesis, University of Wisconsin, Madison, 1964 (Microcard PE 670, University of Oregon, Eugene).

HALE, P. A. "Construction of a Long Serve Test for Beginning Badminton Players (Singles). " Master's thesis, University of Wisconsin, Madison, 1970 (Microcard PE 1133, University of Oregon, Eugene).

HICKS, J. V. "The Construction and Evaluation of a Battery of Five Badminton Skill Tests." Unpublished Doctoral dissertation, Texas Women's University, Denton, 1967.

LOCKHART, A. and F. A. MCPHERSON. "The Development of a Test of Badminton Playing Ability," *Research Quarterly,* XX (1949), pp. 402–5.

MCDONALD, E. D. "The Development of a Skill Test for the Badminton High Clear." Master's thesis, Southern Illinois University, Carbondale, 1968 (Microcard PE 1083, University of Oregon, Eugene).

MILLER, F. A. "A Badminton Wall Volley Test," *Research Quarterly,* XXII (1951), pp. 208–13.

SCOTT, M.G. "Achievement Examinations in Badminton, *Research Quarterly,* XII (1941), pp. 242–53.

SCOTT, M. G. and M. FOX. "Long Serve Test," in *Measurement and Evaluation in Physical Education,* ed. M.G. Scott and E. French. Dubuque, Iowa: Wm. C. Brown Company Publishers, 1959.

THORPE, J. and C. WEST. "A Test of Game Sense in Badminton," *Perceptual and Motor Skills,* XXVIII (1969), pp. 159–69.

Basketball

American Association for Health, Physical Education and Recreation. *Basketabll Skills Test Manual for Boys.* Washington, D. C.: American Association for Health, Physical Education and Recreation, 1966.

American Association for Health, Physical Education and Recreation. *Basketball Skills Test Manual for Girls.* Washington, D. C.: American Association for Health, Physical Education and Recreation, 1966.

DYER, J. T., J. C. SCHWEIG, and S.L. APGAR. "A Basketball Motor Ability Test for College Women and Secondary School Girls," *Research Quarterly,* X (1939), pp. 128–47.

EDGREN, H. D. "An Experiment in the Testing of Ability and Progress in Basketball." *Research Quarterly,* III (1932), pp. 159–71.

GLASSOW, R. B., V. COLVIN, and M. M. SCHWARTZ. "Studies Measuring Basketball Playing Ability of College Women," *Research Quarterly,* IX (1938), pp. 60–68.

JOHNSON, L. W. "Objective Tests in Basketball for High School Boys" in H. H.

Clarke, *Application of Measurement to Health and Physical Education.* Englewood Cliffs, N.J.: Prentice-Hall, Inc., 1967, pp. 306–8.

KAY, H. K. "A Statistical Analysis of the Profile Technique for the Evaluation of Competitive Basketball Performance." Unpublished Master's thesis, University of Alberta, Edmonton, Canada, 1966.

LAMBERT, A. T. "A Basketball Skill Test for College Women." Unpublished Master's thesis, University of North Carolina, Greensboro, 1969.

LATCHAW, M. "Measuring Selected Motor Skills in Fourth, Fifth, and Sixth Grades," *Research Quarterly,* XXV, (1954), pp. 439–49.

LEILICH, A. "Leilich Basketball Test," in H. M. Barrow and R. McGee, *A Practical Approach to Measurement in Physical Education.* Philadelphia: Lea & Febiger, 1972, pp. 280–85.

MILLER, W. K. "Achievement Levels in Basketball Skills for Women Physical Education Majors," *Research Quarterly,* XXV (1954), pp. 450–55.

SCHWARTZ, H. "Knowledge and Achievement Tests in Girls' Basketball on the Senior High School Level," *Research Quarterly,* VIII (1937), pp. 152–56.

STROUP, F. "Game Results as a Criterion for Validating Basketball Skill Tests," *Research Quarterly,* XXVI (1955), pp. 353–57.

THORNES, M. B. "An Analysis of a Basketball Shooting Test and Its Relation to Other Basketball Skill Tests." Master's thesis, University of Wisconsin, Madison, 1963 (Microcard PE 694, University of Oregon, Eugene).

YOUNG, G. and H. MOSER. "A Short Battery of Tests to Measure Playing Ability in Women's Basketball," *Research Quarterly,* V (1934), pp. 3–23.

Bowling

MARTIN, J. L. "Bowling Norms for College Men and Women," *Research Quarterly,* XXXI (1960), pp. 113–16.

MARTIN, J. and J. KEOGH. "Bowling Norms for College Students in Elective Physical Education Classes," *Research Quarterly,* XXXV (1964), pp. 325–27.

OLSON, J. K. and M.R. LIBA. "A Device for Evaluating Spot Bowling Ability," *Research Quarterly,* XXXVIII (1967), pp. 193–210.

PHILLIPS, M. and D. SUMMERS. "Bowling Norms and Learning Curves for College Women," *Research Quarterly,* XXI (1950), pp. 377–85.

SCHUNK C. *Test Questions for Bowling.* Philadelphia: W. B. Saunders Company, 1969.

Fencing

BOWER, M. G. "A Test of General Fencing Ability." Unpublished Master's thesis, University of Southern California, Los Angeles, 1961.

Cooper, C. K. "The Development of a Fencing Skill Test for Measuring Achievement of Beginning Collegiate Women Fencers in Using the Advance, Beat, and Lunge." Unpublished Master's thesis, Western Illinois University, Macomb, 1968.

Fein, J. T. "Construction of Skill Tests for Beginning Collegiate Women Fencers." Unpublished Master's thesis, University of Iowa, Iowa City, 1964.

Safrit, M. J. "Construction of a Skill Test for Beginning Fencers." Unpublished Master's thesis, University of Wisconsin, Madison, 1962.

Schutz, H. J. "Construction of an Achievement Scale in Fencing for Women." Unpublished Master's thesis, University of Washington, Seattle, 1940.

Wyrick, W. "A Comparison of the Effectiveness of Two Methods of Teaching Beginning Fencing to College Women." Unpublished Master's thesis, The Woman's College of the University of North Carolina, Greensboro, 1958.

Field Hockey

Friedel, J. W. "The Development of A Field Hockey Skill Test for High School Girls." Master's thesis, Illinois State Normal University, Normal, 1956 (Microcard, PE 289, University of Oregon, Eugene).

Illner, J.A. "The Construction and Validation of a Skill Test for the Drive in Field Hockey." Master's thesis, Southern Illinois University, Carbondale, 1968 (Microcard PE 1075, University of Oregon, Eugene).

Perry, E. L. "An Investigation of Field Hockey Skills Tests for College Women." Unpublished Master's thesis, Pennsylvania State University, University Park, 1969.

Schmithals, M. and E. French. "Achievement Tests in Field Hockey for College Women," Research Quarterly, XI (1940) pp. 84–92.

Strait, C. J. "The Construction and Evaluation of a Field Hockey Skills Test." Unpublished Master's thesis, Smith College, Northampton, Mass., 1960.

Football

American Association for Health, Physical Education and Recreation. Football Skills Test Manual. Washington, D.C.: American Association for Health, Physical Education and Recreation, 1966.

Borleske, S. E. "Achievement of College Men in Touch Football" in F. W. Cozens, "Ninth Annual Report of the Committee on Curriculum Research of the College Physical Education Association," Research Quarterly, VIII (1937), pp. 73–78.

McElroy, H. N. "A Report on Some Experimentation with a Skill Test," Research Quarterly, IX (1938), pp. 82–88.

Golf

BROWN, H. S. "A Test Battery for Evaluating Golf Skills," *Texas Association for Health, Physical Education and Recreation Journal,* (May 1969), pp. 4–5, 28–29.

CLEVETT, M. A. "An Experiment in Teaching Methods of Golf," *Research Quarterly,* II (1931), pp. 104–12.

COCHRANE, J. F. "The Construction of Indoor Golf Skills Test as a Measure of Golfing Ability." Unpublished Master's thesis, University of Minnesota, Minneapolis, 1960.

McKEE, M. E. "A Test for the Full Swinging Shot in Golf," *Research Quarterly,* XXI (1950), pp. 40–46.

NELSON J. K. "An Achievement Test in Golf," in *Practical Measurements for Evaluation in Physical Education.* eds. B. L. Johnson and J. K. Nelson. Minneapolis: Burgess Publishing Company, 1969.

VANDERHOOF, E. R. "Beginning Golf Achievement Tests." Master's thesis, State University of Iowa, Iowa City, 1956 (Microcard PE 306, University of Oregon, Eugene).

WATTS, H. "Construction and Evaluation of a Target on Testing the Approach Shot in Golf." Unpublished Master's thesis, University of Wisconsin, Madison, 1942.

WEST, C. and J. THORPE. "Construction and Validation of an Eight-iron Approach Test," *Research Quarterly,* XXXIX, No. 4 (1968) pp. 1115–20.

Gymnastics

BOWERS, C. O. "Gymnastics Skill Test for Beginning to Low Intermediate Girls and Women." Master's thesis, Ohio State University, Columbus, 1965 (Microcard PE 734, University of Oregon, Eugene)

FAULKNER, J. and N. LOKEN. "Objectivity of Judging at the National Collegiate Athletic Association Gymnastic Meet: A Ten-year Follow-up Study," *Research Quarterly,* XXXIII (1962), pp. 485–86.

Handball

CORNISH, C. "A Study of Measurement of Ability in Handball," *Research Quarterly,* XX (1949), pp. 215–22.

GRIFFITH, M. A. "An Objective Method of Evaluating Ability in Handball Singles." Unpublished Master's thesis, Ohio State University, Columbus, 1960.

MONTOYE, H. J. and J. BROTZMANN. "An Investigation of the Validity of Using the Results of a Doubles Tournament as a Measure of Handball Ability," *Research Quarterly,* XXII (1951), pp. 214–18.

Pennington, G. G. "A Measure of Handball Ability," *Research Quarterly,* XXXVIII (1967), pp. 247–53.

Ice Hockey

Merrifield, H. H. and G. A. Walford. "Battery of Ice Hockey Skill Tests," *Research Quarterly,* XL (1969), pp. 146–52.

Ice Skating

Carriere, D. L. "An Objective Figure Skating Test for Use in Beginning Classes." Unpublished Master's thesis, University of Illinois, Urbana, 1969.

Leaming, T. W. "A Measure of Endurance of Young Speed Skaters." Unpublished Master's thesis, University of Illinois, Urbana, 1959.

Recknagel, D. "A Test for Beginners in Figure Skating," *Journal of Health and Physical Education,* XVI (1945), pp. 91–92.

Lacrosse

Hodges, C. V. "Construction of an Objective Knowledge Test and Skill Tests in Lacrosse for College Women." Master's thesis, University of North Carolina, Greensboro, 1967 (Microcard PE 1074, University of Oregon, Eugene).

Lutze, M. C. "Achievement Tests in Beginning Lacrosse for Women." Unpublished Master's thesis, State University of Iowa, Iowa City, 1963.

Wilke, B. J. "Achievement Tests for Selected Lacrosse Skills of College Women." Unpublished Master's thesis, University of North Carolina, Greensboro, 1967.

Skiing

Rogers, H. M. "Construction of Objectively Scored Skill Tests for Beginning Skiers." Unpublished Master's thesis, University of Colorado, Boulder, 1960.

Wolfe, J. E. and H. H. Merrifield, "Predictability of Beginning Skiing Success from Basic Skill Tests in College Age Females." Paper presented at the National American Association for Health, Physical Education and Recreation Convention in Detroit, Michigan, April 1971.

Soccer

BAILEY, C. I. and F. L. TELLER. *Test Questions for Soccer*. Philadelphia: W. B. Saunders Company, 1969.

BONTZ, J. "An Experiment in the Construction of a Test for Measuring Ability in Some of the Fundamental Skills Used by Fifth and Sixth Grade Children in Soccer." Unpublished Master's thesis, State University of Iowa, Iowa City, 1942.

HEATH, M. L. and E. G. RODGERS. "A Study in the Use of Knowledge and Skill Tests in Soccer," *Research Quarterly*, III (1932), pp. 33–43.

JOHNSON, J. R. "The Development of a Single-item Test as a Measure of Soccer Skill." Microcarded Master's thesis, University of British Columbia, 1963.

MCDONALD, L. G. "The Construction of a Kicking Skill Test as an Index of General Soccer Ability." Unpublished Master's thesis, Springfield College, Springfield, Mass. 1951.

MCELROY, H. N. "A Report on Some Experimentation with a Skill Test," *Research Quarterly*, IX, (1938), pp. 82–88.

SCHAUFELE, E. F. "Schaufele Soccer Volleying Test," in H.M. Barrow and R. McGee, *A Practical Approach to Measurement in Physical Education*. Philadelphia: Lea & Febiger, 1972, pp. 298–300.

TOMLINSON, R. "Soccer Skill Test," *Soccer-Speedball Guide—July 1964–July 1966*. Washington, D. C.; Division of Girls and Women's Sports, American Association for Health, Physical Education and Recreation, 1964.

WARNER, G.F.H. "Warner Soccer Test," *Newsletter of the National Soccer Coaches Association of America*, VI (1950), pp. 13–22.

WHITNEY, A.H. and H. CHAPIN. "Soccer Skill Testing for Girls," *Soccer-Speedball Guide—July 1946–July 1948*. Washington, D.C.: National Section on Women's Athletics, American Association for Health, Physical Education and Recreation, 1946.

Softball

American Association for Health, Physical Education and Recreation. *Softball Skills Test Manual for Boys*, Washington, D.C.: American Association for Health, Physical Education and Recreation, 1967

American Association for Health, Physical Education and Recreation. *Softball Skills Test Manual for Girls*. Washington, D.C.: American Association for Health, Physical Education and Recreation, 1967.

BROER, M.R. "Reliability of Certain Skill Tests for Junior High School Girls," *Research Quarterly*, XXIX (1958), pp. 139–43.

DAVIS, R. "The Development of an Objective Softball Batting Test for College Women" in M.G. Scott and E. French, *Measurement and Evaluation in Physical Education*. Dubuque, Iowa: Wm. C. Brown Company, Publisher, 1959.

DEXTER, G. "Check List for Rating Softball Batting Skills," *Teachers Guide to Physical Education for Girls in High School.* Sacramento, California State Department of Education, 1957, p. 316.

ELROD, J.M. "Construction of a Softball Skill Test Battery for High School Boys." Unpublished Master's thesis, Louisiana State University, Baton Rouge, 1969.

FOX, M.G. and O.G. YOUNG. "A Test of Softball Batting Ability," *Research Quarterly,* XXV (1954), pp. 26–27.

FRINGER, M.N. "Fringer Softball Battery" in H.M. Barrow and R. McGee, *A Practical Approach to Measurement in Physical Education.* Philadelphia: Lea & Febiger, 1972 pp. 302–7.

KEHTEL, C.H. "The Development of a Test to Measure the Ability of a Softball Player to Field a Ground Ball and Successfully Throw It at a Target." Unpublished Master's thesis, University of Colorado, Boulder, 1958.

O'DONNELL, D.J. "Validation of Softball Skill Tests for High School Girls." Unpublished Master's thesis, Indiana University, Bloomington, 1950.

Research Committee, Central Association for Physical Education of College Women. "Fielding Test," in M.G. Scott and E. French, *Measurement and Evaluation in Physical Education.* Dubuque, Iowa: Wm. C. Brown Company Publishers, 1959.

SAFRIT, M.J. and A. PAVIS. "Overarm Throw Skill Testing," in *Selected Softball Articles,* eds., J. Felshin and C. O'Brien. Washington, D.C.: Division of Girls' and Women's Sports, American Association for Health, Physical Education and Recreation, 1969.

SCOTT, M.G. and E. FRENCH. "Softball Repeated Throws Test," in M.G. Scott and E. French, *Measurement and Evaluation in Physical Education.* Dubuque, Iowa: Wm. C. Brown Company Publishers, 1959.

SHICK, J. "Battery of Defensive Softball Skills Tests for College Women," *Research Quarterly,* XLI, No. 1 (1970), pp. 82–87.

SOPA, A. "Construction of an Indoor Batting Skills Test for Junior High School Girls." Unpublished Master's thesis, University of Wisconsin, Madison, 1967.

THOMAS, J. "Skill Tests," in *Softball-Volleyball Guide—July 1947–July 1949.* Washington, D.C.: National Section on Women's Athletics, American Association for Health, Physical Education and Recreation, 1947.

Speedball

BUCHANAN, R.E. "A Study of Achievement Tests in Speedball for High School Girls." Unpublished Master's thesis, State University of Iowa, Iowa City, 1942.

SMITH, G. "Speedball Skill Tests for College Women," in H.M. Barrow and R. McGee, *A Practical Approach to Measurement in Physical Education.* Philadelphia: Lea & Febiger, 1972.

Stunts and Tumbling

COTTERAL, B. and D. COTTERAL. "Scale for Judging Quality of Performance in Stunts and Tumbling," *The Teaching of Stunts and Tumbling*. New York: The Ronald Press Company, 1936.

EDWARDS, V.M. *Test Questions for Tumbling*. Philadelphia: W.B. Saunders Company, 1969.

Swimming

BENNETT, L.M. "A Test of Diving for Use in Beginning Classes," *Research Quarterly*, XIII (1942), pp. 109–15.

CHAPMAN, P.A. "A Comparison of Three Methods of Measuring Swimming Stroke Proficiency." Master's thesis, University of Wisconsin, Madison, 1965 (Microcard PE 738, University of Oregon, Eugene).

FOX, M.G. "Swimming Power Test," *Research Quarterly*, XXVIII (1957), pp. 233–37.

HEWITT, J.E. "Swimming Achievement Scales for College Men," *Research Quarterly*, XIX (1948), pp. 282–89.

HEWITT, J.E. "Achievement Scale Scores for High School Swimming," *Research Quarterly*, XX (1949), pp. 170–79.

MUNT, M.R. "Development of an Objective Test to Measure the Efficiency of the Front Crawl for College Women." Unpublished Master's thesis, University of Michigan, Ann Arbor, 1964.

ROSENTSWIEG, J. "A Revision of the Power Swimming Test," *Research Quarterly*, XXXIX (1968), pp. 818–19.

WILSON, C.T. "Coordination Tests in Swimming," *Research Quarterly*, V (1934), pp. 81–88.

WILSON, M.R. "Wilson Achievement Test for Intermediate Swimming," in H.M. Barrow and R. McGee, *A Practical Approach to Measurement in Physical Education*. Philadelphia: Lea & Febiger, 1972, pp. 313–19.

Table Tennis

MOTT, J.A. and A. LOCKHART. "Table Tennis Backboard Test," *Journal of Health and Physical Education*, XVII (1946), pp. 550–52.

Tennis

BENTON, R. "Teaching Tennis by Testing," in *Selected Tennis and Badminton*

Articles, ed., D. Davis. Washington, D.C.: Division of Girls' and Women's Sports, American Association for Health, Physical Education and Recreation, 1963.

BROER, M.R. and D.M. MILLER. "Achievement Tests for Beginning and Intermediate Tennis," *Research Quarterly,* XXI (1950), pp. 303–13.

COBANE, E. "Test for the Service," in *Tennis and Badminton Guide—June 1962– June 1964.* Washington, D.C.: Division of Girls' and Women's Sports, American Association for Health, Physical Education and Recreation, 1962.

DIGENNARO, J. "Construction of Forehand Drive, Backhand Drive, and Service Tennis Tests," *Research Quarterly,* XL (1969), pp. 496–501.

DYER, J.T. "Revision of the Backboard Test of Tennis Ability," *Research Quarterly,* IX, (1938), pp. 25–31.

EDWARDS, J. "A Study of Three Measures of the Tennis Serve." Master's thesis, University of Wisconsin, Madison, 1965 (Microcard PE 746, University of Oregon, Eugene).

FELSHIN, J. and E. SPENCER. "Evaluation Procedures for Tennis," in *Selected Tennis and Badminton Articles,* ed. D. Davis. Washington, D.C.: Division of Girls' and Women's Sports, American Association for Health, Physical Education and Recreation, 1963.

HEWITT, J.E. "Revision of the Dyer Backboard Tennis Test," *Research Quarterly,* XXXVI (1965), pp. 153–57.

HEWITT, J.E. "Classification Tests in Tennis," *Research Quarterly,* XXXIX (1968), pp. 552–55.

HUBBELL, N.C. "A Battery of Tennis Skill Tests for College Women." Unpublished Master's thesis, Texas Women's University, Denton, 1960.

HULAC, G.M. "Hulac Rating Scale for the Tennis Serve," in H.M. Barrow and R. McGee, *A Practical Approach to Measurement in Physical Education.* Philadelphia: Lea & Febiger, 1972, pp. 325–26.

HULBERT, B.A. "A Study of Tests for the Forehand Drive in Tennis." Master's thesis, University of Wisconsin, Madison, 1966 (Microcard PE 818, University of Oregon, Eugene).

JOHNSON, J. "Tennis Serve of Advanced Women Players," *Research Quarterly,* XXVIII (1957), pp. 123–31.

JOHNSON, J. "Tennis Knowledge Test," in *Selected Tennis and Badminton Articles,* ed. D. Davis. Washington, D.C.: Division of Girls' and Women's Sports, American Association for Health, Physical Education and Recreation, 1963.

KEMP, J. and M.F. VINCENT. "Kemp-Vincent Rally Test of Tennis Skill," *Research Quarterly,* XXXIX (1968), pp. 1000–1004.

MALINAK, N.R. "The Construction of an Objective Measure of Accuracy in the Performance of the Tennis Serve." Unpublished Master's thesis, University of Illinois, Urbana, 1961.

RONNING, H.E. "Wall Tests for Evaluating Tennis Ability." Master's thesis, Washington State University, Pullman, 1959 (Microcard PE 441, University of Oregon, Eugene).

Scott, M.G. "Achievement Examinations for Elementary and Intermediate Tennis Classes," *Research Quarterly,* XII (1941), pp. 40–49.

Scott, M.G. and E. French. "Scott-French Revision of the Dyer Wallboard Test," *Measurement and Evaluation in Physical Education.* Dubuque, Iowa: Wm. C. Brown Company, Publishers, 1959, pp. 222–25.

Volleyball

American Association for Health, Physical Education and Recreation. *Volleyball Skills Test Manual.* Washington, D.C.: American Association for Health, Physical Education and Recreation, 1967.

Bassett, G., R.B. Glassow, and M. Locke. "Studies in Testing Volleyball Skills," *Research Quarterly,* VIII (1937), pp. 60–72.

Blackman, C.J. "The Development of a Volleyball Test for the Spike." Unpublished Master's thesis, Southern Illinois University, Carbondale, 1968.

Brady, C.F. "Preliminary Investigation of Volleyball Playing Ability," *Research Quarterly,* XVI (1945), pp. 14–17.

Broer, M.A. "Reliability of Certain Skill Tests for Junior High School Girls," *Research Quarterly,* XXIX (1958), pp. 139–45.

Brumbach, W.B. "Brumbach Service Test," in B.L. Johnson and J.K. Nelson. *Practical Measurements for Evaluation in Physical Education.* Minneapolis: Burgess Publishing Company, 1969, pp. 365–66.

Clifton, M. "Single Hit Volley Test for Women's Volleyball," *Research Quarterly,* XXXIII (1962), pp. 208–11.

Crogan, C. "A Simple Volleyball Classification Test for High School Girls," *The Physical Educator,* IV (1943), pp. 34–37.

Cunningham, P. and J. Garrison. "High Wall Volley Test for Women," *Research Quarterly,* XXXIX (1968), pp. 486–90.

French, E.L. and B.I. Cooper. "Achievement Tests in Volleyball for High School Girls," *Research Quarterly,* VIII (1937), pp. 150–57.

Helmen, R.M. "Development of Power Volleyball Skill Tests for College Women." Paper presented at the Research Section of the 1971 American Association for Health, Physical Education and Recreation National Convention, Detroit, Michigan.

Jackson, P.L. "A Rating Scale for Discriminating Relative Playing Performance of Skilled Female Volleyball Players." Master's thesis, University of Alberta, Edmonton, 1966 (Microcard PE 931, University of Oregon, Eugene).

Kessler, A. "The Validity and Reliability of the Sandefur Volleyball Spiking Test." Unpublished Master's thesis, California State College, Long Beach, 1968.

Kronquist, R.A. and W.B. Brumbach. "A Modification of the Brady Volleyball Skill Test for High School Boys," *Research Quarterly,* XXXIX (1968), pp. 116–20.

Latchaw, M. "Measuring Selected Motor Skills in Fourth, Fifth, and Sixth

Grades," *Research Quarterly,* XXV (1954), pp. 439–49.

LIBA, M.R. and M.R. STAUFF. "A Test for the Volleyball Pass," *Research Quarterly,* XXXIV (1963), pp. 56–63.

LONDEREE, B.R. and E.C. EICHOLTZ. "Reliabilities of Selected Volleyball Skill Tests." Paper presented at the Research Section of the 1970 American Association for Health, Physical Education and Recreation National Convention, Seattle, Washington.

LOPEZ, D. "Serve Test," in *Volleyball Guide—July 1957–July 1959.* Washington, D.C.: Division of Girls' and Women's Sport, American Association for Health, Physical Education and Recreation, 1957.

MOHR, D.R. and M.J. HAVERSTICK. "Repeated Volleys Tests for Women's Volleyball," *Research Quarterly,* XXVI (1955), pp. 179–84.

RUSSELL, N. and E. LANGE. "Achievement Tests in Volleyball for Junior High School Girls," *Research Quarterly,* XI (1940), pp. 33–41.

RYAN, M.F. "A Study of Tests for the Volleyball Serve." Master's thesis, University of Wisconsin, Madison, 1969 (Microcard PE 1040, University of Oregon, Eugene).

SLAYMAKER, T. and V.H. BROWN. *Test Questions for Power Volleyball.* Philadelphia: W.B. Saunders Company, 1969,

SNAVELY, M. "Volleyball Skill Tests for Girls," in *Selected Volleyball Articles,* ed. A. Lockhart. Washington, D.C.: Division of Girls' and Women's Sport, American Association for Health, Physical Education and Recreation, 1960.

THORPE, J. and C. WEST. "A Volleyball Skills Chart with Attainment Levels for Selected Skills," *Volleyball Guide,—July 1967–July 1969.* Washington, D.C.: Division of Girls' and Women's Sport, American Association for Health, Physical Education and Recreation, 1967.

WATKINS, A. "Skill Testing for Large Groups," in *Selected Volleyball Articles,* ed. A. Lockhart. Washington, D.C.: Division of Girls' and Women's Sports, American Association for Health, Physical Education and Recreation, 1960.

WEST, C. "A Comparative Study between Height and Wall Volley Test Scores as Related to Volleyball Playing Ability of Girls and Women." Unpublished Master's thesis, The Woman's College of the University of North Carolina, Greensboro, 1957.

Wrestling

YETTER, H. "A Test of Wrestling Aptitude: A Preliminary Explanation." Unpublished Master's thesis, University of Wisconsin, Madison, 1963.

B

tables

TABLE B-1 • Squares and square roots of numbers from 1 to 1,000*

Number	Square	Square root	Number	Square	Square root
1	1	1.0000	21	4 41	4.5826
2	4	1.4142	22	4 84	4.6904
3	9	1.7321	23	5 29	4.7958
4	16	2.0000	24	5 76	4.8990
5	25	2.2361	25	6 25	5.0000
6	36	2.4495	26	6 76	5.0990
7	49	2.6458	27	7 29	5.1962
8	64	2.8284	28	7 84	5.2915
9	81	3.0000	29	8 41	5.3852
10	1 00	3.1623	30	9 00	5.4772
11	1 21	3.3166	31	9 61	5.5678
12	1 44	3.4641	32	10 24	5.6569
13	1 69	3.6056	33	10 89	5.7446
14	1 96	3.7417	34	11 56	5.8310
15	2 25	3.8730	35	12 25	5.9161
16	2 56	4.0000	36	12 96	6.0000
17	2 89	4.1231	37	13 69	6.0828
18	3 24	4.2426	38	14 44	6.1644
19	3 61	4.3589	39	15 21	6.2450
20	4 00	4.4721	40	16 00	6.3246

*H. Sorenson, *Statistics for Students of Psychology and Education* (New York: Mc-Graw-Hill Book Company, 1936), Table K. By permission of the author and publisher.

TABLE B-1   (Continued)

Number	Square	Square root	Number	Square	Square root
41	16 81	6.4031	83	68 89	9.1104
42	17 64	6.4807	84	70 56	9.1652
43	18 49	6.5574	85	72 25	9.2195
44	19 36	6.6332	86	73 96	9.2736
45	20 25	6.7082	87	75 69	9.3274
46	21 16	6.7823	88	77 44	9.3808
47	22 09	6.8557	89	79 21	9.4340
48	23 04	6.9282	90	81 00	9.4868
49	24 01	7.0000	91	82 81	9.5394
50	25 00	7.0711	92	84 64	9.5917
51	26 01	7.1414	93	86 49	9.6437
52	27 04	7.2111	94	88 36	9.6954
53	28 09	7.2801	95	90 25	9.7468
54	29 16	7.3485	96	92 16	9.7980
55	30 25	7.4162	97	94 09	9.8489
56	31 36	7.4833	98	96 04	9.8995
57	32 49	7.5498	99	98 01	9.9499
58	33 64	7.6158	100	1 00 00	10.0000
59	34 81	7.6811	101	1 02 01	10.0499
60	36 00	7.7460	102	1 04 04	10.0995
61	37 21	7.8102	103	1 06 09	10.1489
62	38 44	7.8740	104	1 08 16	10.1980
63	39 69	7.9373	105	1 10 25	10.2470
64	40 96	8.0000	106	1 12 36	10.2956
65	42 25	8.0623	107	1 14 49	10.3441
66	43 56	8.1240	108	1 16 64	10.3923
67	44 89	8.1854	109	1 18 81	10.4403
68	46 24	8.2462	110	1 21 00	10.4881
69	47 61	8.3066	111	1 23 21	10.5357
70	49 00	8.3666	112	1 25 44	10.5830
71	50 41	8.4261	113	1 27 69	10.6301
72	51 84	8.4853	114	1 29 96	10.6771
73	53 29	8.5440	115	2 32 25	10.7238
74	54 76	8.6023	116	1 34 56	10.7703
75	56 25	8.6603	117	1 36 89	10.8167
76	57 76	8.7178	118	1 39 24	10.8628
77	59 29	8.7750	119	1 41 61	10.9087
78	60 84	8.8318	120	1 44 00	10.9545
79	62 41	8.8882	121	1 46 41	11.0000
80	64 00	8.9443	122	1 48 84	11.0454
81	65 61	9.0000	123	1 51 29	11.0905
82	67 24	9.0554	124	1 53 76	11.1355

TABLE B-1   (continued)

Number	Square	Square root	Number	Square	Square root
125	1 56 25	11.1803	167	2 78 89	12.9228
126	1 58 76	11.2250	168	2 82 24	12.9615
127	1 61 29	11.2694	169	2 85 61	13.0000
128	1 63 84	11.3137	170	2 89 00	13.0384
129	1 66 41	11.3578	171	2 92 41	13.0767
130	1 69 00	11.4018	172	2 95 84	13.1149
131	1 71 61	11.4455	173	2 99 29	13.1529
132	1 74 24	11.4891	174	3 02 76	13.1909
133	1 76 89	11.5326	175	3 06 25	13.2288
134	1 79 56	11.5758	176	3 09 76	13.2665
135	1 82 25	11.6190	177	3 13 29	13.3041
136	1 84 96	11.6619	178	3 16 84	13.3417
137	1 87 69	11.7047	179	3 20 41	13.3791
138	1 90 44	11.7473	180	3 24 00	13.4164
139	1 93 21	11.7898	181	3 27 61	13.4536
140	1 96 00	11.8322	182	3 31 24	13.4907
141	1 98 81	11.8743	183	3 34 89	13.5277
142	2 01 64	11.9164	184	3 38 56	13.5647
143	2 04 49	11.9583	185	3 42 25	13.6015
144	2 07 36	12.0000	186	3 45 96	13.6382
145	2 10 25	12.0416	187	3 49 69	13.6748
146	2 13 16	12.0830	188	3 53 44	13.7113
147	2 16 09	12.1244	189	3 57 21	13.7477
148	2 19 04	12.1655	190	3 61 00	13.7840
149	2 22 01	12.2066	191	3 64 81	13.8203
150	2 25 00	12.2474	192	3 68 64	13.8564
151	2 28 01	12.2882	193	3 72 49	13.8924
152	2 31 04	12.3288	194	3 76 36	13.9284
153	2 34 09	12.3693	195	3 80 25	13.9642
154	2 37 16	12.4097	196	3 84 16	14.0000
155	2 40 25	12.4499	197	3 88 09	14.0357
156	2 43 36	12.4900	198	3 92 04	14.0712
157	2 46 49	12.5300	199	3 96 01	14.1067
158	2 49 64	12.5698	200	4 00 00	14.1421
159	2 52 81	12.6095	201	4 04 01	14.1774
160	2 56 00	12.6491	202	4 08 04	14.2127
161	2 59 21	12.6886	203	4 12 09	14.2478
162	2 62 44	12.7279	204	4 16 16	14.2829
163	2 65 69	12.7671	205	4 20 25	14.3178
164	2 68 96	12.8062	206	4 24 36	14.3527
165	2 72 25	12.8452	207	4 28 49	14.3875
166	2 75 56	12.8841	208	4 32 64	14.4222

TABLE B-1   (Continued)

Number	Square	Square root	Number	Square	Square root
209	4 36 81	14.4568	251	6 30 01	15.8430
210	4 41 00	14.4914	252	6 35 04	15.8745
211	4 45 21	14.5258	253	6 40 09	15.9060
212	4 49 44	14.5602	254	6 45 16	15.9374
213	4 53 69	14.5945	255	6 50 25	15.9687
214	4 57 96	14.6287	256	6 55 36	16.0000
215	4 62 25	14.6629	257	6 60 49	16.0312
216	4 66 56	14.6969	258	6 65 64	16.0624
217	4 70 89	14.7309	259	6 70 81	16.0935
218	4 75 24	14.7648	260	6 76 00	16.1245
219	4 79 61	14.7986	261	6 81 21	16.1555
220	4 84 00	14.8324	262	6 86 44	16.1864
221	4 88 41	14.8661	263	6 91 69	16.2173
222	4 92 84	14.8997	264	6 96 96	16.2481
223	4 97 29	14.9332	265	7 02 25	16.2788
224	5 01 76	14.9666	266	7 07 56	16.3095
225	5 06 25	15.0000	267	7 12 89	16.3401
226	5 10 76	15.0333	268	7 18 24	16.3707
227	5 15 29	15.0665	269	7 23 61	16.4012
228	5 19 84	15.0997	270	7 29 00	16.4317
229	5 24 41	15.1327	271	7 34 41	16.4621
230	5 29 00	15.1658	272	7 39 84	16.4924
231	5 33 61	15.1987	273	7 45 29	16.5227
232	5 38 24	15.2315	274	7 50 76	16.5529
233	5 42 89	15.2643	275	7 56 25	16.5831
234	5 47 56	15.2971	276	7 61 76	16.6132
235	5 52 25	15.3297	277	7 67 29	16.6433
236	5 56 96	15.3623	278	7 72 84	16.6733
237	5 61 69	15.3948	279	7 78 41	16.7033
238	5 66 44	15.4272	280	7 84 00	16.7332
239	5 71 21	15.4596	281	7 89 61	16.7631
240	5 76 00	15.4919	282	7 95 24	16.7929
241	5 80 81	15.5242	283	8 00 89	16.8226
242	5 85 64	15.5563	284	8 06 56	16.8523
243	5 90 49	15.5885	285	8 12 25	16.8819
244	5 95 36	16.6205	286	8 17 96	16.9115
245	6 00 25	15.6525	287	8 23 69	16.9411
246	6 05 16	15.6844	288	8 29 44	16.9706
247	6 10 09	15.7162	289	8 35 21	17.0000
248	6 15 04	15.7480	290	8 41 00	17.0294
249	6 20 01	15.7797	291	8 46 81	17.0587
250	6 25 00	15.8114	292	8 52 64	17.0880

TABLE B-1   (Continued)

Number	Square	Square root	Number	Square	Square root
293	8 58 49	17.1172	335	11 22 25	18.3030
294	8 64 36	17.1464	336	11 28 96	18.3303
295	8 70 25	17.1756	337	11 35 69	18.3576
296	8 76 16	17.2047	338	11 42 44	18.3848
297	8 82 09	17.2337	339	11 49 21	18.4120
298	8 88 04	17.2627	340	11 56 00	18.4391
299	8 94 01	17.2916	341	11 62 81	18.4662
300	9 00 00	17.3205	342	11 69 64	18.4932
301	9 06 01	17.3494	343	11 76 49	18.5203
302	9 12 04	17.3781	344	11 83 36	18.5472
303	9 18 09	17.4069	345	11 90 25	18.5742
304	9 24 16	17.4356	346	11 97 16	18.6011
305	9 30 25	17.4642	347	12 04 09	18.6279
306	9 36 36	17.4929	348	12 11 04	18.6548
307	9 42 49	17.5214	349	12 18 01	18.6815
308	9 48 64	17.5499	350	12 25 00	18.7083
309	9 54 81	17.5784	351	12 32 01	18.7350
310	9 61 00	17.6068	352	12 39 04	18.7617
311	9 67 21	17.6352	353	12 46 09	18.7883
312	9 73 44	17.6635	354	12 53 16	18.8149
313	9 79 69	17.6918	355	12 60 25	18.8414
314	9 85 96	17.7200	356	12 67 36	18.8680
315	9 92 25	17.7482	357	12 74 49	18.8944
316	9 98 56	17.7764	358	12 81 64	18.9209
317	10 04 89	17.8045	359	12 88 81	18.9473
318	10 11 24	17.8326	360	12 96 00	18.9737
319	10 17 61	17.8606	361	13 03 21	19.0000
320	10 24 00	17.8885	362	13 10 44	19.0263
321	10 30 41	17.9165	363	13 17 69	19.0526
322	10 36 84	17.9444	364	13 24 96	19.0788
323	10 43 29	17.9722	365	13 32 25	19.1050
324	10 49 76	18.0000	366	13 39 56	19.1311
325	10 56 25	18.0278	367	13 46 89	19.1572
326	10 62 76	18.0555	368	13 54 24	19.1833
327	10 69 29	18.0831	369	13 61 61	19.2094
328	10 75 84	18.1108	370	13 69 00	19.2354
329	10 82 41	18.1384	371	13 76 41	19.2614
330	10 89 00	18.1659	372	13 83 84	19.2873
331	10 95 61	18.1934	373	13 91 29	19.3132
332	11 02 24	18.2209	374	13 98 76	19.3391
333	11 08 89	18.2483	375	14 06 25	19.3649
334	11 15 56	18.2757	376	14 13 76	19.3907

TABLE B-1   (Continued)

Number	Square	Square root	Number	Square	Square root
377	14 21 29	19.4165	419	17 55 61	20.4695
378	14 28 84	19.4422	420	17 64 00	20.4939
379	14 36 41	19.4679	421	17 72 41	20.5183
380	14 44 00	19.4936	422	17 80 84	20.5426
381	14 51 61	19.5192	423	17 89 29	20.5670
382	14 59 24	19.5448	424	17 97 76	20.5913
383	14 66 89	19.5704	425	18 06 25	20.6155
384	14 74 56	19.5959	426	18 14 76	20.6398
385	14 82 25	19.6214	427	18 23 29	20.6640
386	14 89 96	19.6469	428	18 31 84	20.6882
387	14 97 69	19.6723	429	18 40 41	20.7123
388	15 05 44	19.6977	430	18 49 00	20.7364
389	15 13 21	19.7231	431	18 57 61	20.7605
390	15 21 00	19.7484	432	18 66 24	20.7846
391	15 28 81	19.7737	433	18 74 89	20.8087
392	15 36 64	19.7990	434	18 83 56	20.8327
393	15 44 49	19.8242	435	18 92 25	20.8567
394	15 52 36	19.8494	436	19 00 96	20.8806
395	15 60 25	19.8746	437	19 09 69	20.9045
396	15 68 16	19.8997	438	19 18 44	20.9284
397	15 76 09	19.9249	439	19 27 21	20.9523
398	15 84 04	19.9499	440	19 36 00	20.9762
399	15 92 01	19.9570	441	19 44 81	21.0000
400	16 00 00	20.0000	442	19 53 64	21.0238
401	16 08 01	20.0250	443	19 62 49	21.0476
402	16 16 04	20.0499	444	19 71 36	21.0713
403	16 24 09	20.0749	445	19 80 25	21.0950
404	16 32 16	20.0998	446	19 89 16	21.1187
405	16 40 25	20.1246	447	19 98 09	21.1424
406	16 48 36	20.1494	448	20 07 04	21.1660
407	16 56 49	20.1742	449	20 16 01	21.1896
408	16 64 64	20.1990	450	20 25 00	21.2132
409	16 72 81	20.2237	451	20 34 01	21.2368
410	16 81 00	20.2485	452	20 43 04	21.2603
411	16 89 21	20.2731	453	20 52 09	21.2838
412	16 97 44	20.2978	454	20 61 16	21.3073
413	17 05 69	20.3224	455	20 70 25	21.3307
414	17 13 96	20.3470	456	20 79 36	21.3542
415	17 22 25	20.3715	457	20 88 49	21.3776
416	17 30 56	20.3961	458	20 97 64	21.4009
417	17 38 89	20.4206	459	21 06 81	21.4243
418	17 47 24	20.4450	460	21 16 00	21.4476

TABLE B-1   (Continued)

Number	Square	Square root	Number	Square	Square root
461	21 25 21	21.4709	503	25 30 09	22.4277
462	21 34 44	21.4942	504	25 40 16	22.4499
463	21 43 69	21.5174	505	25 50 25	22.4722
464	21 52 96	21.5407	506	25 60 36	22.4944
465	21 62 25	21.5639	507	25 70 49	22.5167
466	21 71 56	21.5870	508	25 80 64	22.5389
467	21 80 89	21.6102	509	25 90 81	22.5610
468	21 90 24	21.6333	510	26 01 00	22.5832
469	21 99 61	21.6564	511	26 11 21	22.6053
470	22 09 00	21.6795	512	26 21 44	22.6274
471	22 18 41	21.7025	513	26 31 69	22.6495
472	22 27 84	21.7256	514	26 41 96	22.6716
473	22 37 29	21.7486	515	26 52 25	22.6936
474	22 46 76	21.7715	516	26 62 56	22.7156
475	22 56 25	21.7945	517	26 72 89	22.7376
476	22 65 76	21.8174	518	26 83 24	22.7596
477	22 75 29	21.8403	519	26 93 61	22.7816
478	22 84 84	21.8632	520	27 04 00	22.8035
479	22 94 41	21.8861	521	27 14 41	22.8254
480	23 04 00	21.9089	522	27 24 84	22.8473
481	23 13 61	21.9317	523	27 35 29	22.8692
482	23 23 24	21.9545	524	27 45 76	22.8910
483	23 32 89	21.9773	525	27 56 25	22.9129
484	23 42 56	22.0000	526	27 66 76	22.9347
485	23 52 25	22.0227	527	27 77 29	22.9565
486	23 61 96	22.0454	528	27 87 84	22.9783
487	23 71 69	22.0681	529	27 98 41	23.0000
488	23 81 44	22.0907	530	28 09 00	23.0217
489	23 91 21	22.1133	531	28 19 61	23.0434
490	24 01 00	22.1359	532	28 30 24	23.0651
491	24 10 81	22.1585	533	28 40 89	23.0868
492	24 20 64	22.1811	534	28 51 56	23.1084
493	24 30 49	22.2036	535	28 62 25	23.1301
494	24 40 36	22.2261	536	28 72 96	23.1517
495	24 50 25	22.2486	537	28 83 69	23.1733
496	24 60 16	22.2711	538	28 94 44	23.1948
497	24 70 09	22.2935	539	29 05 21	23.2164
498	24 80 04	22.3159	540	29 16 00	23.2379
499	24 90 01	22.3383	541	29 26 81	23.2594
500	25 00 00	22.3607	542	29 37 64	23.2809
501	25 10 01	22.3830	543	29 48 49	23.3024
502	25 20 04	22.4054	544	29 59 36	23.3238

TABLE B-1   (Continued)

Number	Square	Square root	Number	Square	Square root
545	29 70 25	23.3452	587	34 45 69	24.2281
546	29 81 16	23.3666	588	34 57 44	24.2487
547	29 92 09	23.3880	589	34 69 21	24.2693
548	30 03 04	23.4094	590	34 81 00	24.2899
549	30 14 01	23.4307	591	34 92 81	24.3105
550	30 25 00	23.4521	592	35 04 64	24.3311
551	30 36 01	23.4734	593	35 16 49	24.3516
552	30 47 04	23.4947	594	35 28 36	24.3721
553	30 58 09	23.5160	595	35 40 25	24.3926
554	30 69 16	23.5372	596	35 52 16	24.4131
555	30 80 25	23.5584	597	35 64 09	24.4336
556	30 91 36	23.5797	598	35 76 04	24.4540
557	31 02 49	23.6008	599	35 88 01	24.4745
558	31 13 64	23.6220	600	36 00 00	24.4949
559	31 24 81	23.6432	601	36 12 01	24.5153
560	31 36 00	23.6643	602	36 24 04	24.5357
561	31 47 21	23.6854	603	36 36 09	24.5561
562	31 58 44	23.7065	604	36 48 16	24.5764
563	31 69 69	23.7276	605	36 60 25	24.5967
564	31 80 96	23.7487	606	36 72 36	24.6171
565	31 92 25	23.7697	607	36 84 49	24.6374
566	32 03 56	23.7908	608	36 96 64	24.6577
567	32 14 89	23.8118	609	37 08 81	24.6779
568	32 26 24	23.8328	610	37 21 00	24.6982
569	32 37 61	23.8537	611	37 33 21	24.7184
570	32 49 00	23.8747	612	37 45 44	24.7385
571	32 60 41	23.8956	613	37 57 69	24.7588
572	32 71 84	23.9165	614	37 69 96	24.7790
573	32 83 29	23.9374	615	37 82 25	24.7992
574	32 94 76	23.9583	616	37 94 56	24.8193
575	33 06 25	23.9792	617	38 06 89	24.8395
576	33 17 76	24.0000	618	38 19 24	24.8596
577	33 29 29	24.0208	619	38 31 61	24.8797
578	33 40 84	24.0416	620	38 44 00	24.8998
579	33 52 41	24.0624	621	38 56 41	24.9199
580	33 64 00	24.0832	622	38 68 84	24.9399
581	33 75 61	24.1039	623	38 81 29	24.9600
582	33 87 24	24.1247	624	38 93 76	24.9800
583	33 98 89	24.1454	625	39 06 25	25.0000
584	34 10 56	24.1661	626	39 18 76	25.0200
585	34 22 25	24.1868	627	39 31 29	25.0400
586	34 33 96	24.2074	628	39 43 84	25.0599

TABLE B-1   (Continued)

Number	Square	Square root	Number	Square	Square root
629	39 56 41	25.0799	671	45 02 41	25.9037
630	39 69 00	25.0998	672	45 15 84	25.9230
631	39 81 61	25.1197	673	45 29 29	25.9422
632	39 94 24	25.1396	674	45 42 76	25.9615
633	40 06 89	25.1595	675	45 56 25	25.9808
634	40 19 56	25.1794	676	45 69 76	26.0000
635	40 32 25	25.1992	677	45 83 29	26.0192
636	40 44 96	25.2190	678	45 96 84	26.0384
637	40 57 69	25.2389	679	46 10 41	26.0576
638	40 70 44	25.2587	680	46 24 00	26.0768
639	40 83 21	25.2784	681	46 37 61	26.0960
640	40 96 00	25.2982	682	46 51 24	26.1151
641	41 08 81	25.3180	683	46 64 89	26.1343
642	41 21 64	25.3377	684	46 78 56	26.1534
643	41 34 49	25.3574	685	46 92 25	26.1725
644	41 47 36	25.3772	686	47 05 96	26.1916
645	41 60 25	25.3969	687	47 19 69	26.2107
646	41 73 16	25.4165	688	47 33 44	26.2298
647	41 86 09	25.4362	689	47 47 21	26.2488
648	41 99 04	25.4558	690	47 61 00	26.2679
649	42 12 01	25.4755	691	47 74 81	26.2869
650	42 25 00	25.4951	692	47 88 64	26.3059
651	42 38 01	25.5147	693	48 02 49	26.3249
652	42 51 04	25.5343	694	48 16 36	26.3439
653	42 64 09	25.5539	695	48 30 25	26.3629
654	42 77 16	25.5734	696	48 44 16	26.3818
655	42 90 25	25.5930	697	48 58 09	26.4008
656	43 03 36	25.6125	698	48 72 04	26.4197
657	43 16 49	25.6320	699	48 86 01	26.4386
658	43 29 64	25.6515	700	49 00 00	26.4575
659	43 42 81	25.6710	701	49 14 01	26.4764
660	43 56 00	25.6905	702	49 28 04	26.4953
661	43 69 21	25.7099	703	49 42 09	26.5141
662	43 82 44	25.7294	704	49 56 16	26.5330
663	43 95 69	25.7488	705	49 70 25	26.5518
664	44 08 96	25.7682	706	49 84 36	26.5707
665	44 22 25	25.7876	707	49 98 49	26.5895
666	44 35 56	25.8070	708	50 12 64	26.6083
667	44 48 89	25.8263	709	50 26 81	26.6271
668	44 62 24	25.8457	710	50 41 00	26.6458
669	44 75 61	25.8650	711	50 55 21	26.6646
670	44 89 00	25.8844	712	50 69 44	26.6833

TABLE B-1 (Continued)

Number	Square	Square root	Number	Square	Square root
713	50 83 69	26.7021	755	57 00 25	27.4773
714	50 97 96	26.7208	756	57 15 36	27.4955
715	51 12 25	26.7395	757	57 30 49	27.5136
716	51 26 56	26.7582	758	57 45 64	27.5318
717	51 40 89	26.7769	759	57 60 81	27.5500
718	51 55 24	26.7955	760	57 76 00	27.5681
719	51 69 61	26.8142	761	57 91 21	27.5862
720	51 84 00	26.8328	762	58 06 44	27.6043
721	51 98 41	26.8514	763	58 21 69	27.6225
722	52 12 84	26.8701	764	58 36 96	27.6405
723	52 27 29	26.8887	765	58 52 25	27.6586
724	52 41 76	26.9072	766	58 67 56	27.6767
725	52 56 25	26.9258	767	58 82 89	27.6948
726	52 70 76	26.9444	768	58 98 24	27.7128
727	52 85 29	26.9629	769	59 13 61	27.7308
728	52 99 84	26.9815	770	59 29 00	27.7489
729	53 14 41	27.0000	771	59 44 41	27.7669
730	53 29 00	27.0185	772	59 59 84	27.7849
731	53 43 61	27.0370	773	59 75 29	27.8029
732	53 58 24	27.0555	774	59 90 76	27.8209
733	53 72 89	27.0740	775	60 06 25	27.8388
734	53 87 56	27.0924	776	60 21 76	27.8568
735	54 02 25	27.1109	777	60 37 29	27.8747
736	54 16 96	27.1293	778	60 52 84	27.8927
737	54 31 69	27.1477	779	60 68 41	27.9106
738	54 46 44	27.1662	780	60 84 00	27.9285
739	54 61 27	27.1846	781	60 99 61	27.9464
740	54 76 00	27.2029	782	61 15 24	27.9643
741	54 90 81	27.2213	783	61 30 89	27.9821
742	55 05 64	27.2397	784	61 46 56	28.0000
743	55 20 49	27.2580	785	61 62 25	28.0179
744	55 35 36	27.2764	786	61 77 96	28.0357
745	55 50 25	27.2947	787	61 93 69	28.0535
746	55 65 16	27.3130	788	62 09 44	28.0713
747	55 80 09	27.3313	789	62 25 21	28.0891
748	55 95 04	27.3496	790	62 41 00	28.1069
749	56 10 01	27.3679	791	62 56 81	28.1247
750	56 25 00	27.3861	792	62 72 64	28.1425
751	56 40 01	27.4044	793	62 88 49	28.1603
752	56 55 04	27.4226	794	63 04 36	28.1780
753	56 70 09	27.4408	795	63 20 25	28.1957
754	56 85 16	27.4591	796	63 36 16	28.2135

TABLE B-1   **(Continued)**

Number	Square	Square root	Number	Square	Square root
797	63 52 09	28.2312	839	70 39 21	28.9655
798	63 68 04	28.2489	840	70 56 00	28.9828
799	63 84 01	28.2666	841	70 72 81	29.0000
800	64 00 00	28.2843	842	70 89 64	29.0172
801	64 16 01	28.3019	843	71 06 49	29.0345
802	64 32 04	28.3196	844	71 23 36	29.0517
803	64 48 09	28.3373	845	71 40 25	29.0689
804	64 64 16	28.3049	846	71 57 16	29.0861
805	64 80 25	28.3725	847	71 74 09	29.1033
806	64 96 36	28.3901	848	71 91 04	29.1204
807	65 12 49	28.4077	849	72 08 01	29.1376
808	65 28 64	28.4253	850	72 25 00	29.1548
809	65 44 81	28.4429	851	72 42 01	29.1719
810	65 61 00	28.4605	852	72 59 04	29.1890
811	65 77 21	28.4781	853	72 76 09	29.2062
812	65 93 44	28.4956	854	72 93 16	29.2233
813	66 09 69	28.5132	855	73 10 25	29.2404
814	66 25 96	28.5307	856	73 27 36	29.2575
815	66 42 25	28.5482	857	73 44 49	29.2746
816	66 58 56	28.5657	858	73 61 64	29.2916
817	66 74 89	28.5832	859	73 78 81	29.3087
818	66 91 24	28.6007	860	73 96 00	29.3258
819	67 07 61	28.6082	861	74 13 21	29.3428
820	67 24 00	28.6356	862	74 30 44	29.3598
821	67 40 41	28.6531	863	74 47 69	29.3769
822	67 56 84	28.6705	864	74 64 96	29.3939
823	67 73 29	28.6880	865	74 82 25	29.4100
824	67 89 76	28.7054	866	74 99 56	29.4279
825	68 06 25	28.7228	867	75 16 89	29.4449
826	68 22 76	28.7402	868	75 34 24	29.4618
827	68 39 29	28.7576	869	75 51 61	29.4788
828	68 55 84	28.7750	870	75 69 00	29.4958
829	68 72 41	28.7924	871	75 86 41	29.5127
830	68 89 00	28.8097	872	76 03 84	29.5296
831	69 05 61	28.8271	873	76 21 29	29.5466
832	69 22 24	28.8444	874	76 38 76	29.5635
833	69 38 89	28.8617	875	76 56 25	29.5804
834	69 55 56	28.8791	876	76 73 76	29.5973
835	69 72 25	28.8964	877	76 91 29	29.6142
836	69 88 96	28.9137	878	77 08 84	29.6311
837	70 05 69	28.9310	879	77 26 41	29.6479
838	70 22 44	28.9482	880	77 44 00	29.6648

TABLE B-1   (Continued)

Number	Square	Square root	Number	Square	Square root
881	77 61 61	29.6816	923	85 19 29	30.3809
882	77 79 24	29.6985	924	85 37 76	30.3974
883	77 96 89	29.7153	925	85 56 25	30.4138
884	78 14 56	29.7321	926	85 74 76	30.4302
885	78 32 25	29.7489	927	85 93 29	30.4467
886	78 49 96	29.7658	928	86 11 84	30.4631
887	78 67 69	29.7825	929	86 30 41	30.4795
888	78 85 44	29.7993	930	86 49 00	30.4959
889	79 03 21	29.8161	931	86 67 61	30.5123
890	79 21 00	29.8329	932	86 86 24	30.5287
891	79 38 81	29.8496	933	87 04 89	30.5450
892	79 56 64	29.8664	934	87 23 56	30.5614
893	79 74 49	29.8831	935	87 42 25	30.5778
894	79 92 36	29.8998	936	87 60 96	30.5941
895	80 10 25	29.9166	937	87 79 69	30.6105
896	80 28 16	29.9333	938	87 98 44	30.6268
897	80 46 09	29.9500	939	88 17 21	30.6431
898	80 64 04	29.9666	940	88 36 00	30.6594
899	80 82 01	29.9833	941	88 54 81	30.6757
900	81 00 00	30.0000	942	88 73 64	30.6920
901	81 18 01	30.0167	943	88 92 49	30.7083
902	81 36 04	30.0333	944	89 11 36	30.7246
903	81 54 09	30.0500	945	89 30 25	30.7409
904	81 72 16	30.0666	946	89 49 16	30.7571
905	81 90 25	30.0832	947	89 68 09	30.7734
906	82 08 36	30.0998	948	89 87 04	30.7896
907	82 26 49	30.1164	949	90 06 01	30.8058
908	82 44 64	30.1330	950	90 25 00	30.8221
909	82 62 81	30.1496	951	90 44 01	30.8383
910	82 81 00	30.1662	952	90 63 04	30.8545
911	82 99 21	30.1828	953	90 82 09	30.8707
912	83 17 44	30.1993	954	91 01 16	30.8869
913	83 35 69	30.2159	955	91 20 25	30.9031
914	83 53 96	30.2324	956	91 39 36	30.9192
915	83 72 25	30.2490	957	91 58 49	30.9354
916	83 90 56	30.2655	958	91 77 64	30.9516
917	84 08 89	30.2820	959	91 96 81	30.9677
918	84 27 24	30.2985	960	92 16 00	30.9839
919	84 45 61	30.3150	961	92 35 21	31.0000
920	84 64 00	30.3315	962	92 54 44	31.0161
921	84 82 41	30.3480	963	92 73 69	31.0322
922	85 00 84	30.3645	964	92 92 96	31.0483

TABLE B-1   (Continued)

Number	Square	Square root	Number	Square	Square root
965	93 12 25	31.0644	983	96 62 89	31.3528
966	93 31 56	31.0805	984	96 82 56	31.3688
967	93 50 89	31.0966	985	97 02 25	31.3847
968	93 70 24	31.1127	986	97 21 96	31.4006
969	93 89 61	31.1288	987	97 41 69	31.4166
970	94 09 00	31.1448	988	97 61 44	31.4325
971	94 28 41	31.1609	989	97 81 21	31.4484
972	94 47 84	31.1769	990	98 01 00	31.4643
973	94 67 29	31.1929	991	98 20 81	31.4802
974	94 86 76	31.2090	992	98 40 64	31.4960
975	95 06 25	31.2250	993	98 60 49	31.5119
976	95 25 76	31.2410	994	98 80 36	31.5278
977	95 45 29	31.2570	995	99 00 25	31.5436
978	95 64 84	31.2730	996	99 20 16	31.5595
979	95 84 41	31.2890	997	99 40 09	31.5753
980	96 04 00	31.3050	998	99 60 04	31.5911
981	96 23 61	31.3209	999	99 80 01	31.6070
982	96 43 24	31.3369	1000	100 00 00	31.6228

TABLE B-2 · Critical Values of the Correlation Coefficient*

df = n-2	α = .10	.05	.02	.01
1	.988	.997	.9995	.9999
2	.900	.950	.980	.990
3	.805	.878	.934	.959
4	.729	.811	.882	.917
5	.669	.754	.833	.874
6	.622	.707	.789	.834
7	.582	.666	.750	.798
8	.549	.632	.716	.765
9	.521	.602	.685	.735
10	.497	.576	.658	.708
11	.476	.553	.634	.684
12	.458	.532	.612	.661
13	.441	.514	.592	.641
14	.426	.497	.574	.623
15	.412	.482	.558	.606
16	.400	.468	.542	.590
17	.389	.456	.528	.575
18	.378	.444	.516	.561
19	.369	.433	.503	.549
20	.360	.423	.492	.537
21	.352	.413	.482	.526
22	.344	.404	.472	.515
23	.337	.396	.462	.505
24	.330	.388	.453	.496
25	.323	.381	.445	.487
26	.317	.374	.437	.479
27	.311	.367	.430	.471
28	.306	.361	.423	.463
29	.301	.355	.416	.456
30	.296	.349	.409	.449
35	.275	.325	.381	.418
40	.257	.304	.358	.393
45	.243	.288	.338	.372
50	.231	.273	.322	.354
60	.211	.250	.295	.325
70	.195	.232	.274	.302
80	.183	.217	.256	.283
90	.173	.205	.242	.267
100	.164	.195	.230	.254

*Table B-2 is taken from Table V.A. of Fisher and Yates, *Statistical Methods for Research Workers,* published by Oliver & Boyd, Edinburgh. By permission of the authors and publishers.

TABLE B-3 • The F distribution*

$$alpha = .05$$

$v_1 = $ d.f. of numerator $v_2 = $ d. f. of denominator

v_2 \ v_1	1	2	3	4	5	6	7	8	9	10
1	161.4	199.5	215.7	224.6	230.2	234.0	236.8	238.9	240.5	241.9
2	18.51	19.00	19.16	19.25	19.30	19.33	19.35	19.37	19.38	19.40
3	10.13	9.55	9.28	9.12	9.01	8.94	8.89	8.85	8.81	8.79
4	7.71	6.94	6.59	6.39	6.26	6.16	6.09	6.04	6.00	5.96
5	6.61	5.79	5.41	5.19	5.05	4.95	4.88	4.82	4.77	4.74
6	5.99	5.14	4.76	4.53	4.39	4.28	4.21	4.15	4.10	4.06
7	5.59	4.74	4.35	4.12	3.97	3.87	3.79	3.73	3.68	3.64
8	5.32	4.46	4.07	3.84	3.69	3.58	3.50	3.44	3.39	3.35
9	5.12	4.26	3.86	3.63	3.48	3.37	3.29	3.23	3.18	3.14
10	4.96	4.10	3.71	3.48	3.33	3.22	3.14	3.07	3.02	2.98
11	4.84	3.98	3.59	3.36	3.20	3.09	3.01	2.95	2.90	2.85
12	4.75	3.89	3.49	3.26	3.11	3.00	2.91	2.85	2.80	2.75
13	4.67	3.81	3.41	3.18	3.03	2.92	2.83	2.77	2.71	2.67
14	4.60	3.74	3.34	3.11	2.96	2.85	2.76	2.70	2.65	2.60
15	4.54	3.68	3.29	3.06	2.90	2.79	2.71	2.64	2.59	2.54
16	4.49	3.63	3.24	3.01	2.85	2.74	2.66	2.59	2.54	2.49
17	4.45	3.59	3.20	2.96	2.81	2.70	2.61	2.55	2.49	2.45
18	4.41	3.55	3.16	2.93	2.77	2.66	2.58	2.51	2.46	2.41
19	4.38	3.52	3.13	2.90	2.74	2.63	2.54	2.48	2.42	2.38
20	4.35	3.49	3.10	2.87	2.71	2.60	2.51	2.45	2.39	2.35
21	4.32	3.47	3.07	2.84	2.68	2.57	2.49	2.42	2.37	2.32
22	4.30	3.44	3.05	2.82	2.66	2.55	2.46	2.40	2.34	2.30
23	4.28	3.42	3.03	2.80	2.64	2.53	2.44	2.37	2.32	2.27
24	4.26	3.40	3.01	2.78	2.62	2.51	2.42	2.36	2.30	2.25
25	4.24	3.39	2.99	2.76	2.60	2.49	2.40	2.34	2.28	2.24
26	4.23	3.37	2.98	2.74	2.59	2.47	2.39	2.32	2.27	2.22
27	4.21	3.35	2.96	2.73	2.57	2.46	2.37	2.31	2.25	2.20
28	4.20	3.34	2.95	2.71	2.56	2.45	2.36	2.29	2.24	2.19
29	4.18	3.33	2.93	2.70	2.55	2.43	2.35	2.28	2.22	2.18
30	4.17	3.32	2.92	2.69	2.53	2.42	2.33	2.27	2.21	2.16
40	4.08	3.23	2.84	2.61	2.45	2.34	2.25	2.18	2.12	2.08
60	4.00	3.15	2.76	2.53	2.37	2.25	2.17	2.10	2.04	1.99
120	3.92	3.07	2.68	2.45	2.29	2.17	2.09	2.02	1.96	1.91
∞	3.84	3.00	2.60	2.37	2.21	2.10	2.01	1.94	1.88	1.83

*E. S. Pearson and H. O. Hartley, *Biometrika Tables for Statisticians* (New York: Cambridge University Press, 1966), vol. I. By permission of the authors and publisher.

TABLE B-3   (Continued)

$$alpha = .05$$

v_1 v_2	12	15	20	24	30	40	60	120	∞
1	243.9	245.9	248.0	249.1	250.1	251.1	252.2	253.3	254.3
2	19.41	19.43	19.45	19.45	19.46	19.47	19.48	19.49	19.50
3	8.74	8.70	8.66	8.64	8.62	8.59	8.57	8.55	8.53
4	5.91	5.86	5.80	5.77	5.75	5.72	5.69	5.66	5.63
5	4.68	4.62	4.56	4.53	4.50	4.46	4.43	4.40	4.36
6	4.00	3.94	3.87	3.84	3.81	3.77	3.74	3.70	3.67
7	3.57	3.51	3.44	3.41	3.38	3.34	3.30	3.27	3.23
8	3.28	3.22	3.15	3.12	3.08	3.04	3.01	2.97	2.93
9	3.07	3.01	2.94	2.90	2.86	2.83	2.79	2.75	2.71
10	2.91	2.85	2.77	2.74	2.70	2.66	2.62	2.58	2.54
11	2.79	2.72	2.65	2.61	2.57	2.53	2.49	2.45	2.40
12	2.69	2.62	2.54	2.51	2.47	2.43	2.38	2.34	2.30
13	2.60	2.53	2.46	2.42	2.38	2.34	2.30	2.25	2.21
14	2.53	2.46	2.39	2.35	2.31	2.27	2.22	2.18	2.13
15	2.48	2.40	2.33	2.29	2.25	2.20	2.16	2.11	2.07
16	2.42	2.35	2.28	2.24	2.19	2.15	2.11	2.06	2.01
17	2.38	2.31	2.23	2.19	2.15	2.10	2.06	2.01	1.96
18	2.34	2.27	2.19	2.15	2.11	2.06	2.02	1.97	1.92
19	2.31	2.23	2.16	2.11	2.07	2.03	1.98	1.93	1.88
20	2.28	2.20	2.12	2.08	2.04	1.99	1.95	1.90	1.84
21	2.25	2.18	2.10	2.05	2.01	1.96	1.92	1.87	1.81
22	2.23	2.15	2.07	2.03	1.98	1.94	1.89	1.84	1.78
23	2.20	2.13	2.05	2.01	1.96	1.91	1.86	1.81	1.76
24	2.18	2.11	2.03	1.98	1.94	1.89	1.84	1.79	1.73
25	2.16	2.09	2.01	1.96	1.92	1.87	1.82	1.77	1.71
26	2.15	2.07	1.99	1.95	1.90	1.85	1.80	1.75	1.69
27	2.13	2.06	1.97	1.93	1.88	1.84	1.79	1.73	1.67
28	2.12	2.04	1.96	1.91	1.87	1.82	1.77	1.71	1.65
29	2.10	2.03	1.94	1.90	1.85	1.81	1.75	1.70	1.64
30	2.09	2.01	1.93	1.89	1.84	1.79	1.74	1.68	1.62
40	2.00	1.92	1.84	1.79	1.74	1.69	1.64	1.58	1.51
60	1.92	1.84	1.75	1.70	1.65	1.59	1.53	1.47	1.39
120	1.83	1.75	1.66	1.61	1.55	1.50	1.43	1.35	1.25
∞	1.75	1.67	1.57	1.52	1.46	1.39	1.32	1.22	1.00

TABLE B-3   (Continued)

$$alpha = .01$$

V_2 \ V_1	1	2	3	4	5	6	7	8	9	10
1	4052	4999.5	5403	5625	5764	5859	5928	5981	6022	6056
2	98.50	99.00	99.17	99.25	99.30	99.33	99.36	99.37	99.39	99.40
3	34.12	30.82	29.46	28.71	28.24	27.91	27.67	27.49	27.35	27.23
4	21.20	18.00	16.69	15.98	15.52	15.21	14.98	14.80	14.66	14.55
5	16.26	13.27	12.06	11.39	10.97	10.67	10.46	10.29	10.16	10.05
6	13.75	10.92	9.78	9.15	8.75	8.47	8.26	8.10	7.98	7.87
7	12.25	9.55	8.45	7.85	7.46	7.19	6.99	6.84	6.72	6.62
8	11.26	8.65	7.59	7.01	6.63	6.37	6.18	6.03	5.91	5.81
9	10.56	8.02	6.99	6.42	6.06	5.80	5.61	5.47	5.35	5.26
10	10.04	7.56	6.55	5.99	5.64	5.39	5.20	5.06	4.94	4.85
11	9.65	7.21	6.22	5.67	5.32	5.07	4.89	4.74	4.63	4.54
12	9.33	6.93	5.95	5.41	5.06	4.82	4.64	4.50	4.39	4.30
13	9.07	6.70	5.74	5.21	4.86	4.62	4.44	4.30	4.19	4.10
14	8.86	6.51	5.56	5.04	4.69	4.46	4.28	4.14	4.03	3.94
15	8.68	6.36	5.42	4.89	4.56	4.32	4.14	4.00	3.89	3.80
16	8.53	6.23	5.29	4.77	4.44	4.20	4.03	3.89	3.78	3.69
17	8.40	6.11	5.18	4.67	4.34	4.10	3.93	3.79	3.68	3.59
18	8.29	6.01	5.09	4.58	4.25	4.01	3.84	3.71	3.60	3.51
19	8.18	5.93	5.01	4.50	4.17	3.94	3.77	3.63	3.52	3.43
20	8.10	5.85	4.94	4.43	4.10	3.87	3.70	3.56	3.46	3.37
21	8.02	5.78	4.87	4.37	4.04	3.81	3.64	3.51	3.40	3.31
22	7.95	5.72	4.82	4.31	3.99	3.76	3.59	3.45	3.35	3.26
23	7.88	5.66	4.76	4.26	3.94	3.71	3.54	3.41	3.30	3.21
24	7.82	5.61	4.72	4.22	3.90	3.67	3.50	3.36	3.26	3.17
25	7.77	5.57	4.68	4.18	3.85	3.63	3.40	3.32	3.22	3.13
26	7.72	5.53	4.64	4.14	3.82	3.59	3.42	3.29	3.18	3.09
27	7.68	5.49	4.60	4.11	3.78	3.56	3.39	3.26	3.15	3.06
28	7.64	5.45	4.57	4.07	3.75	3.53	3.36	3.23	3.12	3.03
29	7.60	5.42	4.54	4.04	3.73	3.50	3.33	3.20	3.09	3.00
30	7.56	5.39	4.51	4.02	3.70	3.47	3.30	3.17	3.07	2.98
40	7.31	5.18	4.31	3.83	3.51	2.29	3.12	2.99	2.89	2.80
60	7.08	4.98	4.13	3.65	3.34	3.12	2.95	2.82	2.72	2.63
120	6.85	4.79	3.95	3.48	3.17	2.96	2.79	2.66	2.56	2.47
∞	6.63	4.61	3.78	3.32	3.02	2.80	2.64	2.51	2.41	2.32

TABLE B-3 (Continued)

$$alpha = .01$$

V_1 V_2	12	15	20	24	30	40	60	120	∞
1	6106	6157	6209	6235	6261	6287	6313	6339	6366
2	99.42	99.43	99.45	99.46	99.47	99.47	99.48	99.49	99.50
3	27.05	26.87	26.69	26.60	26.50	26.41	26.32	26.22	26.13
4	14.37	14.20	14.02	13.93	13.84	13.75	13.65	13.56	13.46
5	9.89	9.72	9.55	9.47	9.38	9.29	9.20	9.11	9.02
6	7.72	7.56	7.40	7.31	7.23	7.14	7.06	6.97	6.88
7	6.47	6.31	6.16	6.07	5.99	5.91	5.82	5.74	5.65
8	5.67	5.52	5.36	5.28	5.20	5.12	5.03	4.95	4.86
9	5.11	4.96	4.81	4.73	4.65	4.57	4.48	4.40	4.31
10	4.71	4.56	4.41	4.33	4.25	4.17	4.08	4.00	3.91
11	4.40	4.25	4.10	4.02	3.94	3.86	3.78	3.69	3.60
12	4.16	4.01	3.86	3.78	3.70	3.62	3.54	3.45	3.36
13	3.96	3.82	3.66	3.59	3.51	3.43	3.34	3.25	3.17
14	3.80	3.66	3.51	3.43	3.35	3.27	3.18	3.09	3.00
15	3.67	3.52	3.37	3.29	3.21	3.13	3.05	2.96	2.87
16	3.55	3.41	3.26	3.18	3.10	3.02	2.93	2.84	2.75
17	3.46	3.31	3.16	3.08	3.00	2.92	2.83	2.75	2.65
18	3.37	3.23	3.08	3.00	2.92	2.84	2.75	2.66	2.57
19	3.30	3.15	3.00	2.92	2.84	2.76	2.67	2.58	2.49
20	3.23	3.09	2.94	2.86	2.78	2.69	2.61	2.52	2.42
21	3.17	3.03	2.88	2.80	2.72	2.64	2.55	2.46	2.36
22	3.12	2.98	2.83	2.75	2.67	2.58	2.50	2.40	2.31
23	3.07	2.93	2.78	2.70	2.62	2.54	2.45	2.35	2.26
24	3.03	2.89	2.74	2.66	2.58	2.49	2.40	2.31	2.21
25	2.99	2.85	2.70	2.62	2.54	2.45	2.36	2.27	2.17
26	2.96	2.81	2.66	2.58	2.50	2.42	2.33	2.23	2.13
27	2.93	2.78	2.63	2.55	2.47	2.38	2.29	2.20	2.10
28	2.90	2.75	2.60	2.52	2.44	2.35	2.26	2.17	2.06
29	2.87	2.73	2.57	2.49	2.41	2.33	2.23	2.14	2.03
30	2.84	2.70	2.55	2.47	2.39	2.30	2.21	2.11	2.01
40	2.66	2.52	2.37	2.29	2.20	2.11	2.02	1.92	1.80
60	2.50	2.35	2.20	2.12	2.03	1.94	1.84	1.73	1.60
120	2.34	2.19	2.03	1.95	1.86	1.76	1.66	1.53	1.38
∞	2.18	2.04	1.88	1.79	1.70	1.59	1.47	1.32	1.00

index